The Landscape of
Homeopathic Medicine
CASE TAKING
*Best practise and creating meaning
in the consultation room*

Volume 1

Alastair C. Gray

Homeopathic Essence

THE LANDSCAPE OF HOMEOPATHIC MEDICINE CASE TAKING

First Edition: 2010
Second Edition: 2014
2nd Impression: 2014

All rights reserved. No part of this book may be reproduced, stored in a retrieval system or transmitted, in any form or by any means, mechanical, photocopying, recording or otherwise, without any prior written permission of the publisher.

© with the author

Published by Kuldeep Jain for
Homeopathic Essence
An Imprint of
B. JAIN PUBLISHERS (P) LTD.
1921/10, Chuna Mandi, Paharganj, New Delhi–110 055 (INDIA)
Tel.: +91-11-4567 1000; Fax: +91-11-4567 1010
Email: info@bjain.com; Website: www.bjain.com

Printed in India by
Yash Printographics, Noida

ISBN: 978-81-319-3299-5

Foreword

It is a pleasure to write a foreword for Alastair Gray's volume on case-taking. It would be misleading to suppose that Alastair has written solely about case taking. Rather, as the title of this book suggests, he has scanned the landscape of homoeopathy and has sketched his impressions in great detail, affording us an overview of the many diverse approaches to the vast terrain of homoeopathy. In this context, taking the case is only a lens through which one may view the whole art, searching for a 'best practice' definition, the noble destination of Alastair's voyage.

I will start with a few words about Alastair, since my impression of him has some bearing on this book. I first met Al as a student at the Dynamis School in 1994. I remember the year vividly, for that was the 'unfortunate' year chosen to prove *Plutonium nitricum*. They bore this burden well, and Alastair's proving left a vivid impression, illuminating the hidden nature of this incredible substance. In his proving, Al had repeated 'double dreams'; at first he would dream of an event such as a race or burglary as an observer from a vantage point high above. Later on that night he would dream the same dream again, but this time as a participant in the event.

It occurs to me that Alastair has taken a similar approach here. While surveying the homoeopathic landscape he has at first sketched a broad overview, later on delving into the details that make this a scholarly as well as an insightful book. This was always Al's skill; to examine a subject from many points of view without being attached to any one teaching other than the most logical choice. In his foreword he calls this critical thinking. It is this critical thinking that defines the higher levels of knowledge which is so often lacking in homoeopathy these days. As the profession undergoes a lengthy period of uncontrolled expansion, a few logical boundaries become necessary.

Case taking is not the most controversial aspect of homoeopathy; that distinction lies with other aspects such as case analysis or classical versus non classical approaches. Nevertheless case taking tends to shape itself around a particular methodology, a case of the foot molding to the shoe. Once we adapt our case taking techniques to our prescribing techniques, prejudice enters the process. Freedom from prejudice is the one and only point Hahnemann recommends when taking a case, a point to which much lip service is paid to but which so easily vanishes in the quest for methodology; methodology has a goal, and a goal is never free.

It is the patient rather than the practitioner that should dictate the case taking outline; this is the essence of individualization. Any form, routine or framework impedes the natural flow of a case and its unique information. Worse still are the various case taking methodologies that enslave themselves to 'finding the remedy', either by questioning along the lines of a remedy, or the more subtle but none less dangerous questioning along the lines of a 'system'. To be truly free from prejudice there should be no goal in mind, no aim. We take the case in order to perceive the patient, not the remedy, miasm, segment or sensation. This is the highest form of the art. Shifting our focus from patient to result blurs our vision. Goal-'less' case taking should be our meditation, action in non action, doing without trying.

To quote Chuang Tzu

When an archer is shooting for nothing, he has all his skill.
If he shoots for a brass buckle, he is already nervous.
If he shoots for a prize of gold, he goes blind or sees two targets --
He is out of his mind! His skill has not changed. But the prize divides him.
He cares. He thinks more of winning than of shooting--
And the need to win drains him of power.
(Translation Thomas Merton 19:4, p. 158)

Taking the case is a dance for two: We follow the patient just as we are led in the waltz; passive, but not inactive. Following, but not dragged. Gradually, as the case unfolds and clarifies we subtly shift roles; from being led in the dance we become the gentle leader, guiding them to the dark corners that have not yet been illuminated. Following the passive receiving of free flowing information we navigate our patient, finally making sure all bases are covered, head to toe. This sequence is reflected in Hahnemann's directions for case taking in Paragraphs 83 to 100; from Zen to data collection. Finding the balance and timing of these is an art.

When I was a first year student of homoeopathy, I read Pierre's Schmidt's book on Chronic Disease, in which he emphasizes being silent during the process of case taking, as Hahnemann instructs in Paragraph 84. I took this on board. At the time I was also studying Chinese medicine, and we were given an exercise to take each other's case. While most of the students asked 'the eight questions', I decided to practice my newly discovered 'silent method'. I vividly remember how my partner was at first puzzled by my silence, then angry, then told me all her troubles. Nature abhors a vacuum. I practiced this method for years, keeping silent through many torturous moments until the poor patients were forced out of their shell. Years later I realized how violent this silence could be. I understood that being silent means being silent in myself, not striving for a result.

When the patient feels this empty and relaxed presence, they are happy to dance. Helping this dance along with a kind word, an anecdote, a friendly joke or a well placed comment enhances rather than disturbs this silence. As in any dance, the most important thing is timing and rhythm. If we can effortlessly 'match' the patient's tempo, volume and frequency, we will have our case.

One final tip from my wife, Camilla. If you have been taking a long case and the landscape is still barren, without a strand of totality or a characteristic symptom to hang on to, pray. It usually works; after all, we are praying to the same source which the patient prays to.

In travelling this landscape Alastair has surveyed it all; history, methodology, technique and controversy, all with a fresh and aptly critical eye. I congratulate him for writing this volume, and look forward to the rest of the series.

Jeremy Sherr
April 10th 2010

Introduction to the Series

- Critical Thinking
- The Need for Clarity
- Scope of Practice
- Homeopathy in Trouble and Under Attack
- The Change in Emphasis within Homeopathic Education
- Research

Introduction to the Series

Critical Thinking

This is the first in a series of books casting a critical eye over the discipline of homeopathic medicine. It is important to note that the critical evaluation is coming from one who is inside the profession. Usually the critiques come from without and often lack an understanding of the historical and other contextual issues. The most important word in that previous sentence was 'critical'. In some parts of the world 'critical' means to criticize. In other parts critical means to reflect and ponder. In the scientific and academic world critical analysis, critical reflection and critical evaluation are the solid underpinnings and foundations of any meaningful area of enquiry. It is not necessarily a personal or professional attack.

The Need for Clarity

In this series of books, seven aspects of the practice of homeopathic medicine are examined, reflected on, deconstructed, critically evaluated and described. This last point, 'described' is crucial. Homeopathic medicine from the inside is a stimulating and exciting discipline to be a part of. From the outside it can seem bewildering. Not only because some of the fundamentals of the art and science of homeopathy are difficult to describe in what is clearly and unequivocally a biomedical world. But it is overwhelmingly confusing because of the certain different styles of practice that homeopaths have. This is not just about bedside manner. The user of homeopathy in India may not be so concerned about the method used by the prescriber. The choice of going to this practitioner or that doctor is a simple one. But in the Western world, in Europe, the US, in Australia and New Zealand homeopathy struggles at times because of its breadth and startling difference in the way in which it is carried out.

Scope of Practice

One of the challenges of the profession is that there is no clear scope of practice, clear guidelines on best practice, or exclusivity of title, as at the moment in those countries where homeopathy is unregulated anyone can call themselves a homeopath. This issue of scope practice is a serious problem in the homeopathic world. For a physician, clear directives can be given in medical school on how to take a case. In physiotherapy there is a clear path and guidelines. For an auditor going into a business or an educational auditor going into a college there are clear questions to ask and a protocol. Homeopathy has a breadth that makes this very difficult. Because homeopathy is the application of an idea, not merely the distribution of medicines, there is a massive range of application. Homeopathy means, 'similar suffering'. This is the origin of the word that Hahnemann coined. That thing in nature that can create symptoms in a healthy person will have the capacity to remove those symptoms in a patient. That is the proposition, yet ask members of the general public what constitutes homeopathic medicine, generally they will identify the issue of the infinitesimal dose, or the fact that homeopaths use serial dilutions of poisons as their therapeutic interventions. Yet the reality is that the infinitesimal dose is secondary to the principle law of homeopathy which is that of the application of similars. This broad scope is the crux of the issue. Homeopathy simply has a massive scope of practice. It is its greatest boon and its largest catastrophe. In a nutshell, there is no symptom of any patient on the planet for which there is not a substance somewhere in nature that has the capacity to create that same symptom in a healthy person. No other profession has such a wide terrain. Homeopaths assert that they can cure everything from depression, heartache, teething pain, lice and herpes. From the perspective of other professions these are bold claims indeed. Furthermore, there is general bewilderment from those looking towards the homeopathic profession that in addition to making these claims there are no agreed guidelines of method or case taking.

It is only possibly the psychological arts and sciences that has anything close to the largeness of scope that homeopaths have. On the one hand you have Psychiatry with its very specific doses of drugs to manage the neuro-chemistry of a patient and it's measurable outcomes, and at the other end of the spectrum you have Somatic Therapy, Gestalt Therapy or Neuro-linguistic Programming. That is a broad scope of strategies and theories orientated to create change in a patient.

In the Western world homeopathy experienced a massive amount of growth in the 1980's and 90's. Private colleges sprang up across Europe, New Zealand, Australia, the US and the unlikeliest of places. Those classrooms were full of the most diverse range of students from interested housewives through to immunologists, physicians, historians, nurses and hippies. Credit where it's due. This was for the most part due to be charismatic and solid work of George Vithoulkas who taught, wrote, published, and raised the awareness of thousands worldwide. A great many were drawn to his lectures and seminars and books. That is a far cry from what we see today at the end of the first decade of the 21st century. Classrooms are still full but they are smaller classrooms. Students are committed but there's no doubt that the student of 2013 is different from the student of 1983.

Homeopathy in Trouble and Under Attack

Modern students hear their teachers talk about the disarray, the decline and the attacks from the outside. Skeptics rallying outside chemists in the UK that stock remedies is but the latest. Homeopathic students these days hear their teachers talking about disunity and an implosion from the inside. Comparisons are made to the decline of homeopathy in the US in the early part of the 20th century, 100 years ago where, from a healthy profession with students, colleges and hospitals, within a generation homeopathy was almost was swept away and what remained was a cottage industry trembling under the shadow of the Flexner Report.

The internal divisions aside, from the outside there are a number of obvious criticisms of homeopathic medicine. Never have they been more sharply defined and focussed than in the UK over the last five years. In no particular order, there were the malaria claims exposed in the print media where, homeopaths were said to be claiming to be able to protect travelers in tropical climates against malaria. Since then systematic and orchestrated attacks have been launched about non-evidence-based medicine (i.e. homeopathy) being free to the public and delivered in the National Health Service (NHS). Furthermore the profession has withstood criticisms of homeopathy taught in universities, a 'non-science' being taught in science degrees. It couldn't possibly work, therefore it doesn't work, has been the cynical message.

All of these recent events have fed perceptions driven by the opponents of homeopathy that it is in the business of taking advantage of vulnerable people, flogging meaningless medicine without conscience, practicing pseudo-science without rigour. How do these perceptions come about? Without doubt ignorance and prejudice on behalf of some, but equally without doubt because of average prescribing, poor practice, negative publicity, because homeopaths have been lazy and have lacked significant academic rigour. With the upsurge in the ability to publish quickly and easily, and with the ability to blog and have an opinion about everything, a great deal of what has emerged in the homeopathic body of literature in the last 20 years has been at the softer end of the spectrum. A word search on 'homeopathy' in Google leads to some bewildering sites and opinions. The number of peer reviewed industry journals are few. This has to change if the profession is to make any progress. These books are an attempt to right the balance, not in a way that is uncritical and reactionary but in a grounded way that seeks to place aspects of homeopathy in their true context.

This volume examines the landscape of homeopathic case taking in all of its complexity. To students of homeopathy and those questioning homeopathy this book seeks to describe and identify the varieties that exist within the profession, and just why they are there. Because this discipline spans 200 years and involves a literature base that takes into account the whole globe there is no shortage of variety.

Later volumes will describe the landscape of homeopathic method. In a similar way it will go into detail and describe the variety of homeopathic prescribing techniques and why they are different. A volume will be devoted to and will identify the therapeutic suggestions, and the specific interventions for a number of named conditions. In addition the landscape of the homeopathic theory of chronic disease will be examined. Called miasmatic theory, this book will delve into the variety of ways of perceiving the true cause of disease that started with Hahnemann and has many colourful manifestations today. Moreover a volume will examine the landscape of homeopathic materia medica, the compilation of our books on remedy indications, and furthermore describe homeopathic philosophy in depth. It is timely given that the seminal book, the *Organon of Medicine* was published 200 years ago recently. These works will focus on the homeopathic community and profession, all at once taking into account the history, the personalities and the evolution of this discipline and ask, 'How Did We Get To This Place?'

My own approach to homeopathy is one based on a grounded strategy. 'Feet on the ground head in the clouds' (Sherr 1994), is the best and natural posture to adopt in practice. Homeopathy attracts individualistic people. It attracts creative people, and people that are on their third careers. It attracts people that have been in nursing, or the corporate world and are looking for something else. It also attracts people that are great healers not necessarily great researchers or technicians and certainly not scientists. Homeopathic colleges experience their greatest attrition because of medical sciences subjects not homeopathic ones.

That does not mean my approach to homeopathic medicine is dry by any means. But it does mean one thing in particular and not all homeopaths will be in agreement. After 20 years of practice and 15 years of teaching I'm no longer of the opinion that the homeopathic remedy is the most crucial thing in a positive curative intervention. There has been a heavy emphasis on the remedy as the thing that does the work in the 200 year history of homeopathy. The emphasis has been on the simillimum, the Holy Grail, the silver bullet, the perfect remedy. This detracts from the ultimate skill behind practicing homeopathy. Moreover the idea is divorced from the reality at the coal face of homeopathic practice. It is the therapeutic relationship, and the ability of a homeopath to listen and receive a full case that is at the heart of the good prescription. It is this relationship between the practitioner and the patient that is the true emphasis. When I was in my role as head of the homeopathy department at Endeavour College of Natural Health it was the educational and pedagogical focus. This is not to detract from knowledge of materia medica, theory or philosophy but to right an imbalance.

The Change in Emphasis within Homeopathic Education

I was a part of a great team that worked tirelessly to develop the degree curriculum at Endeavour in Australia. While nothing is ever perfect, it is very good. In addition, I worked on the degree submission at Cyberjaya University College of Medical Sciences in Malaysia. Benchmarking against the University of Central Lancashire's undergraduate degree, to my mind these efforts have taken homeopathic medicine education a few necessary steps forward. Not all like them or appreciate them. To some they are a threat. They are competition, and they definitely raise the standards to a level that means that some will not be able to attain what is necessary. It is never the intention to exclude, nevertheless what was being clearly identified within our profession more than most in the last decade is that we have a lack of participants able to research well and think critically.

Worse, homeopathic education is in a mess. In the colleges there is a disconnect between professional standards, in other words what is agreed upon as the necessary skills to develop in order to competently practice homeopathic medicine, and the level to which these subjects are taught. Diplomas and advanced diplomas get clogged with massive amounts of critical thinking and cognitive skills that are educationally well ahead of the award they are offering. There is huge over-assessment. Outside the colleges, homeopathic education is driven by entrepreneurs not educators, large personalities with an angle attempt to keep students coming back with the next thing.

We have thousands upon thousands of cured cases, that are passed on from practitioner to teacher, teacher to student, and over the years many of these have found their way into our journals. Uncomfortable and distressing as it is, in the 21st century, in the biomedical world in which we live, these constitute nothing but anecdotal evidence. In the cold world of science anecdotal evidence sits at the very bottom of the evidence hierarchy. At the top of the evidence hierarchy is the gold standard randomly controlled double-blind trial. There are some but precious few of these in homeopathy and just one of these trials counts for more than thousands upon thousands of anecdotal stories. Practicing homeopaths find this an unhappy situation to find themselves in. Some deal with it by saying, 'Well that cold scientific world is stuffed and they can have it. We don't have to play their games and play in that biomedical sandpit. We will do our own thing'. Some decide to become more medically orientated and attempt to conduct homeopathic trials attempting to demonstrate homeopathy's efficacy but these are often of poor quality. A third group argue that by engaging with research and questioning rigorously the false emphasis of the evidence hierarchy, homeopathy and homeopaths will be able to be accepted into an academic world on their own terms with their own methods validated and appreciated. Moreover, the other health and complementary health professionals are asked to provide evidence for what they do. Homeopaths are not a breed apart. The steps of a) asking a question, b) searching for evidence to answer it, c) critically appraising the evidence, d) integrating the evidence into clinical practice, e) evaluating how the steps from a - d went, (Hoffmann 2010) is actually not that demanding.

Research

Research is therefore at the centre of the upgrade from the traditional homeopathic qualification, which is the diploma or advanced diploma to a degree in complementary medicine and especially homeopathic medicine. These degree courses now place homeopathy within the context of the history of healing. From Galen through to Vesalius, from Freud through to the world of evidence-based medicine, a homeopathic degree now emphasizes critical reflection, evaluation and analysis. Questioning and reflecting, criticizing and arguing about the things taught in natural medicine colleges is essentially saying to students, 'Don't believe everything that is told to you, validate it. Think about it. Reflect on it. Is it right? Is it congruent?' What we see is that students coming out of these programs are smart, they don't accept anything just because it's been told to them by someone with a reputation. Students are encouraged to not project impossible qualities onto their lecturers. The cult of the guru, that has infected the profession of homeopathy and continues to do so is discouraged. In the attempt to create a generation of homeopaths with new skills to research and critically think, they are able to take their seat beside practitioners from multiple other modalities. Degrees are not just extra unnecessary classes. Too often degrees have been clip-on's to courses and they involve beefing up medical sciences and irrelevant subjects that others want to see. What is needed is a cogent, coherent, upward spiral of learning grounded in reality.

These seven books are an attempt to raise the bar, ground homeopathic education, encourage debate, critical reflection and research. They are also orientated to professional homeopaths to reflect on what they do, what they learned, what underlying assumptions they carry, where indolence and laziness are a feature of their working lives and maintain their professional development where ever they are. When I learnt homeopathy I thought what I was learning was homeopathy. What I now know is that I was being taught a style of homeopathy underpinned by a number of philosophical points of view and assumptions. This is to not say that these assumptions are wrong or that style homeopathy was wrong. It seems to me therefore that it is important to realise that different styles of case taking relate to different ways of practising homeopathy and it is important to understand where one comes from to follow best practice. Flexibility in moving from one style of homeopathy and one style of case taking relevant to that style of homeopathy, is a necessary professional reality depending on where and how one is prescribing. What is crucial is questioning, becoming familiar with and understanding the underpinning assumptions, the sacred cows that go with whatever style of practice one chooses.

Alastair Gray
Gold Coast Australia 2013

Acknowledgements

It has been said that writing a book is just like giving birth to an elephant. This book would not have been possible but for some great nursing and midwifery from a number of friends and colleagues. A number of thanks are in order. Firstly, the 'Landscape' series was conceived on a journey from Brussels to Amsterdam. Thanks to Dale Emerson and Nishant Jain for that road trip.

In the course of completing this book I have received fantastic editorial and research support from Julia Harte. She contributed considerably to Chapter Seven and her excellent critical eye for detail throughout the book was needed to offset my lack of it. Further editorial support has come from Nikki Waterhouse, Annalisa Turner and Tim Gray. Thanks to them all for unpacking my unusual sentence structure and their patience in reminding me that I can't always get what I want, how I want. Thanks to Lisa Buzassyova for the ongoing support in the clinic and practice.

Thanks also to Rajan Sankaran for the opportunity and permission to publish our discussion that took place in 2009, while he was in Byron Bay giving his seminar. For the cover design and photography, my sincere gratitude to Philip Ritchie and Eyconology Design, and to Alex Craig for the other photography.

Acknowledgements

Profound thanks to my friends and colleagues in Sydney, Ken D'Aran, David Levy, Peter Tumminello, Carmen Nicotra, and to Susanna Shelton in New Zealand. Over the years they have been a source of inspiration and professional and personal support. To a large degree it is from the ongoing stimulating conversations, arguments and tantrums, that clarity of thought has come. They may recognize in the text, some of the interactions that have taken place in the classroom, hallway, on the phone, at the tennis net, over dinner or driving to work.

Thanks also to Kate Chatfield, Ian Townsend and Jean Duckworth at the University of Central Lancashire. The experience of completing the Masters of Science, plus the great stimulation from my colleagues there, has been responsible for the refocussing of my thinking, practice and teaching of homeopathy.

Contributors

Dr Parag Singh and Dr Harsh Nigam gave assistance in the researching for this book. Through the identification of the more colourful historical contributions in the landscape of case taking that went into the creation of this book they laid some solid foundations.

Dr Parag Singh completed his BHMS in 1993 and did his MD from National Institute of Homeopathy, Calcutta in December 1996. He has been practicing classical homeopathy since 1997 at his private clinic and has an interest in literary research work in the field of homeopathy.

Dr Harsh Nigam, has an MBBS and an MD (Physiology) degree. He obtained his membership of the British Homeopathic Association from the Royal London Homeopathic Hospital. He has been practising homeopathy since 1993. His works include 'Principles and Practice of Homeopathic Case Management', and 'Lectures on Homeopathic Philosophy with Classroom Notes and Word Index'.

Ben Gadd researched and wrote Chapter ten in this book. He runs a homeopathic practice in inner south-east Melbourne, Australia. Prior to becoming a homeopath he worked as a registered nurse in a variety of mental health settings. He lectures at the Melbourne campus of Endeavour College of Natural Health, and has a strong interest in the application of research to clinical practice.

Publisher's Note to 2nd edition

The first edition of this book on *Case Taking* has received a great response from readers in the past four years and we would like to thank them all for the same. We are now happy to bring forth the second edition of this eminent work. A whole new index has been added to the book for easy reference of students and practitioners alike, and the book comes with additional information and perspectives. This book is part of a series from B. Jain to give voice to expert opinion and the evaluation of views on a range of different subjects from Hahnemann's time to the present. We hope this book will be of invaluable help to every homoeopath and it will soon find it's place on their desks and shelves.

Publisher's Note to 1st edition

In the 200 years of homeopathy many books have been published on various aspects of homeopathic practice, the ways to it and the different approaches to it. All the stalwarts gave different ways of practicing homeopathy, their views about case taking, prescription, remedy selection, miasms and so on. The amount of information is enormous. But the difficulty is that in spite of such a huge amounts of data there is no place where we can find all this information together, and there is no guideline which will help us understand what to do with this data and when to apply it. All the diverse approaches to the science of homeopathy and its principles are correct but what is required is the understanding of its application in the correct way.

To solve this major hurdle of a homeopathic practitioner **B. Jain Archibel** has picked up this project in order to clear all the confusions regarding this vast body of information and its usage. This project is being conducted and coordinated by Alastair Gray who has clinical experience of more than 20 years and a teaching experience of 15 years. He has also completed a lot of work on the proving of new and old homeopathic drugs and has contributed to the homeopathic literature. He is being assisted by researchers and contributors from different fields who are working on this project with him. This project is called 'The Landscape of Homeopathic Medicine' where seven topics about homeopathic practice will be discussed in seven books. The first one is on *Case Taking,* the very first step of homeopathic practice.

Here, Alastair has covered all the concepts of case taking from the stalwarts starting from Dr Hahnemann to the current day teachers like Brian Kaplan and Rajan Sankaran. The concept of the Landscape of Homeopathic Medicine is not just to bring out all the facts but also critically analyze the same in the context of what is meant and how it should be applied.

We hope that this work is read by all homeopathic practitioners and students and we are sure that they will find it very useful for their practice.

B. Jain Archibel

Contents

Foreword	iii
Introduction to the Series	vii
Acknowledgements	xx
Contributors	xxii
Publisher's Note to 2nd edition	xxiv
Publisher's Note to 1st edition	xxv

Chapters

Introduction to Case Taking

1. Introduction	**3**
• The Need for Best Practice	5
• This Book	7
• Requirements of the Case Taker?	12
• Literature Review	12

Part One
Information Gathering to Find the Medicine

2. Hahnemann	**23**
• The Directives	27
• Main Aphorisms	28
Other Aphorisms	39
• Hahnemann's World – Why He Gave those Instructions	42

- The Key Concepts – What Hahnemann Asks us to Look for — 44
  - Totality — 44
  - Peculiarity — 53
- What is Required? — 56
  - Non-Prejudice — 56
  - Sound Senses — 62
  - Attention in Observing — 63
  - Fidelity in Tracing the Picture of the Disease — 65
- Hahnemann's Directives for Case Taking in Specific Situations — 65
- Further Directives of Hahnemann — 69
- Summary of Hahnemann's General Directives for Best Practice — 72
  - What to Do — 72
  - What Not to Do — 78
- Hahnemann's Main Writings — 78
- Core Requirements for Case Taking from Hahnemann — 79

3. Post Hahnemann — 81

- Consolidation — 85
- Clarity — 86
- Böenninghausen's Instructions on Case Taking and Forming a Complete Image — 87
- Other Authors — 91
  - Dunham — 91
  - Bidwell — 93
  - Guernsey — 95

Farrington	95
Hering	95
Hughes	96
Burnett, Cooper and Clarke	97
Boger	100
Nash	102
T. F. Allen	103
H. C. Allen	105

4. Kent — **109**
- Classical — 114
- Repertory, Types, The Person not the Disease — 115
- Swedenborg — 116
- Mind — 117
- Kent's Instructions on Case Taking — 119
- The Science of Case Taking for the Lower Plane of Homeopathy — 120
- The Art of Case Taking for the Higher Plane of Homeopathy — 122
- What the Homeopath Needs — 125
    - Tact and Timing — 128
- Kent and Peculiarity — 131
- Hysteria, Exaggeration and the Irish — 132

5. Post Kentian Approaches — **135**
- Schmidt — 140
- Tyler — 155
- Wright-Hubbard — 157
- Roberts — 160

- Close — 163
- Getting Mental Symptoms — 167

6. Best Practice Gathering Information — 171
- Before Opening Your Mouth Remember — 177
- The Purpose of Case Taking — 181
- Attitude — 181
- Method and Steps of Case Taking — 183
- First Serve — 184
- Observation — 187
- Questioning and Silence — 191
- Physical Examination — 192
- Recording — 194
- Own Words — 196
- Importance and Underlining — 197
- Legalities — 197
- Time Management and Endings — 198
- To Questionnaire or Not — 198
- Difficulties and Specific Situations in Taking the Case — 200
- The Last Word and Great Advice — 212
- Being a Beginner — 214

Part Two
Getting to the Centre, Making Meaning and Learning from Other Disciplines to Find the Medicine

7. Post Jungian Approaches to Case Taking: Homeopathy and Wounded Souls — 219

- Introduction — 223
- Historical Context — 226
- Post-Jungian Approaches to Case Taking in Homeopathy — 228
- Dream Work — 231
- Tattoos — 234
- Psychology and Psychotherapy — 235
- Art Therapy and Sandplay — 235
- Archetypes, Myths, Fairy Tales, Stream of Consciousness and Metaphor — 237
- To Jung or Not to Jung — 239
- Questioning — 242
- Disclaimer — 246
- Developing the Necessary Case Taking Skills — 247
- Looking for Clues without Scaring your Client or Acting too Weird — 248
- Conclusion — 249
- Doing Nothing — 250

8. Learning and Borrowing from other Disciplines — 253
- Introduction — 257
- Police — 259
- Human Resources — 260
- Borrowing from Psychological Approaches — 260
- A Relationship Not an Event — 261
- Rogers — 262
- Empathy — 265
- Unconditional Positive Regard — 266

- Congruence — 267
- Authenticity — 268
- Other Strategies and Techniques — 270
- Humour and Provocation — 270
- Borrowing Further — 273

9. Sankaran and Sensation — 277
- Introduction — 281
- Debate — 283
- Case Taking from the Beginning; Spirit of Homeopathy — 286
- The Purpose, the Method and the Techniques — 286
- Sensation and Going Beyond Delusion — 298
- The Levels — 299
- Sensation is Non-human Specific — 302
- Case Taking in a New Light — 304
- Conclusion — 304

Part Three
Patient-Centered Medicine and the Relationship

10. The Therapeutic Relationship in Homeopathy – Ben Gadd — 327
- Why a Therapeutic Relationship? — 331
- What Patients Want from a Consultation — 332
- Common Elements in the Therapeutic Relationship — 333
- Homeopathy and Psychotherapy — 336

- Homeopathic and Allopathic Consultations — 338
- Placebo — 340
- Empathy — 343
- Patient-centredness — 345
- Therapeutic Alliance and Compassion — 347
- Impact of Homeopathic Process and Philosophy of Disease — 350

11. Conclusions — 357

- Healthy Schizophrenia — 360
- Linear Case Taking — 360
    - Best Practice — 361
    - Beautiful Silence — 364
    - Spontaneity and Transparent Responses — 366
    - Projections, Assumptions, Speculation — 367
    - Closing the Texbooks and Analyze Later — 367
    - Sleuthing for the Case — 368
    - Other Case Taking Concepts — 369
    - Fishing — 370
    - Poker — 371
    - Steaming the Mussel — 372
    - Clear Education and Answering Questions — 373
- Getting to the Centre of the Case — 373
    - Psychoanalytic — 375
    - Jungian — 376
    - Synthetic Case Taking Skills — 377
- Improving Clinical Case Taking Skills - Predilection and Practice — 378

- The Role of Intuition 379
- Random Directives before Case Taking 381
- Reflective Questions for the Homeopath 381
- Reflective Questions for the Client 384
- Patient-Centred, Person-Centred and the Relationship 385
    - Self Disclosure 386
- Final Conclusions Case Taking 389

Appendices 393
References 425
Index 447

Introduction to Case Taking

Chapter 1

Introduction

- The Need for Best Practice
- This Book
- Requirements of the Case Taker?
- Literature Review

In this chapter you will:

1. Understand the need for homeopathic medicine to develop evidence and best practice guidelines.
2. Describe what has occurred historically.
3. Identify the need to engage in a meaningful attempt to deconstruct and redevelop aspects of homeopathic practice.

Chapter 1
Introduction

The Need for Best Practice

In the last two or three decades the major milestones in homeopathic literature are about the science of homeopathy, the art of homeopathy, or the spirit of homeopathy. More recently attention has turned to best practice in homeopathy and it is with that in mind that this book seeks to synthesize, describe and articulate the skills of homeopathic case taking; how to get the right information needed to make an accurate prescription. This is not a book about homeopathic reasoning. It is not a book about homeopathic method. This is a book that seeks to describe the landscape of homeopathic case taking. A broad landscape approach is necessary because there are simply so many different opinions. As a consequence it limits its scope to the receiving of information in the homeopathic context. In this book there is no discussion of the relative merits of different homeopathic methods, but the reality is that it is not so easy to separate homeopathic case taking from the style of prescribing advocated. If we are to look at the technique of homeopathic medicine advocated by Scholten for example, it is impossible to speak about what he does in the consultation room and the information that he gets out of clients without referring to his preferred method. Nevertheless this book attempts to identify why homeopaths ask the things they do, how to get the right information needed for those styles, how to massage information out of clients, how to be an effective case taker. This book argues that getting the right information out of a patient is a crucial part of the process of homeopathy. This is about how homeopaths get their information. With this defined scope, this book may be useful for users of homeopathic medicine. But overwhelmingly this is a book for students and practitioners of the art and science of homeopathy.

The reason for this book is that there is still no agreement on best practice. The different schools think they do it, but as yet there is still no congruence of thought on just how we gather information and just what is the information we need. The different schools require different information. In this there are clear parallels with psychotherapy. Just as Cognitive Behavioural Therapy can be perceived as measurable, dry, yet effective with its statistically verifiable world of outcomes and specific changes, homeopathy has its equivalent. It is entirely possible to give a homeopathic remedy based on statistical possibility of creating the most likely change given the information provided. A specific prescription based on collated data, an organ affinity prescription or a traditional Böenninghausen prescription, with its almost mathematical simplicity based on a complete symptom may be the most effective. This is a different approach than a totality prescription based on perhaps some bland information in the case.

In psychotherapy for example, very different approaches, Person Centred Therapy or Somatic Therapy are tolerated and exist and are respected side by side. Homeopathy too has these more organic synthetic styles of prescribing and intervening. But there is an uneasiness in the coexistence. In these psychological disciplines it is well-known that one's philosophy and one's approach impacts on the questions asked and obviously the answers given. One of the paradoxes in homeopathic medicine is that we are attempting to extract that which we can then use to find a simillimum. But we don't know what that information is going to be. Of all the things the person says what is the important bit? What is the crucial information going to be? Taking a good case is the essential element that is agreed upon and common to all the approaches and the different styles of homeopathy that are practiced today. Some say it is half the job. One of the principles that is articulated in this book is that it is far more than that. In fact it is everything. A case well taken will determine an easily found remedy.

In this book we explore the best ways to get the information we need. It will be argued that it is not a linear process and nor is there any one strategy which is to be adopted. Talking to children, teenagers, men, women, reluctant patients, loquacious patients, anxious patients all require different approaches and sympathies. The contemporary homeopath needs to learn the different techniques of extracting information out of any client in an appropriate and safe way, at the same time getting what is needed but respecting the boundaries and sensitivities of the client. Those familiar with homeopathy may also look on this book as an historical development of homeopathic thought as our work has evolved in the last 200 years.

This Book

This is a book in three clear parts. The first part is a historical journey from the beginning through to the end of the 19th-century. It looks at the directives made by the prominent homeopaths of the time and places them within the context of Hahnemannian homeopathy. It describes best practice on how to gather information, what is the best information, what to do and what not to do. These instructions are much more orientated to medical practitioners in medical contexts, almost biomedical situations.

The second part of the book attempts to create a context for what has happened with those directives in homeopathic medicine since that time. After the great influx of European homeopaths into the east coast of America in the mid-1800s, the rise of the homeopathic colleges and the great homeopathic years of the 19th-century with its strong personalities and expansion, homeopathy in the US began to become marginalized in the first part of the 20th century (Winston 1999). Patients flocked back to orthodox practitioners with their drugs and new surgical techniques. More marginal patients, those falling through the cracks of the medical system and those with conditions more emotional and mental rather than physical became the bulk of clients seen by homeopaths. Into the 1900's with Freud, Jung and the rise of psychoanalysis and psychotherapy, homeopaths borrowed from that developing field and completely changed the process of homeopathic case taking marking a shift away from the style Hahnemann and the homeopaths of the 19th century had advocated and used. To the modern student this is a confusing situation. Teachers of homeopathy all around the world have wrestled with what is the best way to describe best practice to a homeopathic student given this historical evolution. After all, in the education programs of other disciplines it is a nonsense to start with the directives of the founder of the profession. No one talks about the first lawyer, the first accountant or the first economist. But in homeopathy everyone starts with Hahnemann. In modern osteopathic training what is taught is evidence-based best practice. Dr Still may get a mention but a very brief one.

This second part is orientated towards understanding that homeopaths since the turn of the 20th century have attempted to create meaning from the information that they are gathering and engage in a psychological process in a relationship that our founders did not. This is not to say that Hahnemann wasn't interested in his clients but it is to acknowledge that the modern homeopath in the Western world at least engages with their clients in a very different way to the pioneers. From the perspective of the 21st century modern teachers of homeopathy project their own values and perspective back onto the words of Hahnemann. At worst they distort the original meaning and completely see the life, works, and practice of Hahnemann in a projected light. At best they are able to over-reach the original intention and direction of homeopathy by placing those directives in a much more sophisticated framework and with a much deeper perspective.

The third part of this book describes the growing body of evidence and literature in the academic world of homeopathy. Here the homeopathic case taking process will be described in the context of the relationship between the patient and practitioner.

We find ourselves in a situation that is very different from what Hahnemann started with or perhaps intended. The modern student or observer is expected to grasp something very complex. What we see today comes from the building blocks of Hahnemann, Böenninghausen, then developed by Kent and post-Kentians such as Schmidt, plus the English homeopaths from the 1980's and 1990's that taught my generation, as well as those additional techniques and strategies such as psychotherapy, counseling, human resources, that others have brought to the profession. It is very difficult for other people looking at our profession to understand what we do because they don't understand the landscape. They think homeopathy is medical, or they think that it's psychological and they don't necessarily see the nuances or historical progression. Then they are asked to grasp Sankaran's work.

In the teaching of homeopathy or the deconstruction and redevelopment of one's practice it is important to realise that to prescribe well using Böenninghausen homeopathy the homeopath needs to be adept at Böenninghausen style case taking, and those students of these basic building blocks need to be immersed in that style. But if they're differently inclined they can work with a Kentian approach, or still going further the Sankaran method which requires again, a completely different system or style of case taking based on a different philosophy and set of assumptions. In these approaches the emphasis is the remedy as the goal but recently a more humanistic or patient-centred homeopathic approach is evolving moving practitioners to a model of practice and method and the selection of the remedy where the most important thing in the process is the relationship between the patient and practitioner and the homeopathic remedy is as a consequence secondary.

Homeopathy is a diverse and broad profession. It is often said that no two homeopaths are alike. This is especially so when travelling the world and seeing how homeopaths in Ireland differ in their style of practice from homeopaths in Australia,

Brazil, Italy and India. This is the profession's great strength and tremendous weakness. It means that a homeopath from New Zealand with a background in the study of history and no scientific or medical training can engage in a meaningful practice. Clients will present with anxiety, depression, fatigue, premenstrual syndrome or trouble with the prostate. It means that a homeopath from Malaysia, can study for four years and get their degree in medical science, and work in a free clinic providing primary health care to patients with cancer, polio, tuberculosis, hepatitis and gangrene. The homeopath in New Zealand has been educated by homeopaths with a completely different perspective and background to the homeopath educated and practising in Malaysia. There is no value judgement around this whatsoever. Yet it seems to the modern student of homeopathy worldwide that there is a need to distil and identify what is being said to them and from what context it comes. This is the overarching purpose of this book; to provide that context.

In essence this book describes the seismic shifts that have taken place and the changes in direction that homeopaths have taken over the 200 years of our art. As we approach the 200th year of the publication of the *Organon* in 1810, it is a time for reflection on those directives that Hahnemann gave us, the value of them now in the 21st century with the developments that have taken place inside our profession and those developments that have taken place around our profession that have impacted on what we do. Just how have those changes that have taken place in psychotherapy, nursing the developments in medicine, in science and the classification of drugs, medicines and of the animal, vegetable and mineral kingdoms impacted on best practice for homeopaths.

Requirements of the Case Taker?

As well as describing the landscape there is a subtext in this work. As an educator I have had a question for a decade. While we know what we are supposed to get as case takers and do as case takers, what is the most effective way to teach those skills and foster the clear techniques that are necessary? One of the things I will be highlighting in this book is an ongoing list of skills and qualities identified as useful or mandatory. Readers will be encouraged to take an audit of themselves to assess what qualities and pre-requisites they need to strengthen to create confidence and competence.

Literature Review

One of the delights of homeopathy, but also its Achilles heel most clearly defined in this age where everyone has a blog, is that everyone has an opinion. When it comes to case taking homeopaths have not been shy in coming forward. In gathering the resources required for this description of the landscape it was intended to look at the prominent features of that landscape, perhaps Kent, Close, Schmidt, Sankaran, Vithoulkas, Hahnemann. After all why look any further? It was a surprise therefore to realise that virtually every homeopath that has ever picked up a pen has had an opinion or a say on this topic. In the course of a literature review for this manual on case taking these authors provided useful and meaningful material.

Introduction

1.	Agrawal Comparative Study of Chronic Miasms
2.	Allen Chronic Miasms
3.	Bailey Homeopathic Psychology
4.	Bakshi Manual of Psychiatry
5.	Baldwin Organon of the Art of Healing Restated
6.	Ball Understanding Disease
7.	Banerjea Miasmatic Diagnosis
8.	Banerjee Chronic Disease - Its Cause and Cure
9.	Bentley Appearance and Circumstance
10.	Bentley Homeopathic Facial Analysis
11.	Bentley Soul and Survival
12.	Blackie Classical Homeopathy
13.	Böenninghausen 2001 NASH Journal
14.	Böenninghausen Lesser Writings of Böenninghausen
15.	Boericke 2002 NASH Journal
16.	Boericke Homeopathy
17.	Boericke Organon 6th ed.- Hahnemann
18.	Boger Collected Writings of C M Boger - Edited by Robert Bannan
19.	Boger Cyrus Maxwell Böenninghausen's Characteristics and Repertory
20.	Boger Studies in the Philosophy of Healing
21.	Boger Study of Materia Medica and Case Taking
22.	Boger Synoptic Key
23.	Borland Homeopathy in Theory and Practice
24.	Boyd Introduction to Homeopathic Medicine
25.	Bradford Life & Letters of Hahnemann
26.	Burley Identity and Individualism
27.	Carlyon Understanding Homeopathy, Homeopathic Understanding
28.	Cartier Potencia Cincuenta Milesimal en Teoría y Prác
29.	Chand Compendium of Lectures on Homœopathy 1950-1995
30.	Chatterjee Fundamentals of Homeopathy and Valuable Hints for Practice
31.	Chauhan Journey into the Human Core
32.	Choudhury Indications of the Miasms
33.	Cicchetti Dreams, Symbols, and Homeopathy

34.	Clarke Homeopathy Explained
35.	Close Genius of Homeopathy
36.	Cole Classical Homeopathy Revisited
37.	Collins Gem Homeopathy
38.	Cook Samuel Hahnemann, His Life and Times
39.	Coulter 1998 NASH Journal
40.	Creasy The Integrity of Homeopathy
41.	Dancu Homeopathic Vibrations - A Guide for Natural Healing
42.	Das Guide to Hahnemann's Chronic Diseases and Philosophy
43.	Das Synopsis of Homœopathic Ætiology
44.	Das Treatise on Organon of Medicine - Three Volumes
45.	Detinis Mental Symptoms in Homeopathy
46.	Dhawale Principles and Practice of Homeopathy vol. 1
47.	Dudgeon Lectures on the Theory and Practice of Homeopathy
48.	Dunham How to Take the Case
49.	Farrington Lesser Writings
50.	Felix Totality of Symptoms
51.	Flores Eescritos Medicos Menores del Dr Samuel Hahnemann
52.	Foubister Organon of Medicine 6th edition
53.	Foubister Tutorials on Homeopathy
54.	Fraser Using Mappa Mundi in Homeopathy
55.	Fraser Using Philosophy in Homeopathy
56.	Fraser Using Realms in Homeopathy
57.	Fuller Beyond the Veil of Delusions
58.	Gafoor The Art of Interrogation
59.	Ghatak Chronic Disease - Its Cause and Cure
60.	Ghegas Classical Homœopathic Lectures - Volume D
61.	Golden Homeopathic Body-System Prescribing
62.	Grahame Chakra Prescribing and Homeopathy
63.	Grimmer Collected Works of Grimmer
64.	Gutman Homeopathy - The Fundamentals
65.	Gutman Homœopathy: Fundamentals of its Philosophy and the Essence of its Remedies
66.	Haehl Life and Work of Samuel Hahnemann

67.	Hahnemann Chronic Diseases Theoretical Part
68.	Hahnemann Lesser Writings of Samuel Hahnemann
69.	Hahnemann Organon 5th and 6th ed Paris
70.	Hamilyn The Healing Art of Homeopathy – The Organon
71.	Handley In Search of the Later Hahnemann
72.	Hansford The Herdsman's Introduction to Homeopathy
73.	Hempel Science of Therapeutics (2 Vols. Combined)
74.	Henriques Crossroads to Cure
75.	Hering 1994 NASH Journal
76.	Hochstetter Hahnemann Organon - Hochstetter 6th Edition
77.	Kaplan The Homeopathic Conversation
78.	Kent 1995 NASH Journal
79.	Kent Filosofía Homeopatica
80.	Kent Lectures on Homeopathic Philosophy
81.	Kent Lesser Writings
82.	Kent New Remedies, Clinical Cases, Lesser Writings
83.	Kent What the Doctor Needs to Know
84.	Kishore Card Repertory
85.	Koehler The Handbook of Homeopathy
86.	Kramer Practical Guide to Methods of Homeopathic Prescribing
87.	Kulkarani Communication Skills - A practical approach
88.	Kulkarani. Communication Skills in case taking
89.	Kunzli Hahnemann Organon - Kunzli modern translation
90.	Lippe 2003 NASH Journal
91.	McQuinn The Path To Cure
92.	Mangialavore Identifying With Society
93.	Mansoor Case taking - A Developmental Approach
94.	Mansoor Difficulties in Taking Chronic Cases
95.	Master Bedside Organon of Medicine
96.	Master Lacs in Homeopathy
97.	Mast-Heudens The Foundation of the Chronic Miasms in the Practice of Homeopathy
98.	Mathur Principles of Prescribing
99.	Mirman Demystifying Homeopathy

100.	Morrell Hahnemann & Homeopathy
101.	Morrish Homeopathy A Rational Choice in Medicine
102.	Morrish Medicine Flows, Homeopathic Philosophy
103.	Murphy Hahnemann's Organon Of Medicine 6th Edition
104.	Murphy Robin Murphy's Case Analysis and Prescribing Techniques
105.	Nash Expanded Works on Nash
106.	Nash How to Take the Case
107.	Naude/Pendleton/Kunzli Organon 6th ed. (Naude) Hahnemann
108.	Nigam Principles and Practice of Homeopathic Case Management
109.	Norland Signatures Miasms Aids -Spiritual Aspects of Homeopathy
110.	O'Reilly Organon 6th ed.- Hahnemann
111.	Ortega Notes on Miasms
112.	Pacaud and Kratimenos Homeopathy Encyclopedia
113.	Paschero Homeopathy
114.	Patel Art of Case-Taking and Practical Repertorisation
115.	Robbins Evolving Homeopathy
116.	Roberts Homeopathy: Principles and Practice
117.	Roberts Principles and Art of Cure
118.	Rothenberg What Every Homeopath Wants Their Patient to Know - CD
119.	Rowe The Desert World: A Homeopathic Exploration
120.	Rowe The Homeopathic Journey
121.	Roy The Principles of Homeopathic Philosophy
122.	Saine Psychiatric Patients - Hahnemann and Psychological Cases
123.	Saine The Method
124.	Saji Case taking- A Repertorial approach
125.	Sankaran on you tube
126.	Sankaran Substance of Homeopathy
127.	Sankaran The Schema
128.	Sankaran The Spirit of Homeopathy
129.	Sankaran The System of Homeopathy
130.	Sarkar Organon of Medicine
131.	Saxton Miasms as Practical Tools
132.	de Schepper Achieving and Maintaining the Simillimum
133.	de Schepper Advanced Guide for Professional Homeopaths

134.	de Schepper Hahnemann Revisited
135.	de Schepper Human Condition: Critical
136.	de Schepper What About Men?
137.	Schmidt Art of Case Taking
138.	Schmidt Art of Interrogation
139.	Schmidt The hidden Treasure of the last Organon
140.	Shepherd A Physician's Posy
141.	Singh Organon of Medicine
142.	Smith Medical Homeopathy
143.	Sydow Learning Classical Homeopathy
144.	Tiwari Essentials of Repertorization
145.	Tyler Hahnemann's Conception of Chronic Diseases
146.	Ullman Prozac Free Reichenberg
147.	Ullman The Homeopathic Revolution
148.	Vijayakar Predictive Homeopathy Part 1, Suppression
149.	Vithoulkas Talks on Classical Homeopathy
150.	Vithoulkas Science of Homeopathy
151.	Watson A Guide to the Methodologies of Homeopathy
152.	Watson Case Taking and Analysis
153.	Watson Mental and Emotional Health
154.	Watson Running A Successful Practice
155.	Watson The Tao of Homeopathy
156.	Watson Understanding the Miasms
157.	Wauters The Homeopathy Bible
158.	Wesselhoeft Hahnemann Organon - Wesselhoeft
159.	Whitmont 1999 NASH Journal
160.	Whitmont Psyche & Substance
161.	Whitmont The Alchemy of Healing: Psyche and Soma
162.	Winston Heritage of Homeopathic Literature
163.	Wright-Hubbard Homeopathy As Art and Science
164.	Wright-Hubbard A Brief Study Course in Homeopathy

This book is intended to be a distillation but also a celebration of the work and personalities of our predecessors. The description of the landscape comes after numerous years of travel and contact within the homeopathic community around the world. Like most homeopaths my entry into this discipline was eclectic and individual. Having a startling and surprising reaction to a homeopathic intervention for an aspect of my own chronic disease that had troubled me for two decades I began to study. Initially in New Zealand, I soon travelled to the United Kingdom and studied at the School of Homeopathy in Devon with Misha Norland. A combination of his teaching with that of Jeremy Sherr at the Dynamis School plus exposure to other prominent homeopaths of the day set me on the path. Yet it was the coal face of homeopathy when I moved to Sydney, Australia that re-orientated my thinking and my style of prescribing. Soon being asked to teach and wrestling with those questions of how best to deliver information, I began to lecture as much as I was practising dividing my time between clients and the classroom. Homeopathy in Australia, for historical reasons is often taught within the context of naturopathic training and this presented an extra challenge for my homeopathic understanding, an extra layer of complexity teaching homeopathy to biomedical thinkers. Soon, invitations to conferences and to deliver seminars required further re-engineering of my teaching style and the content. For a decade I've had the good fortune to have the opportunity to teach and travel extensively in Asia, India, Malaysia and Thailand, in the US to Colorado, Canada, and to Europe, Ireland, the United Kingdom, Belgium, Holland and Germany. Never letting a good opportunity go by I've interviewed anyone I could get my hands on about their practice, their strategies, their understanding, their successes and failures and the specific details of their thriving practices. A significant amount of the work in this book can be attributed directly to them as well as the books and references it was necessary to research.

The conclusion from those interviews and from this research is overwhelmingly simple. All judgments aside, best practice is determined by the method employed. To do best practice with Hahnemannian homeopathy what is required of the case taker is to do a good job getting the information. But to do best practice with Post Jungian or Sankaran sensation method homeopathy what is required is to make sense of the symptoms, understand the patient, observe and use the brain to make meaning of what has been heard to get to the centre of the problem. To do best practice in humanistic or person-centred homeopathy what is required is that the practitioner is there, fully and contactfully. It is the most amazing privilege to sit and hear someone's story, to take their case. It is everything, all at once a hunt, an inquiry, a meditation, or an opportunity to be with someone and to understand another person at the deepest level.

Part One
Information Gathering to Find the Medicine

Part One

Chapter 2

Hahnemann

- The Directives
- Main Aphorisms
    - Other Aphorisms
- Hahnemann's World - Why He Gave those Instructions
- The Key Concepts - What Hahnemann Asks us to Look for
    - Totality
    - Peculiarity
- What is Required?
    - Non-Prejudice
    - Sound Senses
    - Attention in Observing
    - Fidelity in Tracing the Picture of the Disease
- Hahnemann's Directives for Case Taking in Specific Situations
- Further Directives of Hahnemann
- Summary of Hahnemann's General Directives for Best Practice
    - What to Do
    - What Not to Do
- Hahnemann's Main Writings
- Core Requirements for Case Taking from Hahnemann

In this chapter you will:
1. Learn Hahnemann's guidelines for case taking.
2. Understand their historical context.
3. Comprehend their simplicity and understand the issues that subsequent homeopaths have been left to wrestle with.

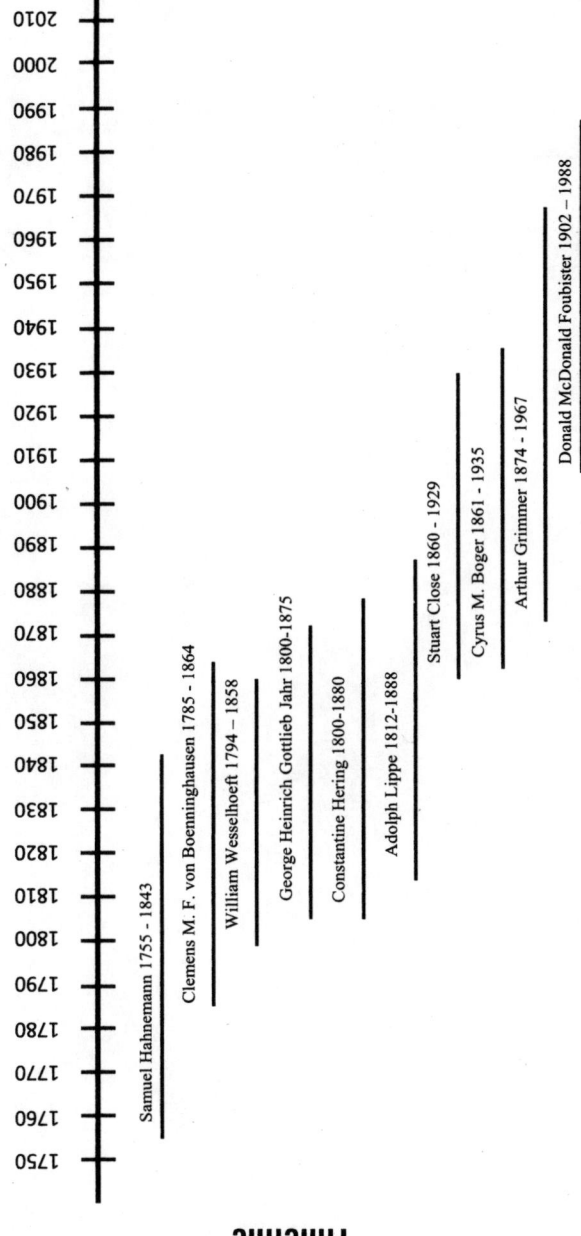

Timeline

- Samuel Hahnemann 1755 - 1843
- Clemens M. F. von Boenninghausen 1785 - 1864
- William Wesselhoeft 1794 – 1858
- George Heinrich Gottlieb Jahr 1800-1875
- Constantine Hering 1800-1880
- Adolph Lippe 1812-1888
- Stuart Close 1860 - 1929
- Cyrus M. Boger 1861 - 1935
- Arthur Grimmer 1874 - 1967
- Donald McDonald Foubister 1902 – 1988

Chapter 2
Hahnemann

The Directives

It all starts with Hahnemann. Any casual reader, or any committed student of homeopathy meets Hahnemann on day one. Battered copies of the *Organon* of Medicine are generally on the bookshelves, close at hand with every serious practitioner of homeopathy. Even 200 years after its first edition, students from all over Europe and the USA will have attended seminars by those such as Jeremy Sherr or in Australia with Ken D'Aran lecturing beautifully on the meaning and wisdom of the *Organon*. Other contemporary presenters do the same. Kent based his postgraduate school lectures on it. Embedded within curriculum in homeopathic undergraduate schools all over the world is time and energy devoted to understanding the fundamentals from Hahnemann.

Nevertheless students of homeopathy are often deeply disturbed when they realise they have to buy this book, this old book in such a strange layout and language. No other branch of study goes back to the source book in such a way; to the original accountant, or the original physiotherapist. In other disciplines knowledge is built, piece by piece and over time. Best practice is accumulated over time. Other professions textbooks are new, glossy and expensive. That said, the reticence is often transformed to profound satisfaction when listening to a lecturer who knows it well, taking you slowly word by word, interpretation by translation through its overt and hidden meanings.

Many believe the book is perfect as is. *Hahnemann's struggle throughout his life was to leave behind a document so perfect on its own so that future generations of genuine medical arts practitioners would have no difficulty and no confusion. The Organon actually is a road map to encourage homeopaths and spoon-feed them to ask specific questions on specific circumstances* (Gray 2010a). When it comes to the case taking directives it all seems essentially straightforward.

Main Aphorisms

§ Eighty Three

> This individualizing examination of a case of disease, for which I shall only give in this place general directions, of which the practitioner will bear in mind only what is applicable for each individual case, demands of the physician nothing but freedom from prejudice and sound senses, attention in observing and fidelity in tracing the picture of the disease.

There is immense clarity in this statement. There are four things that are required of the homeopath, to 1) be free from prejudice, 2) have sound senses, 3) be attentive in observing, and 4) be faithful in outlining the described disease. Three of those seem quite clear and unambiguous, however reflection requires some discussion about prejudice and just what

Hahnemann may have meant by this particular statement. Prejudice for Hahnemann was more about making favourites of remedies and naming diseases, than a posture of unconditional positive regard or neutrality that was emphasized by many in homeopathic training in the 1980's and 1990's.

§ Eighty Four

> The patient details the history of his sufferings; those about him tell what they heard him complain of, how he has behaved and what they have noticed in him; the physician sees, hears, and remarks by his other senses what there is of an altered or unusual character about him. He writes down accurately all that the patient and his friends have told him in the very expressions used by them. Keeping silence himself he allows them to say all they have to say, and refrains from interrupting them unless they wander off to other matters. The physician advises them at the beginning of the examination to speak slowly, in order that he may take down in writing the important parts of what the speakers say.

These are practical instructions. The patient talks, and the homeopath asks those who know the client what they have heard and seen. It sounds clear, but again upon reflection there are a number of assumptions. Not every patient talks. Our clinics are actually full of reluctant clients. Some actually don't like talking or describing their problems. Some are men. Moreover practicing homeopathic medicine in Sydney, Australia or Bristol in England in the 21st century means that the homeopath has to be hesitant before asking those around the patient what they have seen about their behaviour or symptoms. Ethical considerations in the western world seriously impinge upon this particular directive. Kent (1900) concurred:

> Get the nurse, if possible, to repeat the exact words of the patient. If such a thing can be done in acute sufferings it is worth more than the words or expressions of the nurse, the wife for instance, because the more interested and anxious the person is the less likely she will be able to present a truthful image, not that she wants to deceive, but she is dreadfully wrought up and the more she thinks of what he has said the greater his sufferings appear to her and she exaggerates them. It is important to have the statement from one who is disinterested. Two or three of the observers who are intelligent having been consulted and their statements recorded, the physician then notes his own observations. He should describe the urine if there is anything peculiar about that, but if the urine and stool are normal he need not care about the description of these.

The homeopath is encouraged to listen, watch and write down what is unusual about the client. So much about the sentence is misunderstood in the practice of homeopathy. The crucial word to my mind, is 'unusual'. What is unusual for some is completely normal to another. In actual fact there is tremendous ambiguity in the meaning of this aphorism. Unusual in what way, unusual about their appearance, their voice, their personality? Culturally we have tremendous differences in interpretation when looking at the same set of circumstances. In addition, it is often interpreted that Hahnemann meant unusual from when the patient was last healthy. This has some significance when another homeopath interprets it as unusual in the context of their personality or character. A patient in the middle of their consultation looks out the window and says 'I am a weather watcher'. It's a strange thing to say. At the time, in the consultation who knows if this is an important factor when her presenting symptoms are menopausal flushes.

Hahnemann then encourages homeopaths to write accurately all that they have heard. He gives no descriptions however of how best to do that. The advice on keeping silence however is crucial. Allowing the client to have their say and not interrupting is the quintessential professional posture of the homeopath. Keeping silence of course can mean that some clients, especially of the loquacious disposition, wander off onto other matters and he encourages homeopaths, but without describing when, to intervene when it is perceived that they are talking about non-essential details. Much is left to common sense.

In 2010 most people can type faster than they write so the comments advising the physician to encourage the client to speak slowly is less important that it may have been in the age of feather, ink and nib.

§ Eighty Five

> He begins a fresh line with every new circumstance mentioned by the patient or his friends, so that the symptoms shall be all ranged separately one below the other. He can thus add to any one, that may at first have been related in too vague a manner, but subsequently more explicitly explained.

Because some clients describe their symptoms in a disordered way, and because some patients have complicated case presentations, Hahnemann directs the homeopath to start each statement with a new line on the page. In the modern context students rightfully question whether this is appropriate given that the other healing professions such as nursing, physiotherapy, counseling, psychotherapy and of course medicine have a very inflexible opinions about gaps being left on a page; simply it's not recommended.

§ Eighty Six

When the narrators have finished what they would say of their own accord, the physician then reverts to each particular symptom and elicits more precise information respecting it in the following manner; he reads over the symptoms as they were related to him one by one, and about each of them he inquires for further particulars, e.g., at what period did this symptom occur? Was it previous to taking the medicine he had hitherto been using? While taking the medicine? Or only some days after leaving off the medicine? What kind of pain, what sensation exactly, was it that occurred on this spot? Where was the precise spot? Did the pain occur in fits and by itself, at various times? Or was it continued, without intermission? How long did it last? At what time of the day or night, and in what position of the body was it worst, or ceased entirely? What was the exact nature of this or that event or circumstance mentioned - described in plain words?

Aphorism 86 is often forgotten by new and experienced homeopaths alike. Sometimes described as mopping up, this aphorism encourages the listener to go back to each and every symptom and milk that symptom for everything they can get: sensations, modalities concomitants, causations etc. This is a great opportunity to read back to the client what they have just said and ensure its accuracy. It is also an opportunity for the homeopath to indulge in perhaps a little bit of deception to ensure that every aspect of that symptom is extracted. By pretending not to understand fully at this juncture, the patient is required to revisit their symptoms in all aspects and in depth. It is at this point that very specific questions can be asked. It's an opportunity to extract in immense detail the specific kinds of sensations, how they manifested, when they manifested.

Of course the specific language that the client uses to describe the symptoms can sometimes be important in the selection of the medicine itself and Hahnemann encourages us to keep this in the record. The aphorism is so skillfully written because it describes simply something that is so incredibly complex and that takes place on so many levels.

§ Eighty Seven

And thus the physician obtains more precise information respecting each particular detail, but without ever framing his questions so as to suggest the answer to the patient, so that he shall only have to answer yes or no; else he will be misled to answer in the affirmative or negative something untrue, half true, or not strictly correct, either from indolence or in order to please his interrogator, from which a false picture of the disease and an unsuitable mode of treatment must result.

As a consequence of asking open questions the homeopath gets all the information they need. The individual presentation of the symptoms remained characteristically clear and both patient and practitioner avoid the tendency to get stuck on named diseases. Yet further reflection requires that the student and practitioner ask just how questions are to be framed, just how open to make a question to a closed patient. Is it really laziness when the homeopath needs to revert to a closed question when an open one is intimidating to the unsuspecting patient?

§ Eighty Eight

> If in these voluntary details nothing has been mentioned respecting several parts or functions of the body or his metal state, the physician asks what more can be told in regard to these parts and these functions, or the state of his disposition or mind, but in doing this he only makes use of general expressions, in order that his informants may be obliged to enter into special details concerning them.

It sounds simple enough. Having discussed the presenting symptoms then the practitioner asks about the mental state and the functioning of the mind and the disposition. However questions about the specific words used here go to the heart of many of the disputes and schools of thought that divide and delineate our profession. What is a mental state? What is disposition? And crucially which parts of the mental state and disposition did he mean? Did he mean generally? Or did he mean only when the symptoms of the disease were present?

§ Eighty Nine

> When the patient (for it is on him we have chiefly to rely for a description of his sensations, except in the case of feigned diseases) has by these details, given of his own accord and in answer to inquiries, furnished the requisite information and traced a tolerably perfect picture of the disease, the physician is at liberty and obliged (if he feels he has not yet gained all the information he needs) to ask more precise, more special questions.

Just as in Aphorism 86, Hahnemann in Aphorism 89 reiterates the need to go back and fill in the gaps, and completely trace the disease, fully form the picture.

§ Ninety

When the physician has finished writing down these particulars, he then makes a note of what he himself observes in the patient, and ascertains how much of that was peculiar to the patient in his healthy state.

This directive encourages the homeopath to add their personal annotations to the record, especially those observations that are unusual or peculiar. This clarity must be tempered with the legal and ethical obligations of the 21st century. Other complementary health practitioners are required to be succinct, accurate and factual. The homeopathic professional posture is almost the opposite. Moreover just who owns these doodles, observations and thoughts about a patient? What would a judge say about the notes of a homeopath subpoenaed in a court case? When emphasizing this point I draw on an example of case notes from when I had been practicing less than a year. I use this as an exercise in how not to do it. In addition to the fact that they were in pencil and almost illegible it is quite clearly observable that I have made personal comments about the patient's facial features, their smell and their dress sense, and moreover added to the record once the patient had left the room. Imagine standing in front of a judge and justifying those additions to what is a legal document. It's an example of a simple directive that needs to be adapted to the 21st century.

§ Ninety Three

If the disease has been brought on a short time or, in the case of a chronic affection, a considerable time previously, by some obvious cause, then the patient - or his friends when questioned privately - will mention it either spontaneously or when carefully interrogated.

Here Hahnemann reminds us that the cause of the disease must be asked for before beginning the evaluation of the case and the search for a medicine.

§ Ninety Four

While inquiring into the state of chronic disease, the particular circumstances of the patient with regard to his ordinary occupations, his usual mode of living and diet, his domestic situation, and so forth, must be well considered and scrutinized, to ascertain what there is in them that may tend to produce or to maintain disease, in order that by their removal the recovery may be prompted.

It is absolutely within the homeopath's jurisdiction to ask about lifestyle, nutrition, habits, attitudes and opinions. All of these need to be known according to Aphorism 94 so that the homeopath can make a judgment call on whether to remove or negotiate the removal of these perceived obstacles. This is all the more crucial when those symptoms are impacting upon the health and well-being of the client, or maintaining the chronic disease that the client has, or anti-doting the homeopathic prescription. This is one of the greatest arts of the practice of homeopathy. Knowing when to intervene, how to intervene, just what time is it necessary to negotiate the compliance of a patient who has an addiction to pizza, red wine, cigarettes, chocolate, speed, heroin, sugar, salt, television or sex.

§ Ninety Five

In chronic disease the investigation of the signs of disease above mentioned, and of all others, must be pursued as carefully and circumstantially as possible, and the most minute peculiarities must be attended to, partly because in these diseases they are the most characteristic and least resemble those of acute diseases, and if a cure is to be affected they cannot be too accurately noted; partly because the patients become so used to their long sufferings that they pay little or no heed to the lesser accessory symptoms, which are often very pregnant with meaning (characteristic) often very useful in determining the choice of the remedy - and regard them almost as a necessary part of their condition, almost as health, the real feeling of which they have will - nigh forgotten in the sometimes fifteen or twenty years of suffering, and they can scarcely bring themselves to believe that these accessory symptoms, these greater or lesser deviations from the healthy state, can have any connection with their principal malady.

Details are crucial. Individuality is everything. The characteristic minutiae of a patient's symptoms can be gold. This is where Hahnemann encourages us that careful questioning about these lifestyle issues are so important. Because these lifestyle issues can be consequences from, or a part of the patient's acute or chronic disease there must be attention to detail in this regard. And because the homeopath needs to know the progression of the chronic disease in detail they must be prepared to go into the past with specific reference to those times that the health changed in a meaningful way, where the cause of the disease originated from.

§ Ninety Eight

Now, as certainly as we should listen particularly to the patient's description of his sufferings and sensations, and attach credence especially to his own expressions wherewith he endeavors to make us understand his ailments - because in the mouths of his friends and attendants they are usually altered and erroneously stated, - so certainly, on the other hand, in all diseases, but especially in the chronic ones, the investigation of the true, complete picture and its peculiarities demands especial circumspection, tact, knowledge of human nature, caution in conducting the inquiry and patience in an eminent degree.

A forgotten aphorism, and surely an example of Hahnemann's lack of interest in punctuation, or perhaps just a horrid translation, Aphorism 98 reminds us that in order to understand patients peculiarities, sufferings and sensations, the homeopath has to be worldly. It's necessary for the homeopath to have been around, to have been around the block. Classrooms and colleges these days are full of 18-year-olds. But in this aphorism Hahnemann is saying that the homeopath has to know human nature. He implies that timing is everything and crucial in conducting the enquiry. We know that patients leave us when they feel that an inappropriate intervention, or inappropriate question has been launched too early at them. Patience is a virtue and in homeopathic medicine it is an absolute necessity. Timing is everything and the ability to wait till the right time is mandatory.

So having told us that attention to detail, sound senses, a lack of prejudice, and fidelity are the requisite qualities of the engaging homeopath, Hahnemann then tells us that tact, knowledge, caution, timing, and patience are fundamental underpinnings of the homeopath.

How are these things taught? If these are the fundamental qualities of a busy homeopath in 1810 and also in 2013, then how is a director of a college, or the lecturer in the classroom to teach attention to detail. How does one teach fidelity or faithfulness? What textbook teaches tact? Where does one go for the knowledge base on patience? Homeopathic curricula are bursting at the seams with information about remedies, families, groups, kingdoms, methods. Yet in black and white the qualities of the homeopath are not taught in homeopathy school. According to Hahnemann the requisite features of the busy homeopath are learned elsewhere. This is a paradox that homeopathic colleges, curricula and industry leaders are reluctant to embrace. And in the 21st century the evidence is clear. Hahnemann is right. Research confirms (Gray 2009) that the thriving homeopath, and the success of his or her practice is not determined by the great results that they get in the clinic. This is a fallacy. Thriving practice is determined by the qualities of persistence, tenacity, desperation and having a wolf at the door, tact and timing a close second.

Other Aphorisms

§ Five

Useful to the physician in assisting him to cure are the particulars of the most probable exciting cause of the acute disease, as also the most significant points in the whole history of the chronic disease, to enable him to discover its fundamental cause, which is generally due to a chronic miasm. In these investigations, the ascertainable physical constitution of the patient (especially when the disease is chronic), his moral and intellectual character, his occupation, mode of living and habits, his social and domestic relations, his age, sexual function, etc., are to be taken into consideration.

Somewhat controversially Hahnemann mentions the constitution of the patient. He does that in Aphorism five and while on first reading an innocuous statement, it seems to be at odds with many of the other directives that have been given to date. Bewildered and confused students hear that the homeopath must ask about the constitution in one place, but then in another aphorism it is characteristic symptoms only that are to be looked for. Then somewhere else it is strange rare and peculiar symptoms. Yet in some other place it is the mental state. Elsewhere the directive is the disposition. Homeopathic students throw up their hands. Some walk away. Some turn to naturopathy and its perceived simplicity.

In Aphorism five, Hahnemann asks the homeopath to ascertain the moral and intellectual character, the way they live and intimacies around age and sexuality. In these investigations, the ascertainable physical constitution of the patient (especially when the disease is chronic), his moral and intellectual character, his occupation, mode of living, diet and habits, his social and domestic relations, his age and sexual function are to be taken into consideration (Hahnemann 1922 §5, §7, §94, §208). Moreover these accessory circumstances are features contributing to the development of a chronic miasm in a particular direction. These accessory circumstances may tend to produce or to maintain disease and after their removal (if possible, as we cannot always ask the patient to leave their job or wife or husband or their living place) recovery is more likely. Elsewhere in the *Organon*, Hahnemann argues that only after removing these accessory circumstances (for example, morbid obesity, criminality, occupations causing diseases, living in damp or unhygienic or polluted places, addictions, familial, social or marital stresses) can we start tracing the picture of disease as completely as possible in order to be elucidate the most striking and peculiar (characteristic) symptoms (Hahnemann 1922 §209). How to do so is one of the great arts.

§ Forty Two

Nature herself permits, as has been stated, in some cases, the simultaneous occurrence of two (indeed, of three) natural diseases in one and the same body. This complication, however, it must be remarked, happens only in the case of two dissimilar disease, which according to the eternal laws of nature do not remove, do not annihilate and cannot cure one another, but, as it seems, both (or all three) remain, as it were, separate in the organism, and each takes possession of the parts and systems peculiarly appropriate to it, which, on account of the want of resemblance of these maladies to each other, can very well happen without disparagement to the unity of life.

Mention must be made of Aphorism 42 because it mentions careful questioning needs to be conducted to determine if there is more than one disease present in the body at the same time as happens on occasion.

These case taking directives have stood the test of time. While later elaborated upon by Kent, Lippe, Hering, Dunham, Tyler, Close, Roberts, Schmidt and Hubbard-Wright to name a few, his ideas on what to ask for and how to get it have essentially remained unaltered. This has become good practice, best practice, when it comes to getting the information. Only very recently, with the arrival of sensation method, and with homeopathic academics borrowing from person-centered therapies has it been necessary to talk about different information and skills required of the homeopathic case taker.

By relying upon a source book, especially one in another language, and in another language that is 200 years old, that relies upon translation, and sometimes translated by people that were medical specialists not translators, just like the great religions, homeopathy opens itself up to antagonistic postures adopted by strong personalities focusing on interpretations of words written in a distant time. There is the opportunity for opposition, reinterpretation, fundamentalism. It is a great source book but there are more questions than answers. It all began with Hahnemann.

Hahnemann's World – Why He Gave those Instructions

The study of history is such a useful thing. History is not about dates, but about time, and change over time. At its best, history is the study of how this become that - how that situation then becomes this now. Such a perspective can assist us in understanding what was going on for Hahnemann at the time and inform us of the present. He began writing in a meaningful way on homeopathy in the 1790's. Robespierre was fresh in the memory, Napoleon was dancing through Europe, the English and French were at war on land and at sea. Tennessee was admitted into the Union. Germany didn't exist. The Australian colony was 8 years old. I encourage students of homeopathy to watch movies such as *Amadeus*, or Kenneth Branagh's *Frankenstein* to get a feel for medicine as it was practised around the time that Hahnemann was beginning his journey. It's important not to get too idealistic about the past nor air brush or photo-shop it.

What we know for sure is that Hahnemann's journey into homeopathy was a direct reaction against the excesses of medicine as it was practiced at the time. Specifically the use of leeches, bloodletting and primitive surgical interventions were the reasons he cited for looking for something more gentle permanent and rapid.

> I renounced the practice of medicine, that I might not incur the risk of doing injury....it was agony for me to walk in darkness, when I had to heal the sick and to prescribe according to such and such a hypothesis concerning diseases, substances which owed their place in the Materia Medica to an arbitrary decision (Bradford 1895).

Theories as to the cause of disease abounded. The shadow of middle-ages theories of humors was still present. Naming diseases was important. For these reasons his emphasis on the fundamental principles of peculiarity and totality make historical sense. To the willing non-allopathically minded student in the 21st century these points may seem self-evident. Certainly the introduction to the *Organon* should be read in this light.

> Hahnemann remains one of the four epochal figures in the history of the practice medicine. Hippocrates, the Observer, introduced the art of clinical observation as the necessary basis for pathologic diagnosis. Galen, the Disseminator, spread with powerful authority the teachings of Hippocrates over the medical world. Paracelsus, the Assailer, introduced chemical as well as physical analysis into the practice of medicine. Hahnemann, the Experimenter, discovered the symptomatic source of both

pathologic and therapeutic diagnosis and thereby made the practice of medicine scientific. Hahnemann steps in to say, for the first time in all history: Remove the effects and you remove the disease, the cause of the effects. Cessat effectus cessat causa (Krauss in Hahnemann 1922).

The Key Concepts – What Hahnemann Asks us to Look for

Totality

In 1796 'similars' was not a new idea. The seeds of simillimum go back to the Greeks, Rosicrucians and Paracelsus even though Hahnemann argued he knew none of the writings of the great alchemist (Danciger 1987). Nevertheless it challenged conventional wisdom and science as it was known. Similarly, the idea of totality pushed the boundaries. This was a radical concept. To the modern ear, versed in Louise Hay, Deepak Chopra and the other mind/body medicine gurus from the 80's, 90's and 00's, the idea of totality doesn't seem to be so impressive. Hahnemann was saying that the most important thing to look for in the case of disease was the totality of it, the total disease image, especially in the treatment of chronic disease. For him the whole idea of the exercise should be to make a portrait of the disease, which should be the sum, or essence of the characteristic symptoms that constituted the totality of the disease.

> Once the totality of the symptoms that principally determine and distinguish the case - in other words, the image of any kind of disease has been exactly recorded, the most difficult work is done. During the treatment (especially of a chronic disease), the

medical-art practitioner then has the total disease image always before him. He can behold it in all of its parts and lift out the characteristic signs. He can then select from the lists of symptoms of all the medicines which have become known (according to their pure actions) a well aimed similar, artificial disease potence, in the form of a homoeopathically chosen medicinal means, to oppose the total disease image. During treatment (at a follow-up examination of the patient) when medical-art practitioner inquires as to the result of the medicine and the altered condition of the patient, all he needs to do with his new disease findings is refer to the original list of symptoms and omit those that have improved, note what is still present, and add whatever has, perchance, come up in the way of new ailments (Hahnemann 1922 §104).

Debate

It sounds so simple. Look for the totality of symptoms. This is the job of the homeopath. But which symptoms, and which totality? In an acute condition it is perhaps easy to determine. I cut my foot on a piece of glass. I have blood. I have pain. I have a laceration. There is redness and some swelling. This constitutes the totality of symptoms. Prescribe a remedy. Simple. I have got a headache. It's left-sided, pulsates, is better when I lie down, and is worse what I when I get anxious and stressed. This could well constitute the totality of symptoms in this particular case. Give the remedy. Simple.

But it is rarely simple and quite clearly what has happened when it comes to the treatment of chronic diseases over the last 200 years with homeopathy is that different interpretations of this fundamental concept have determined the different ways in which homeopaths have prescribed. Some have argued that Hahnemann clearly meant the totality of characteristic symptoms of the disease. Other homeopaths have argued just as loudly that he did not mean that, he meant the homeopathic state of the patient. Other homeopaths, as we will hear in other chapters, have argued that it is the totality of the person that needs to be treated. The thinking traditionally around this area has been muddled and confused (D'Aran 1997).

Many homeopaths looking at the state of the profession around the world have clear opinions on how things have come to be so. Poor understanding of the basics of homeopathic prescribing are the reason for its troubles they argue. Too much emphasis on speculative methods is blamed. Focussing on aspects of personality or constitution leads to the prescription of bland polycrests that do very little. Patients don't get better and homeopathy gets a bad name. These homeopaths argue that it is a misunderstanding of this point about totality that is at the centre of the issue. Such grand totality's were never Hahnemann's intention. For them, homeopaths are being taught erroneously when it is said that our job is to look at the totality of the symptoms of the person. Case notes and repertorisations become bloated with meaningless information, facts not relevant in the case. The eyes are blue. So what. They felt sad when the cat died. So what.

This is a fundamental point of difference in the various schools that practice homeopathy. To my mind Hahnemann was relatively clear on this point. In Aphorism six he insists we look for the characteristic symptoms in the case. What he doesn't define is 'characteristic'. I will argue in chapter two that subsequent homeopaths, most notably Böenninghausen, defined it for him. A symptom requires a location, a complaint, a modality. A concomitant symptom, a cause, and some sensations can also be useful as well. This represents a complete symptom, the characteristic totality. One of the reasons why I like this interpretation of totality is because to a first-year student it makes perfect sense. Homeopathy seems logical and able to be learned through repetition. It is easily replicated. Confidence in prescribing is a consequence. But this is different to the style of homeopathy taught in different colleges where experts with years and years of clinical experience describe and talk about their very complicated cases where perhaps they had a successful result with a remedy based on a much larger totality. This is advanced work and very difficult to replicate.

It is notoriously difficult to go back into history and to try and work out what someone may have meant with their words. Hahnemann was influenced by inductive logic of Bacon and introduced homeopathy as a science of phenomenology. It can be argued that homeopathic case taking is nothing but the study of the disease phenomenon with the individualizing characteristics for which a remedy can be selected on the similar principle. It is the study of the outwardly reflected picture of the internal essence of the disease. On this point homeopaths all agree. But it has to be acknowledged that there are many different

- Miasmatic
- Particular to general - Böenninghausen.
- General to particular – Kent.
- Keynotes (minimum syndrome of maximum value) - H.C. Allen, Gurensey, Lippe, Nash, Skinner.
- Organopathy – Burnett, Rademacher.
- Constitutional – Grauvolg, Clarke.
- Chronological sequential - Hughes, Woodward.
- Etiological - Burnett, Clarke.
- Anamnesis - Dunham.
- Last appearing or Guiding symptoms – Hering.
- Nosodes – Tyler, Julian, Allen, Burnett.
- Tautopathy – Patel
- Archetype & symbols - Whitmont

kinds of similarity and different approaches to totality, and homeopaths differ when provided with the same set of facts on which to prescribe. In fact they have come up with all sorts of legitimate ways in which to prescribe, all based on their perceived totality.

The approaches in the box above are all meaningful ways of prescribing. But all require a different interpretation of what totality means.

Cause

If knowing totality is important then understanding the cause of the disease is crucial. The case taker must pursue this. The cause in one condition is the height of the keyboard creating the RSI. The cause was the car crash I was in, the grief or the loss. The exciting or precipitating cause of the illness ranks very high in importance. Farrington says that *Arnica* may well cure an illness originating from an injury, even though symptoms of *Arnica* may not be actually present in the case (P. Sankaran 1996). The patient was once a healthy individual and something happened to upset that balance of health. The knowledge of this 'something' - is very important. It might have been an injury, an emotional upset, shock, a loss, greed, disappointment, fright, anxiety or vexation, an exposure to cold damp, heat or sun, an indiscretion in diet or activity, overexertion, suppression of discharges or eruptions, or any one of the numerous influences which excite or activate disease conditions, and which the careful observer can uncover by close and intelligent questioning (P Sankaran 1996). Dixton notes, 'I could cite cures following the finding of causes in history taking from diagnosis too, like a cataract following a suppressed footsweat, a nervous breakdown from an unfortunate love affair, an insanity from a fright, an epilepsy from a head injury, a tuberculosis from a suppressed eczema. But let's stop here by just pointing out again the moral: that it is easy if you take the time to get a complete history of the individual before you make that first prescription' (P. Sankaran 1996).

> Now, as in a disease, from which no manifest exciting or maintaining cause (causa occasionalis) has to be removed, we can perceive nothing but the morbid symptoms, the totality of the symptoms must be the principal, indeed the only thing the physician has to take note of in every case of disease (Hahnemann 1922 §7).

> *When the patient describes or admits that he has become irritable, or suspicious, or jealous, impatient, restless, afraid, nervous, etc., when he has developed any of these negative traits, I suspect that there must have been some shock, disappointment, bad news, etc., some negative or unhappy experience at the back of these and by close and tactful questioning - here some leading questions may be necessary - I am usually able to discover what it is (P Sankaran).*

Homeopathy provides many useful antidotes and interventions for various types of causes, some of which western modern physicians may not comprehend. There is always a cause. Whether it can be identified and found is something else.

Hahnemann encouraged us to first, remove false or psuedo symptoms from the totality of symptoms. These are present due to the accessory circumstances or maintaining cause and generally cease spontaneously after the removal of these trivial causes. He taught that the fundamental cause of all true chronic disease has to be investigated in each individual case by the thorough accumulation of symptoms. The fundamental cause is generally due to a chronic miasm (Hahnemann 1922 §5, §206). There are three types of chronic diseases and it is important in the case taking to be clear what we are dealing with. As we are taking the case an ongoing classification of these symptoms, those caused by medicines or lifestyle is required leaving the symptoms of the chronic disease to be addressed. Symptoms due to miasmatic causes never disappear spontaneously but require anti-miasmatic remedies. After removing these psuedo symptoms we have the numerical totality of all true symptoms of the disease.

Elimination of Maintaining Cause and the Value of Previous History

Asking about the cause is very different to knowing how to remove it.

> There is no sense in treating a patient who has been exposed to chemical fumes and thereby suffers, if he continues to expose himself to it. A traffic policeman having varicose veins will improve little if he continues to stand the whole day. If the patient is under the stress of some strong emotional factors, he must avoid such situations which excite him (P Sankaran 1996). Where the indicated remedy has been correctly chosen, we have to consider the possible obstacles to cure which as, Whitmont says maybe 'living habits, drugs, irreversible or mechanical pathology, psychological factors and the

---

1) Artificial chronic diseases which are caused by an allopathic treatment and the prolonged use of medicines in large doses; disease caused by medicine.

2) Inappropriately named chronic disease which occurs after continual exposure to avoidable noxious influences- indulging in alcohol, addictions, or prolonged abstinence from things that are necessary for the support of life (vitamin or mineral deficiency), unhealthy localities, deprived of exercise or open air, overexertion of body or mind, living in a constant state of worry; disease caused by lifestyle.

3) True natural chronic diseases are those that arise from a chronic miasms - (Hahnemann 2001 §74- §77).

miasmatic background'. This is the art of case management (P. Sankaran 1996).

P. Sankaran mentions,

> I have known several patients who did not show any improvement with the indicated remedy, but who on careful further enquiry revealed that they had earlier suffered from some illness such as Smallpox, Diphtheria, Measles, injury, repeated vaccinations etc., and only after the effects of these previous diseases/causes had been antidoted by suitable homoeopathic medicines such as Variolinum, Diphtherinum, Morbillinum, Arnica, Thuja, etc., these patients had started improving.
>
> In a case Lippe prescribed Lac caninum because ten years earlier patient suffered from an attack of Diphtheria and the character of the attack had been that it had gone from one side to the other and back again. The patient was completely cured of the impotence and infertility. Weisselhoeft writes, 'As far as we know, Lac caninum has no sexual weakness. The fact disturbed Lippe very little in his selection. He looked deeper and found the cause and the remedy. This is true homoeopathic pathology.' Sometimes the origin of the illness might be so remote in time or so early in childhood that it might have been completely forgotten. Yet careful probing might elicit the real source. Foubister in the case of a lady who had ulcerative colitis and who clearly needed Sepia. Sepia however failed to help her but when she received Hypericum which was given because she had developed the condition after a fall on her back, she was cured (P. Sankaran 1996).

Family History, Treatment History and the Importance of Pathology

Patients never seem to arrive when they should in the clinic. We must be prepared to treat the patient at any stage of the disease, be it acute or chronic. This is why Boericke and Boger gave a number of pathological indications for various remedies. 'If characteristic symptoms are available don't take pathological symptoms. But if they are not available, do consider the pathological symptoms' (P. Sankaran 1996). Homeopaths worldwide know that when patients show no response to the remedy which was clearly indicated even after careful enquiry, after eliciting the family history of tuberculosis or cancer in the parents or ancestors, a dose of *Tuberculinum* or *Carcinosin* will lead to improvement. There are innumerable other examples (P. Sankaran 1996).

- Grimmer writes that the four best antidotes to the coal tar drugs like Aspirin are Arnica, Carbo veg., Lachesis and Mag. phos. to be given according to the symptoms present in each individual case.

- Foubister says, the use of an anaesthetic may subvert the harmonious functioning of the organism. So he suggests that it is always wiser to enquire for a history of operations and the undue after-effects of any anaesthetic applied therein. Where the anaesthetic is clearly known, e.g. Chloroform or Ether, a potency of the same may clear up the ill-effects.

- Grimmer, 'One more important source of interference with the homoeopathic remedy is the widespread use of sera and vaccines as protective agents against acute disease. The reaction to these products of diseases is often lasting in its effect and leaves the victims of this practice sick and suffering.'

- Boger used Anthracinum, Psorinum or Sulphur and Hayes suggests Phos.

Peculiarity

In many places throughout the *Organon*, Hahnemann tells us to look for any peculiarity or that which completely distinguishes this from that.

> The more striking, singular, uncommon and peculiar (characteristic) signs and symptoms of the case of disease are chiefly and most solely to be kept in view; for it is more particularly these that very similar ones in the list of symptoms of the selected medicine must correspond to, in order to constitute it the most suitable for effecting the cure. The more general and undefined symptoms: loss of appetite, headache, debility, restless sleep, discomfort, and so forth, demand but little attention when of that vague and indefinite character, if they cannot be more accurately described, as symptoms of such a general nature are observed in almost every disease and from almost every drug (Hahnemann 1922 §153).

Hahnemann advocated the use of singular, uncommon and peculiar (characteristic) signs and symptoms in constructing the characteristic totality of the disease which is the key for individualizing the patient for the final selection of remedy. Yet clearly, what is peculiar for some homeopaths is normal for others.

Just what is peculiar? This is a question I have been asked by students for a decade. My own working definition of peculiar is, 'I have never heard *that* before!' Of course this is extremely subjective because of the life experience or cultural filter that the homeopath is bringing to the consultation and from which he or she is seeing the patient. On the occasions that I have been lecturing in for example Malaysia, and I have presented a case that I presented in Auckland the week before I've been startled by some of the reactions. A patient says, 'I don't drink during the week but on Friday or Saturday I give it a nudge', meaning that they may have four or five drinks which is typical in Ireland, the UK or New Zealand. This has my Malaysian students apoplectic and reaching for the *Nux vomica*. My Australian students don't even hear the patient say that.

Just what is normal? How many drinks is it okay to have? Is smoking dope every now and again a problem? In the practice of homeopathy and wrestling with the idea of just what is a strange, rare and peculiar symptom brings homeopaths right up against their own personal experiences of life, their values, ethics, their morals, and what they feel is right or wrong. What is the right way to live?

A patient says to me, 'I have this embarrassing problem. Sometimes when I am having sex I get a piercing pain at the end of my penis just as I am about to ejaculate. It's strange, it never happens when I'm having sex with men, only when I am having sex with my wife'. This meets my own personal criteria of a strange symptom and one that I need to pursue. I've never heard it before. It is peculiar. But what about the

> In addition, the observant physician will be able to note various small but significant details such as the decubitus, the expression, perhaps a flapping of the alae nasi or twitching somewhere, etc., which will all add up to a totality. I may mention that in a case of pneumonia I was guided to the remedy by a wrinkling of the forehead of the patient. Van Tine has remarked, 'There is no symptom in the sick room without its value, especially in acute and serious cases.'
> (P Sankaran)

22 year old patient in Sydney in the city who says to me, 'I wake up every morning and have two double shots of coffee, I drink most nights, I hate vegetables, and I don't get enough sleep'. To one homeopath this is nothing other than a lifestyle of a 22-year-old and is common and nothing to be concerned about. To another homeopath it's shocking behaviour at the core of the disease and definitely needs to be explored. For one homeopath it's pseudo chronic disease and ignored because it would not provide any guide to the selection of the specific remedy (Dimitriadis 1993). For another it's a feature of the miasmatic disease.

It is difficult in the case taking process to not appear bored by common symptoms. But it is very important that we don't allow that disinterest to appear on our faces or expressions and for the patient to see that. There is nothing more off-putting for a client than to have a homeopath suddenly sit bolt upright in a chair having been slouching just because something has come out of their mouth that appeared interesting. Any patient will suddenly think to themselves, 'What was it that I just said that was so startling?' and the moment is lost.

In the pursuit of peculiarity, what is required of the homeopath is to listen, adopting the posture like an oyster in the ocean allowing everything to come towards it and through it. Eventually, with questioning and waiting there will be one thing that is strange (Hahnemann) that doesn't make sense (Sankaran) or is straight up bizarre. From Hahnemann's time all homeopaths know that peculiarity is to be valued in case taking. Toothache better for cold water, etc. But it means we have to understand what is going on and have some worldliness, know what is normal and what is expected and furthermore, notice these things as they are emerging in the consultation and placed in the context of the circumstances of the client. For excellent examples of fine observation of peculiarity see Dimitiadis in *Homoeopathic Links 1/93*.

What is Required?

Non-Prejudice

In addition to telling us what to look for, Hahnemann articulates the posture we should adopt to get it. Freedom from prejudice is the expression used in homeopathy. Prejudice means judging the present on the basis of past experience, which leads to a fixed rigidity of thinking. The homeopath should not use their own yardsticks and parameters to understand a case. It involves detaching from past experiences, emotions, desires and aversions and physical reactions. The only way to become unprejudiced is to become aware of our prejudices.

> Prejudice and doubt may be overcome by reflection, study, self discipline and auto suggestion by cultivating the scientific spirit (Gafoor 2010).

> The unprejudiced observer...takes note of nothing in every individual disease, except the changes in the health of the body and of the mind (morbid phenomenon, accidents, symptoms), which can be perceived externally by means of the senses... notices only the deviations from the former healthy state of the now diseased individual, which are felt by the patient himself, remarked by those around him and observed by the physician (Hahnemann 1922 §6).

> I was taught that Hahnemann meant, *Don't be a prejudiced person when you are taking the case, don't judge what you hear.* But

looking at the other parts of the *Organon* where Hahnemann discusses prejudice confirms that he meant something else entirely.

In Aphorism 83,

> This individualizing examination of a disease case, for which I am giving only general instructions here (and from which the disease examiner should retain only what is applicable to each single case) demands nothing of the medical-art practitioner except freedom from prejudice and healthy senses, attention while observing and fidelity in recording the image of the disease.

In Aphorism 73a,

> The homoeopathic physician is not caught up in prejudices devised by the ordinary school, which established names for some fevers (outside of which, great teeming nature would not dare produce any others) in order to treat them according to a definite mold. The homoeopathic physician does not acknowledge such names as dungeon fever, bilious fever, typhus fever, putrid fever, nerve fever, or mucous fever; rather, he cures each one according to its own peculiarity, without giving it a fixed name.

In Aphorism 257,

> The genuine medical–art practitioner will know how avoid making favorites of certain medicines that he has happened to find indicated rather often and has used with success. Otherwise, he will often overlook more rarely used medicines that would be more homeopathically fitting and therefore more helpful. By the same token, the medical-art practitioner will not (out of mistrustful weakness) avoid medicines, in his further medical pursuit, that he previously employed with disadvantage because

he had incorrectly selected them (therefore, his own fault) or for other reasons.

In Aphorism 141,

> Of all the provings of the pure actions of simple medicines in altering the human condition, and of the artificial disease states and symptoms that they engender in the healthy person, the most excellent provings remain those that the healthy, unprejudiced, conscientious and fine-feeling physician employs upon himself, with all the care and caution taught here. He knows [is aware] with the greatest certainty that which he has perceived in himself (Hahnemann 1922).

Neutrality

While many have lectured that being unprejudiced meant being neutral and having unconditional positive regard for the patient it seems this is a projection. Hahnemann meant, 'do not think you know something about the disease.' When I was a student a much more liberal interpretation was given to this idea. The discussions around prejudice involved not having opinions or prejudices about people's lifestyle choices, sexual orientation, and bottles of wine they drank, and the social partners they had, what time of day they took tea, with whom they played bridge. It was explained that a homeopath needs to be unprejudiced, and almost have an unattached Buddhist-like approach to case taking. Many times in my student days lecturers described meditating for hours before the patient walked in the room, clearing the mind to ensure that there were no projections on to any client. From the perspective of running a busy city clinic it all seems a little precious and self-indulgent, but this was the interpretation of prejudice at the time and I know that a generation of English homeopaths were taught the same thing in the same way.

> *Common prejudice which emerge during case takings are:*
>
> a) *Thermal reaction: A physician uses his own parameters for comparing the patient's heat & cold tolerance & adaptabilities to various temperatures.*
>
> b) *Likes & dislikes: If physician has craving for sweet he interprets desire for sweet in a patient as a common symptom with less intensity*
>
> c) *Emotions or reactions at the mental plane: If physician himself is loquacious he will not interpret loquacity of patient as a deviation from state of health*
>
> d) *Similar unresolved situations: If physician suffers from involuntary sighing because of past unresolved grief he will consider involuntary sighing in a patient as a common phenomenon & will miss to observe it*
>
> *In addition the physician should guard himself against prejudices arising from:*
>
> a) *Successful experience of a similar clinical condition.*
>
> b) *Limited use of a specific group of medicines & knowledge acquired from the study of materia medica & therapeutics*
>
> c) *Diagnosis (sometimes it may become a problem for some physicians who think of medicines mostly in terms of diagnosis)*
>
> d) *Similar physical make up or bodily reactions (a lady physician while investigating physical attributes did not note some menstrual concomitants because she too had similar expression during menses. An obese physician may over look slight obesity in his patients)*
>
> e) *Similar habits (a physician who smokes & drinks tends to ignore a similar habit in his patients)*
>
> *His experience of life & living (personal benefits and wrong notions) may interfere in investigating and interpreting the information (Tiwari 2000).*

Students at that time were encouraged to meditate, get supervision, and participate in provings to ensure that they stayed at the cutting-edge of their own personal journey and individuation process. The attitude was that it was necessary to be neutral and the therapeutic approach and posture was a balance of open and closed, open hearted but without gushing, leaking or projecting onto the client.

Others such as Close (1924) have argued that being without prejudice meant,

> 'the homeopath should detach himself from his own past experience, his emotions, desires, aversions & physical reactions i.e. to detach from his own self to understand the true language of disease in the form of sign & symptoms. This can be achieved through strong commitment & a constant practice with a desire to serve the fellow beings. The important way to become unprejudiced is to become aware of our prejudice. Prejudice is preconceived idea or notion.

Close (1924) put it this way,

> 'Without prejudice!' Sounds easy but try it. Who of us is without prejudice? The prejudice of a materialistic mind; of pathological theories which seem too often to be antagonistic to homoeopathic principles; of doubt as to the use of the single remedy or of use of any medicine at all; the prejudice of 'a constitutional aversion to work!' Many of us are 'born tired.' We don't like to work. Laziness, selfishness and an 'easy conscience' are responsible for more homoeopathic sins and shortcomings than anything else, for good homoeopathic prescribing means work! These are our worst enemies, and the worst enemies of homeopathy. No man who is in the grip of settled doubt or prejudice can do good work. Nowhere will prejudice show more clearly than in the homoeopathic examination of a patient. If one approaches a case prejudiced in favor of some pathological theory his examination will insensibly, but inevitably, be limited by that theory. Prejudice and doubt may be overcome by reflection, study, self-discipline and auto-suggestion; by cultivating the scientific spirit; by returning often to a consideration of and reflection upon the broad general principles underlying our art with the purpose of reforming methods, strengthening morale and correcting faulty

mental attitude, or point of view. Beliefs and convictions may be strengthened and energy stimulated by reflecting upon the fact that our therapeutic method is efficient and successful because it is based upon immutable law.

From the more modern liberal understanding of prejudice we understand that it is professionally beneficial to have this posture of neutrality. A homeopath said to me,

> I'm struggling with prejudice all the time. Because you're human, it's human nature to judge. But I find, once I've got my homeopath hat on I'm all right with that. But outside I'm judging all the time, but in the clinic I don't.

As for myself I know I am not free from judgement at all. I'm not free from judgement when, the North Shore housewife pulls up in a four wheel drive and is so upset with her husband because, 'he doesn't appreciate me anymore and my life is so boring and empty.' Or the patient that rings me up and says, 'I know I've got an appointment with you this afternoon but I'm in Melbourne, sorry mate.'

There are some patients that I really like and look forward to seeing, and also the opposite. It goes both ways. As soon as I have an opinion I recognise that as judgement and prejudice and I've noticed that actually, I have them all the time. The way that I have reconciled this in myself is to notice when it happens. I think it is the only realistic way we can maintain this posture. I remember being taught by a tutor at my college years ago who advocated we replicate what he did, which was to meditate for an hour before each client, so when the patient came he would be in the moment and free from prejudice and centred, completely present. It is a constant process of observation. A student said,

But the prejudice can happen during the consultation. Something is triggered, you know I had two patients the other day, in a row, and they both had lost their mothers and I don't know and I had lost my mother and that was taking me away and that stuff will come out. And she said she'd lost her mother suddenly and I'd lost my mother suddenly. So, all of a sudden, it's really hard for me not to think 'Oh, I know how she feels, I know how horrible that is, I know how difficult that is.' It may not have been. I found out through that story, she wasn't actually that close to her mother and she was actually dealing with different issues with regards to it. I can't say I was completely unprejudiced, I mean I was sitting there thinking, all of those things, I would probably do all of them. I will be prejudiced and I won't use my senses properly and I'm not observational sometimes.

Sound Senses

As well as non prejudice, Hahnemann encourages that while taking the case, the homeopath sees, listens, takes notice of smell (if any) and examines by adopting various methods of physical examination. In order to obtain a complete picture of the disease one has to know what to notice and where to look in a given case. This requires sound knowledge of materia medica, homeopathic philosophy, anatomy, physiology, pathology, psychology and other social and medical sciences. Not much more needs to be said on this point. All of the case takers senses are to be used to elicit information. Kent agreed, *all the senses must be on the alert in order to perceive that which is similar, and most similar* (Kent 1900 Lecture 22). In order to obtain a complete picture of the disease one has to know what to notice and where to look for it in a given case.

A physician's sense can be called sound only if he is capable of utilizing them in an undisturbed uninterrupted and unbiased way. It depends on the sensitivity and commitment of the physician to his profession (Gafoor 2010).

Attention in Observing

Hahnemann in his essay *Medical Observer* writes, 'True it is, that the careful observer alone can become a true healer of disease'. He mentioned the following points in favor of observation:

a) The medical practitioner requires possessing the capacity and habit of noticing carefully and correctly.

b) He should direct all his thought upon the matter in hand and should come out of his self.

c) Great patience supported by the power of will, should sustain him.

d) The best opportunity for exercising and perfecting our observing faculty is afforded by instituting experiments with medicine upon ourselves.

e) He must restrain himself from poetic fancy, fantastic wit, speculation, overstrained reasoning, forced interpretation and from a tendency to explain things (Hahnemann 1922).

One day in my clinic I was leaning out the window and saw my next client parking his car. It was a very large well used and slightly battered land cruiser and it also had kangaroo bars at the front and wrapping around the roof. And that was the striking thing because there are no kangaroos in Bristol which is where I was living at the time. It was one of the first things I asked about and his response, coupled with where he went in the conversation, the need to protect himself from bad people, from terrorists, from bombs, and have an escape vehicle went a significant way in his eventual prescription of *Mercury* helping his presenting symptom which was snoring. Attention to detail in observing leads to good results.

But there are plenty of examples of poor attention to observation in homeopathic case taking. One of the more spectacular examples from my own practice involved me getting excited about a patient who presented with hayfever and insomnia. Like a good case taker I noticed that the patient was from a northern Scandinavian country, and his favourite food was blood pudding. I also couldn't help noticing that he had a very large bat tattooed on his arm. I asked him about it and followed a line of enquiry. Resisting the impulse to ask if he liked to sleep upside down, I found a remedy for him, prescribed it and made some but not a lot of progress. Over the next few weeks and months I went through a number of remedies as I was trying to relieve some of his symptoms. When on a hot day he came back, perhaps his fifth visit he was wearing a T-shirt that revealed, in addition to the tattoo of the bat, a myriad of others which, had I asked or been more attentive I would have noticed at the outset. Also tattooed on his body were the gates of hell, roses, dolphins, scorpions, spiderwebs, obscure mythical creatures, and other weirdness.

The literature is full of examples of skilled practitioners noticing the minutest details and from the outset Hahnemann encouraged us to notice these peculiarities.

> A careful observer alone can become a true healer of disease. In order accurately to perceive what is to be observed in patients, we have to come out of ourselves and attach ourselves with all powers of concentration upon the subject. Poetic fancy and speculation must, for a while, be suspended and all overstrained reasoning, forced interpretation and tendency to explain away things must be suppressed. His attention should be on the watch that nothing actually present escape his observation and also what he observes be understood exactly as it is. The capability

should be acquired by practice and the best opportunity for exercising and perfecting our observing faculty is afforded by instituting experiments with medicines upon ourselves (Gafoor 2010).

Fidelity in Tracing the Picture of the Disease

Homeopaths should be able to translate their observations into words by using the most appropriate expressions. Notations should be candid and in the patient's own words as far as possible. Intensity, circumstances, association and other details of all expressions must find a place in the record without changing its meaning. Fidelity means faithfulness, and it is interesting that Hahnemann asks us to be faithful in outlining the image just as we would were we tracing a drawing. Faithfulness in tracing the picture of the disease is a lovely choice of words because it's essentially saying that when a homeopath is taking the case, they are drawing a map. A map is a map and it is a representation of the reality, of the territory but it is still a map. It's the grease-proof paper that you drew on and traced the outline of a drawing on the kitchen table when you were a child. It was drawn faithfully. Fidelity is also a term that is heard these days in relation to speakers and sound production. High fidelity means faithfulness to the original source; to the true source to the sound. A homeopath needs to be faithful and loyal in noticing and recording the deviation from health.

Hahnemann's Directives for Case Taking in Specific Situations

There are a few other more minor points that need to be made regarding Hahnemann's instructions for case taking. They relate to specific situations that may occur and what to do in those situations and come from an exploration of his major writings.

Indisposition

If a patient complains of one or more trivial or transient symptoms, that have been only observed a short time previously, the physician should not regard this as a fully developed disease that requires serious medical aid. A simple alteration in the diet and regimen will usually suffice to dispel such an indisposition (Hahnemann 1922 §150). These symptoms also should not be added to the original case taking. Moreover we must not change our previously selected remedy on the basis of these indispositions. The best practice is to give lifestyle advice then wait and watch.

One Sided Disease

A one-sided disease displays only one or two principal symptoms which obscure almost all the others. For the first prescription we have to be guided by these few symptoms and the medicine which, in our judgment, is the most homeopathically indicated should be prescribed. Essentially in this difficult situation we are to do our best. In the next visit for the second prescription we have to regard the whole collection of symptoms that may have emerged and that are now visible as belonging to the disease itself and to treat what has emerged accordingly (Hahnemann 1922 §173-§184).

Local Affections

The exact character of the local affection should be noted. All the changes, sufferings and symptoms observable in the patient's health and which may have been previously noticed when no medicine has been used, should also be considered. All of the above are taken in conjunction to form a complete picture of the disease. The local affection should only be regarded as an inseparable part of the whole, as one of the most considerable and striking symptoms of the whole disease (Hahnemann 1922 §192, §193).

Mental Diseases

In these situations an appropriate professional posture towards the patient must be observed, by way of an auxiliary mental regimen (Hahnemann 1922 §226, §228, §229).

> 1) To furious mania we must oppose calm intrepidity and cool, firm resolution
> 2) To doleful, querulous lamentation, a mute display of commiseration in looks and gestures
> 3) To senseless chattering, a silence not wholly inattentive
> 4) To disgusting and abominable conduct and to conversation of a similar character, total inattention. We must merely endeavour to prevent the destruction and injury of surrounding objects, without reproaching the patient for his acts, and everything must be arranged in such a way that the necessity for any corporeal punishments and tortures whatever may be avoided.
> 5) On the other hand, contradiction, eager explanations, rude corrections and invectives, as also weak, timorous yielding, are quite out of place with such patients.
> 6) Such patients are most of all exasperated and their complaint aggravated by contumely, fraud, and deceptions that they can detect.
> 7) The physician and keeper must always pretend to believe them to be possessed of reason.
> 8) All kinds of external disturbing influences on their senses and disposition should be if possible removed; there are no amusements for their clouded spirit, no salutary distractions, no means of instruction, no soothing effects from conversation, books or other things for the soul that pines or frets in the chains of the diseased body, no invigoration for it, but the care
> 9) The treatment of the violent insane maniac and melancholic can take place only in an institution specially arranged for their treatment but not within the family circle of the patient.

Intermittent Diseases

These diseases present with periodicity i.e. they recur at certain periods. Patients do not have complaints between two attacks and enjoy apparent health. Case taking in such cases should be done in two phases. First, when the patient presents with the attack, it should be treated as an acute complaint. Second, after the patient recovers from the attack, a complete history with other detailed information should be obtained. It should be treated as a chronic disease (Hahnemann 1922 §231).

Alternating Disease

These diseases have more than one group of symptoms, which manifest one at a time. When one group of symptoms dominates, the other group either disappears or becomes less prominent. Nevertheless, one group of symptoms does not form the complete picture of the disease but it is only a part of the whole phenomena. A thorough history of the suffering throughout the year and of different systems and parts should be taken into account. It should be treated as a chronic disease (Hahnemann 1922 §232).

Chronic Disease with Acute Exacerbation

Case taking during acute attacks should be limited to the presenting complaints, characteristic modalities, concomitants and other relevant changes. This constitutes the acute totality. A detailed case taking must be undertaken after the acute exacerbation subsides, to treat the underlying chronic disease.

Further Directives of Hahnemann

1. General instructions regarding case taking

These have been described in detail. However having talked about the directives for case taking Hahnemann also gave instruction into more specific matters.

2. Specific Enquiries

2.1 Enquiries into cases of suspicious character

Through astutely phrased questions or other private inquiries the physician must seek to trace the possible 'dishonoring occasions' of diseases which the patient or his relations do not readily confess at least not of their own free will. To these belong: poisoning or attempted suicide, onanism, debaucheries of common or unnatural lust, overindulgence in liquor, punch or other heating drinks, tea, or coffee, gluttony in general or with particular detrimental foods, infection with a venereal disease, unhappy love, jealousy, domestic discord, vexation, grief over family misfortune, abuses, dogged revenge, offended pride, financial problems, superstitious fear, hunger, or perhaps bodily infirmity in the private parts (a hernia, a prolapse) (Hahnemann 1922 footnote §91).

2.2 Enquiries into women's diseases

In chronic diseases of women, one should pay special attention to such things as pregnancy, infertility, sexual desires, deliveries, miscarriage, breast-feeding, vaginal discharge and the state of the menses and the following should be ascertained:

Does the menstrual period recur at intervals that are too short or too long?
How many days does it last?
Is the flow continuous or interrupted at intervals?
How heavy is it?
How dark is its colour?
Is there leucorrhoea? If so, is it before or after the menstrual flow? How is it constituted? What sensations attend its flow? What is the quantity? Under what conditions does it occur? What brings it on?
Especially, what ailments of body and soul, and what sensations and pains does the patient have before, during and after menstrual period?

2.3 Enquiries into an acute

Investigation of acute diseases is the easiest for the homeopath, because all the phenomena and deviations from health are, for the most part, spontaneously detailed and clear (Hahnemann 1922 footnote §99).

2.4 Enquiries into a serious and rapidly deteriorating disease previously managed by orthodox medicines

If the disease is of a rapid course and serious then it is important not to delay treatment.

2.5 Enquiries into a epidemic and sporadic disease

A careful examination will show that every prevailing epidemic is in many respects a phenomenon of unique character, differing vastly from all previous epidemics therefore never substitute conjecture for actual observation, never taking for granted that the case of disease before him is already wholly or partially known.

2.6 Enquiry into chronic disease

In all diseases, but especially in chronic ones, the investigations of the true, complete picture and its peculiarities demand special circumspection, tact, knowledge of human nature, caution in concluding the enquiry and patience in an eminent degree.

2.7 Enquiry into a case of chronic disease previously on orthodox medicine

The symptoms and feelings of the patient during a previous course of medicine do not furnish the pure picture of disease, but on the other hand, those symptoms and ailments which he suffered from before the use of medicines, or after they had been discontinued for several days, give the true fundamental idea of the original form of the disease and these especially the physician must take note of.

2.8 Enquiry into a case of mental and emotional disease

In these diseases we must be very careful to make ourselves acquainted with the whole of the phenomena. To this collection of symptoms belongs in the first place the accurate description of all the phenomena of the previous so called corporeal disease, before it degenerated into a one-sided and became a disease of the mind and disposition. This can be learned from the report of the patient's friends.

2.9 Enquiry into a case of intermittent disease

The symptoms of the patient's health during the interval when they are free from the intermittent condition must be the chief guide to the most appropriate homeopathic remedy.

3. Some other Enquiries

When the above information is gained, it still remains for the homeopath to assess what kinds of allopathic treatment had up to that date affected or created the chronic disease, and what effects (desired or adverse) these had produced (§207). Furthermore:

- the age of the patient
- the mode of living and diet
- the occupation, the domestic position
- the social relations
- the state of the disposition and mind must next be taken into consideration (§208).

After this is done, the physician should endeavour in repeated conversation with the patient to trace the picture of his disease as completely as possible, according to directions given above, in order to be able to elucidate the most striking and peculiar (characteristic) symptoms in accordance with which he selects the first antipsoric or other remedy having the greatest symptomatic resemblance, for the commencement of the treatment (Hahnemann 1922 §209).

Summary of Hahnemann's General Directives for Best Practice

	What to do
1)	*The symptoms should be written from three sources: Patient's complaints (history of his suffering), attendant's report (what they heard him complaint of, how he has behaved & what they have noticed in him), physician's observation (sees, hears, and remarks by his other senses what there is of an altered or unusual character about).*

2)	Attach credence especially to patient's own expressions because in the mouths of his friends and attendants they are usually altered and erroneously stated. So case taking especially in chronic case demands especial circumspection, tact, knowledge of human nature, caution in conducting the inquiry and patience to an eminent degree. While investigation of acute diseases, or of such as have existed but a short time, is much the easiest for the physician, because all the phenomena and deviations from the health are still fresh in the memory of the patient and his friends, still continue to be novel and striking.
3)	Write down accurately all that the patient and his friends have told him in the very expressions used by them.
4)	The physician advises them at the beginning of the examination to speak slowly, in order that he may take down in writing the important parts of what the speakers say.
5)	Begin a fresh line with every new circumstance mentioned by the patient or his friends, so that the symptoms shall be all ranged separately one below the other. He can thus add to any one, that may at first have been related in too vague a manner, but subsequently more explicitly explained.
6)	When the narrators have finished what they would say of their own accord, the physician then reverts to each particular symptom and elicits more precise information respecting it in the following manner (so that a true complete picture in the language of our materia medica can be traced).
7)	He reads over the symptoms as they were related to him one by one, and about each of them he inquires for further particulars, e.g. at what period did this symptom occur? Was it previous to taking the medicine he had hitherto been using? Whilst taking the medicine? Or only some days after leaving off the medicine? (Because the symptoms and feelings of the patient during a previous course of medicine do not furnish the pure picture of the disease, in chronic disease leave him some days quite without medicine, or in the meantime administer something of an unmedicinal nature, but in acute disease observe the morbid condition, altered though it may be by medicines i.e. the conjoint malady formed by the medicinal and original diseases, and combat it with a suitable homeopathic remedy, so that the patient shall not fall a sacrifice to the injurious drugs he has swallowed.)

8)	What kind of pain, what sensation exactly, was it that occurred on this spot? Where was the precise spot? Did the pain occur in fits and by itself, at various times? Or was it continued, without intermission? How long did it last? At what time of the day or night, and in what position of the body was it worst, or ceased entirely? What was the exact nature of this or that event or circumstance mentioned - described in plain words? (This is how the symptoms have been recorded in our provings.)
9)	If in these voluntary details nothing has been mentioned respecting several parts or functions of the body or his mental state, the physician asks what more can be told in regard to these parts and these functions, or the state of his disposition or mind.
10)	But only makes use of general expressions, in order that his informants may be obliged to enter into special details concerning them. For example, what is the character of his stools? How does he pass his water? How is it with his day and night sleep? What is the state of his disposition, his humour, his memory? How about the thirst? What sort of taste has he in his mouth? What kinds of food and drink are most relished? What are most repugnant to him? Has each its full natural taste, or some other unusual taste? How does he feel after eating or drinking? Has he anything to tell about the head, the limbs, or the abdomen.
11)	When the patient (for it is on him we have chiefly to rely for a description of his sensations, except in the case of feigned diseases) has by these details, given of his own accord and in answer to inquiries, furnished the requisite information and traced a tolerably perfect picture of the disease, the physician is at liberty and obliged (if he feels he has not yet gained all the information he needs) to ask more precise, more special questions.
12)	When the physician has finished writing down these particulars, he then makes a note of what he himself observes in the patient, and ascertains how much of that was peculiar to the patient in his healthy state. (He notices only the deviations from the former healthy state of the now diseased individual).

		For example:
		• How the patient behaved during the visit - whether he was morose, quarrelsome, hasty, lachrymose, anxious, despairing or sad, or hopeful, calm, etc.
		• Whether he was in a drowsy state or in any way dull of comprehension; whether he spoke hoarsely, or in a low tone, or incoherently, or how otherwise did he talk?
		• What as the colour of his face and eyes, and of his skin generally?
		• What degree of liveliness and power was there in his expression and eyes?
		• What was the state of his tongue, his breathing, the smell from his mouth, and his hearing?
		• Were his pupils dilated or contracted?
		• How rapidly and to what extent did they alter in the dark and in the light?
		• What was the character of the pulse?
		• What the condition of the abdomen?
		• How moist or hot, how cold or dry to the touch, was the skin of this or that part, or generally?
		• Whether he lay with head thrown back, with mouth half or wholly open, with the arms placed above the head on his back, or in what other position?
		• What effort did he make to raise himself?
		• And anything else in him that may strike the physician as being remarkable.
	13)	If the disease (acute or chronic) has been brought by some obvious cause, then the patient - or his friends when questioned privately - will mention it either spontaneously or when carefully interrogated.

14)	Any causes of a disgraceful character, which the patient or his friends do not like to confess, at least not voluntarily, the physician must endeavor to elicit by skillfully framing his questions, or by private information. To these belong poisoning or attempted suicide, onanism, indulgence in ordinary or unnatural debauchery, excesses in wine, cordials, punch and other ardent beverages, or coffee, over-indulgence in eating generally, or in some particular food of a hurtful character, infection with venereal disease or itch, unfortunate love, jealousy, domestic infelicity, worry, grief on account of some family misfortune, ill-usage, baulked revenge, injured pride, embarrassment of a pecuniary nature, superstitious fear, hunger, or an imperfection in the private parts, a rupture, a prolapsus, and so forth.
15)	In chronic diseases of females it is especially necessary to pay attention to pregnancy, sterility, sexual desire accouchements, miscarriages, suckling, and the state of the menstrual discharge. Menses, short intervals, or is delayed beyond the proper time, how many days it lasts, whether its flow is continuous or interrupted, what is its general quantity, how dark is its colour, whether there is leucorrhoea (whites) before its appearance or after its termination, but especially by what bodily or mental ailments, what sensations and pains, it is preceded, accompanied or followed (Concomitant), if there is leucorrhoea, what is its nature, what sensations attend its flow, in what quantity it is, and what are the conditions and occasions under which it occurs?
16)	The so-called hypochondriacs and other persons of great sensitiveness and impatient of suffering, portray their symptoms in too vivid colours and, in order to induce the physician to give them relief, describe their ailments in exaggerated expressions. (A pure fabrication of symptoms and sufferings will never be met with in hypochondriacs).
17)	This very exaggeration of their expressions becomes of itself an important symptom in the list of features of which the portrait of the disease is composed.
18)	The case is different with insane persons and rascally feigners of disease.

19)	Other individuals of an opposite character, however, partly from indolence, partly from false modesty, partly from a kind of mildness of disposition or weakness of mind, refrain from mentioning a number of their symptoms, describe them in vague terms, or allege some of them to be of no consequence.
20)	In epidemic and sporadic diseases it is quite immaterial whether or not something similar has ever appeared in the world before under the same or any other name. The physician must any way regard the pure picture of every prevailing disease as if it were something new and unknown.
21)	A careful examination will show that every prevailing disease is in many respects a phenomenon of a unique character, differing vastly from all previous epidemics with the exception of those epidemics resulting from a contagious principle that always remains the same, such as smallpox, measles.
22)	The whole extent of such an epidemic disease and the totality of its symptoms cannot be learned from one single patient, but is only to be perfectly deduced (abstracted) and ascertained from the sufferings of several patients of different constitutions.
23)	In the same manner the miasmatic chronic maladies which always remain the same in their essential nature especially the psora must be investigated, as to the whole sphere of their symptoms.
24)	When the totality of the symptoms that specially mark and distinguish the case of disease is once accurately sketched the most difficult part of the task is accomplished.
25)	He can investigate it in all its parts and can pick out the characteristic symptoms, in order to oppose to these, that is to say, to the whole malady itself.
26)	In the next visit after taking the remedy the fresh examination of the patient only needs to strike out of the list of the symptoms noted down at the first visit those that have become ameliorated, to mark what still remain, and add any new symptoms that may have supervened.

	What not to do
1)	Keeping silence himself he allows them to say all they have to say, and refrains from interrupting them, unless they wander off to other matters. Because every interruption breaks the train of thought of the narrators and all they would have said at first does not again occur to them in precisely the same manner after that (series of disease phenomenon will be missed).
2)	Don't frame questions so as to suggest the answer to the patient, so that he shall only have to answer yes or no; else he will be misled to answer in the affirmative or negative something untrue, half true, or not strictly correct, either from indolence or in order to please his interrogator, from which a false picture of the disease and an unsuitable mode of treatment must result. For instance, the physician should not ask, was not this or that circumstance present?

	Hahnemann's Main Writings
1)	School leaving essay in 1775 in Latin. The wonderful structure of the human hand
2)	Aetiology and Therapeutics of Spasmodic Affections. Thesis for his MD was written in Latin, Erlangen
3)	Treatment of Chronic Ulcers, 1782 Gommern
4)	A Treatise on Forensic Detection of Poisoning by Arsenic, 1786 Dresden
5)	The Treatise on Syphilis, 1788 Locowitz
6)	An Account of the Case of Insanity (of Klockenbring), 1792 Georgenthal
7)	Friend of Health, 1792 and 1795 Valschleben and Koenigslutter
8)	Pharmaceutical Lexicon, 1795 Valschleben and Koenigslutter
9)	Essay on a New Principle for ascertaining the curative powers of drugs, 1796 Koenigslutter
10)	Are the obstacles to the attainment of simplicity and certainty in practical medicine insurmountable? 1792 Koenigslutter
11)	Essay on the Treatment of Fevers and Periodical Diseases, 1798
12)	Essay on the Antidotes, 1799
13)	Effects of Coffee, 1803 Dessau

14)	Aesculapius in the Balance, 1805 Torgau
15)	Medicine of Experience, 1805 Torgau
16)	Materia Medica of A.von Haller, 1806
17)	Fragmenta de viribus medicamentorum positives Sive in sano copore humano observatis, 1806
18)	On the Value of Speculative Systems, 1808 Torgau
19)	Observations on the 3 Current Systems of Medicine
20)	Organon of the Rational Healing Science, 1810 Torgau
21)	Reine Arzneimittellahre (Materia Medica Pura), 1811 Leipsig
22)	The Treatment of Typhus Fever, 1814
23)	The thesis De Helleborismo Veterum was defended in 1812
24)	The Spirit of Homeopathic Doctrine, 1812
25)	How do small doses of such very attenuated medicines still possess great power, 1829 Coethen
26)	Chronische Krankheiten (Chronic Diseases), 1828 (till 1838) Coethen (and Paris)
27)	Allopathy, a warning to all sick persons, 1831 Coethen
28)	4 Articles on Cholera, 1830, 1831 Coethen
29)	Organon (2nd Edition) 1819 (Leipzig) & 3rd, 4th and 5th Edition in 1824, 1829 and 1833, Coethen (Organon of Medicine)

Core Requirements for Case Taking from Hahnemann

Be Silent
Be Faithful
Watch for Detail
Observe Acutely
Use Tact
Use Timing

Chapter 3

Post Hahnemann

- Consolidation
- Clarity
- Böenninghausen's Instructions on Case Taking and Forming a Complete Image
- Other Authors
    - Dunham
    - Bidwell
    - Guernsey
    - Farrington
    - Hering
    - Hughes
    - Burnett, Cooper and Clarke
    - Boger
    - Nash
    - T. F. Allen
    - H. C. Allen

In this chapter you will:
1. Become familiar with the writings on case taking by some of Hahnemann's contemporaries and those who survived him.
2. Understand how in the years after Hahnemann's death his followers adapted his directives.
3. Identify the historical precedents which still have their implications for homeopathy today.

Timeline

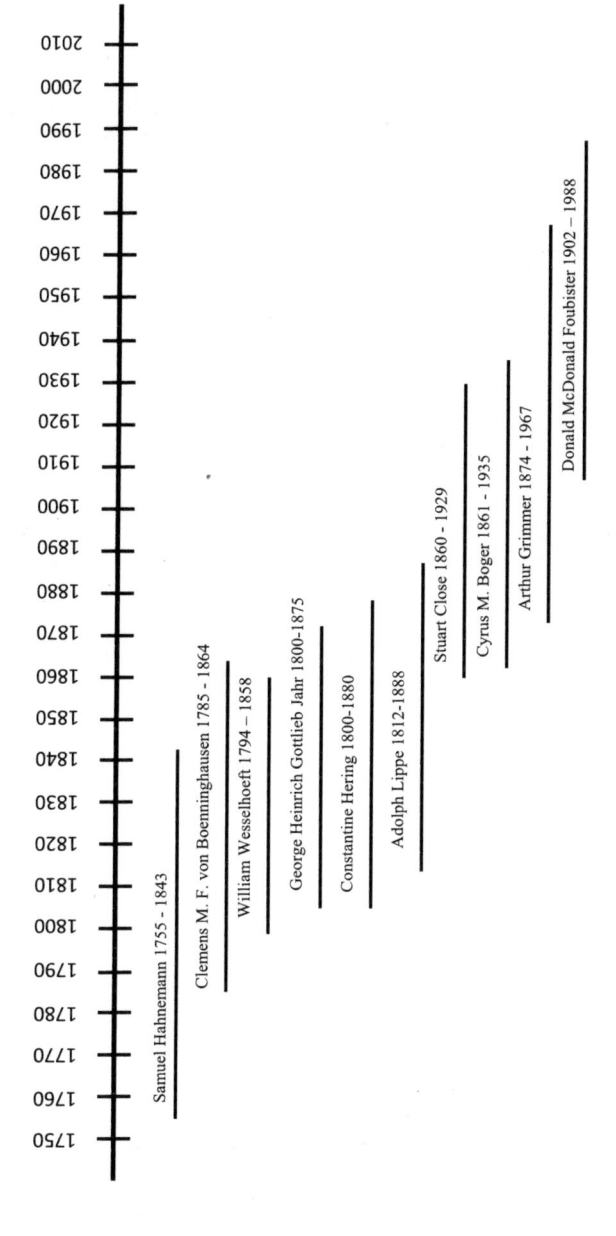

- Samuel Hahnemann 1755 - 1843
- Clemens M. F. von Boenninghausen 1785 - 1864
- William Wesselhoeft 1794 – 1858
- George Heinrich Gottlieb Jahr 1800-1875
- Constantine Hering 1800-1880
- Adolph Lippe 1812-1888
- Stuart Close 1860 - 1929
- Cyrus M. Boger 1861 - 1935
- Arthur Grimmer 1874 - 1967
- Donald McDonald Foubister 1902 – 1988

Chapter 3
Post Hahnemann

When it is well done, the patient is half cured already. (Adolph Lippe)

Consolidation

After such clarity, the passage of time notwithstanding, it is hard to imagine what could be added to the conversation after Hahnemann. Nevertheless in the historical development there is a natural gap, or at the very least a chapter, that examines attitudes to case taking from Hahnemann through to Kent. While what occurred was a continuation of the tradition, many subsequent homeopaths and leaders in the profession emphasized one aspect while others emphasized another. Bidwell said this. Boger that. Nash up. Lippe down. Thompson (1924) specifically mentioned in the *Bureau of Homoeopathy* the importance of the pulse in case taking. Essentially they all contributed to the literature by emphasizing aspects of case evaluation and analysis after the case taking was complete. Hahnemann had seen case taking as the individualising examination of a case of disease, a unique art of getting into conversation, observation and collecting information from patients as well as from bystanders to understand the patient and employ the homeopathic diagnostic framework. Depending on the circumstances and patient's condition sometimes the observation by physician or narration by patient or information by attendants alone may be sufficient to define the problem of the patient.

Clarity

One of Hahnemnan's contemporaries and favourites was Böenninghausen. Baron Clemens Maria Franz von Böenninghausen (1785-1864) was born in the Netherlands on a family estate of his father. The family traced its lineage through Westphalian and Austrian ancestry. He graduated from the Dutch university at Groningen with the degree of Doctor of Civil and Criminal law, and thereafter for several years he filled increasingly influential positions at the court of Louis Napoleon, King of Holland, remaining in the Dutch Civil Service until the resignation of the King in 1810, when he too retired from the Dutch service. In 1812 he married and went to one of the family estates in what later became western Prussia. He devoted much thought developing the state agriculturally, and became greatly interested in agriculture and allied sciences, particularly botany. He formed the first agricultural society in the western part of Germany. At the reorganization of the Prussian provinces of Rhineland and Westphalia in 1816 he was offered the position of President of the Provincial Court of Justice for the Westphalia district. His agricultural and botanical writings brought him recognition and two prominent botanists of the day each named a genus of plants after him.

In 1827 he developed tuberculosis. Weihe who was the first homeopathic physician in the province of Rhineland and Westphalia sent some *Pulsatilla*. His recovery was gradual but constant, so that by the end of the summer he was considered to be cured. He became an immediate convert and surprisingly began writing on the subject immediately and did his best to create an interest in homeopathy among the physicians with whom he came in contact. He quickly identified the need for an index to cope with the rising number of remedies and he began work on a repertory. From 1830 Böenninghausen was in close touch with Hahnemann, until his death. (Winston 1999, www.wholehealthnow.com).

Böenninghausen's Instructions on Case Taking and Forming a Complete Image

While giving instructions to the patient about writing the case history he emphasized the following:

1. Get a general image of the patient
2. Then a brief mention should be made of former sicknesses, then kind of treatment and the medicines used.
3. Then the present disease
4. Then a complete register of all the morbid symptoms
5. Every symptom should be clear and complete with internal sensations
6. Exact location with modalities
7. Natural sequence in the symptoms
8. Every new symptom in a new line.

Böenninghausen's method as it has come to be known, described the two natures of the case, the main symptoms and the side symptoms. After the case was taken, the next step was to sort it into the main symptoms (those of the major complaint) and the side symptoms (those other symptoms that apparently are unconnected to the major symptoms). Erroneously, it has been taught for a century in some parts that a complete symptom had a Sensation, Location, Modality and Concomitant. Hering and Boger point out that those four characteristics describe a complete case. A complete symptom, in fact, has only the Sensation, Location, and Modality. A concomitant will have all three as well, and it becomes a concomitant by its nature of being another symptom in the case (other than the main symptom), even though it may appear unrelated to the main complaint (Winston 2001, Dimitriadis 2000).

> Böenninghausen's complete symptom consisted of a
> 1. Complaint (objective – what / subjective – sensation) fully qualified by it's precise
> 2. Location
> 3. Modalities

The Hahnemann/Böenninghausen approach started with the presenting complaint. Appropriate questions would be, 'What does it feel like? Where is it located and extend to? What makes it better or worse?' The next concern was, 'What else can you tell me about condition or other history?' In the Hahnemannian tradition as articulated by Böenninghausen a symptom is a finding. A complete symptom comprises an objective phenomena (ulcer), a subjective experience of it, a sensation (burning pain), a location (left leg), and any modifications or modalities (it feels better with applying heat to the part).

It did not necessarily need a pathological label. This is a point that requires clarification. Locations and modalities are not so much symptoms in themselves, but rather defining components of a symptom which may render it complete. Thus they are distinguishing features rather than symptoms. Gypser, Dimitriadis and D'Aran have all emphasized that Böenninghausen's method required,

1. What (Complaint/Sensation)
2. Where (Location)
3. How (Modifications)

This constitutes a legitimate homeopathic diagnosis. Only distinguishing complaints need be considered according to clarity and completeness. A case of disease may therefore be individualised through its group of significant complaints in unique combination. Once a case is complete, then its corresponding remedy can be identified. The remedy is identified and the homeopathic diagnosis is complete. A 'Lachesis ulcer' therefore becomes the homeopathic diagnosis. A complete case comprises of one or more complete symptoms. If each complaint shares common modalities then these modalities that link one condition to another represents a common thread suggesting that all complaints are one disease that should be resolved with the one medicine.

Concomitant Symptoms

These are symptoms that are secondary to the main complaint. They may be very important if they share the same modalities since this strengthens the homeopathic diagnosis and thus the choice of medicine that will influence both the main complaint and the secondary complaint as they represent the same susceptibility. Concomitant symptoms may appear to be an isolated part of a symptom that has no completeness and thus is somehow associated with the main complaint but seems illogical or apparently disconnected. This may then really be an individualising component of the main complete symptom and can identify a unique remedy choice. In this system if each complaint has no clear relationship or shared modality then the most disturbing or important complete symptom must be prescribed on. Then as each complaint improves the next will present itself in its own completeness and so on till all complaints are resolved and balance and homeostasis is returned. Such a clear system requires simple yet rigorous questioning to ensure that each symptom, the main and the side symptom have this completeness.

Some of Böenninghausen's Works

- *The Cure of Cholera and its Preventatives - 1831*
- *Repertory of the AntiPsoric Medicines, preface by Hahnemann - 1832 or 1833*
- *Summary View of the Chief Sphere of Operation of the Antiposric Remedies and of their Characteristic Peculiarities, as an appendix to their Repertory - 1833*
- *Contributions to a Knowledge of the Peculiarities of the Homeopathic Remedies - 1833*
- *Homeopathic Diet and a Complete Image of a Disease - 1833*
- *Homeopathy, a Manual for the Non-Medical Public - 1834*
- *Repertory of the Medicines which are not Antipsoric - 1835*
- *Attempt at Showing the Relative Kinship of Homeopathic Medicines - 1836*
- *Therapeutic Manual for the Homeopathic Physicians, for the use at the sickbed and in the study of Materia Medica Pura. - 1846*
- *Brief Instructions for the Non-Physicians as to the Prevention and Cure of Cholera - 1849*

- *The Two Sides of the Human Body and Relationships. Homeopathic Studies.* - 1853
- *The Homeopathic Domestic Physician in Brief Therapeutic Diagnosis. An Attempt.* - 1860
- *The Homeopathic Treatment of Whooping Cough in its Various Forms.* - 1860
- *The Aphorisms of Hippocrates, with Notes by a Homeopath.* - 1863

Other Authors

Dunham

Böenninghausen's contemporaries emphasized other aspects of the work. Carroll Dunham in *'Homoeopathy the Science of Therapeutics* wrote, *'But it must never be forgotten that without the characteristics,... there can be no individualisation, and without this there can be no accurate homeopathic prescription'* (Dunham 1877).

He emphasized more than others the significance of physical examination. *The physician discovered that the patient had, years ago, received a gun-shot wound in the thigh. A close examination confirms that it still lay imbedded in the muscles of the thigh. An exploratory operation was performed and the ball was removed and the patient had no more convulsions* (Dunham 1877). He argued that old symptoms can be used only with the greatest care, for so many of them may have arisen from poor living, the abuse of drugs, or the acquisition of some other miasm.

In 'Lectures on Materia Medica' under the chapter 'Symptoms their study or how to take the case,' Dunham says,
1) To take the case requires great knowledge of human nature, of the history of disease and of the materia medica.

> 2. Our summary of the symptoms must cover not merely the moment of time at which we observe the patient, but also some previous time during which the symptoms may have been different from those of the present time
>
> 3. Because at some particular moment, the symptoms of a case and of a drug may appear to be very similar; but if we compare the succession and order of the symptoms, we may notice a marked difference. We look among drug provings for a similar series of phenomena.
>
> 4. It shows how much an extensive knowledge of the Materia Medica aids us in taking the case.
>
> 5. Individualizing symptoms are the trifling symptoms (not the pathognomic one), arising probably from the peculiarity of the individual patient.
>
> 6. Is it essential that the pathognomonic symptom of the case should be present among the symptoms of the drug? Theoretically, it certainly is. Practically, in the present rudimentary condition of our provings, it is not.

Dunham gives many instances where such mistakes have been made, and only a wide knowledge of drugs, of the habits of the people, and the special conditions under which many occupations are carried on, enables the homeopath to avoid errors (Dunham 1877).

A few cases from Dunham:

a) Alternating symptoms: a case presented with headache in winter and diarrhoea in summer. He prescribed Aloes in the winter, on the strength of the summer diarrhoea, and cured both.

b) History of suppression: in a case of deafness since suppression of milk-crust, Mezereum was prescribed for the milk-crust, and the deafness never returned.

c) Past mental disposition: in a case of epilepsy, Platina was prescribed on the strength of previous strong passion and peculiar disposition; imperious and high stepping.

d) Family history: Agaricus was prescribed in a case of supposed uterine disease treated by caustics and presenting with aching in the heels. The whole family had spinal meningitis; two brothers had died, and a sister was paraplegic. Agaricus cured the uterine disease (Dunham 1878).

> Carroll Dunham (1828-1877) was born in New York in 1828, graduated from Columbia University in 1847 and his MD at the college of Physicians and Surgeons of New York in 1850. While in Dublin he received a dissecting wound which nearly killed him, but he cured himself with the help of a homeopathic medicine - Lachesis. He visited various homeopathic hospitals in Europe and then went to Munster where he came in contact with Böenninghausen. Dunham practiced in Brooklyn and was a prolific writer. For twenty-five years, he regularly contributed articles and from 1860 he was editor of the 'American Homœopathic Review.' In 1865 he accepted the professorship of Materia Medica in the New York Homœopathic Medical College (www.hpathy.com, www.wholehealthnow.com, www.homeoint.org) His contributions; Lectures on Materia Medica and Homeopathy, The Science of Therapeutics.

Bidwell

Bidwell (1915) the author of *How to Use the Repertory* mentioned the importance of the 'Homeopath's Trinity'. He advocated the instructions given in Organon (Hahnemann 1922 §83-104). He puts it strongly as, *I will say with utmost belief that less than one man in a hundred practicing homeopathy today knows how to take a case properly.* He advocated:

1.	Value of symptoms
2.	Individualized diseased patient.
3.	Close observation
4.	Masked Symptoms
5.	Past History
6.	Original Symptoms
7.	The physician should not be in a hurry

Case

Case who was one of the greatest prescribers of his time discussed case taking in his book *Some Clinical Experiences of E. E. Case* (1916);

> That the symptoms of the case have been carefully taken, giving us, as expressed in the appropriate language of Hahnemann; The outwardly reflected image of the inner nature of the disease; that is, of the suffering vital force.

He identified rightly that homeopaths often find those symptoms confusing, often conflicting, and too great in number.

> Some are peculiar to the constitution of the patient; some are resultant from former disease; some are functional; others are pathological, really diseased conditions of the organs; still others are sympathetic, the result of those diseased conditions; many may be due to the action of drugs already administered; some may be purely imaginary. We have been taught to give that remedy which has produced all the symptoms of the patient and achieved the highest numerical totality in the repertory, it frequently happens that we cannot find a remedy whose pathogenesis contains them all. Some of you doubtless have worked out a case, as I have often done, with a repertory, and found that the symptoms led not to a single, but to several remedies, one seeming to be just as applicable as another, a disheartening result after hours of faithful study. Shall we employ the remedy which covers the greatest number of symptoms, a purely numerical comparison or can we select some special symptoms which have more weight than others in making the choice?

Guernsey

Emphasizing peculiar symptoms, Guernsey argued the mentals were the most important. Known for his keynote prescribing skills, he was an adept in detecting the symptoms peculiar to a drug, and claimed that when one of these was present in a case of sickness, others belonging to the drug would be found, which would make its choice as the curative remedy probable. Brilliant results sometimes follow this method of prescribing, also many failures. It was surely a different approach to Hahnemann.

Farrington

Similarly to Guernsey, Farrington emphasized highly characteristic symptoms that ran like a red thread through the whole profile of a remedy as containing the 'universal' quality of symptoms in his work.

Hering

Happy is that physician, who, having made his diagnosis, can forget it while prescribing.

Hering emphasized a thorough knowledge of pathology so that homeopaths could separate the symptoms of the disease itself from those belonging to the individual suffering from disease, for it was upon the latter alone that the prescription should be based. His great statement on case taking, *To listen, to write, to question, to coordinate.*

Constantine Hering was born at Oschath in Saxony on 1 January 1800. At the age of seventeen, he became interested in medicine and joined the University of Leipzig, where he became the favourite pupil of Dr. Henrich Robbi a critic of Hahnemann. He received his diploma as Doctor of Medicine,

> **Hering's Contributions**
>
> Domestic Physician
>
> Guiding Symptoms
>
> He wrote many articles, monographs, and books. He was the chief editor of the 'North America Homeopathic Journal', 'The Homeopathic News', 'The American Journal of Homeopathic Materia Medica' and the journal of his own college.
>
> He proved 72 drugs, including Lachesis, Cantharis, Colchicum, Iodium, Mezereum, Sabadilla, Sabina, Psorinum, Nux-mosch, Crotalus, Apis, Hydrophobinum, Phytolacca, Platina, Glonine, Gelsemium, Kalmia, Ferrum met, Flouric acid, Phosphoric acid (Winston 1999). http://www.hpathy.com/biography/c-hering.asp, Julian, www.homeoint.org

Surgery, and Obstetrics in 1826 after his introduction to homeopathy from a dissecting wound (experience) and his academic attempts to disprove it (intellectual). Hering left Germany for the West Indies and finally arrived at Philadelphia in 1833. He established a homeopathic school at Allentown, Pennsylvania, commonly known as the Allentown Academy. He remained in constant contact with Hahnemann until his death.

Hughes

Richard Hughes was of the opinion that we should observe the sequence of appearance of symptoms both during proving as well as during case taking. The remedy selected should be the one which has produced a similar sequence of symptoms in the proving. His case taking therefore emphasized this aspect. The proving remedy creates a primary action and a secondary action. This should be mirrored in the chronology of the patient's disease. The remedy should not only match the symptoms but also the sequence. Hughes objected to Hahnemann's approach of writing proving symptoms in his materia medica in anatomical schema. Hughes noted the original proving symptoms with the appearance of the different symptoms as they occurred in chronological time (Hughes 1868).

Burnett, Cooper and Clarke

Another English homeopath, Clarke in his, *Dr. Skinner's Grand Characteristics* wrote,

> If practice depended entirely on books, the multiplication of these would soon make practice impossible; fortunately, there are many features of homeopathy which tend to simplification of practice and none knew this better than Thomas Skinner. When for instance, we have a feverish patient who turns deadly pale and faints on any attempt to rise from the horizontal posture, we have no need to make an hour's search in repertories...... The patient is crying out for Aconite. That symptom is a 'grand characteristic' in the phraseology of Skinner. This term has the same meaning as Lippe's Keynotes, and Nash's Leaders. Clarke emphasized in the literature this idea of the characteristic and constitution. This was to have numerous consequences for case taking.

John Henry Clarke MD (1853 – November 24, 1931) was English. He was a prominent classical homeopath and disturbingly a vocal anti-semite. He wrote several articles on Christianity that had a militant flavour. Clarke was a busy practitioner. As a physician he not only had his own clinic in Piccadilly, London, but he also was a consultant at the London Homeopathic Hospital. For many years, he was the editor of The Homeopathic World. He wrote many books, his best known were Dictionary of Practical Materia Medica and Repertory of Materia Medica. Also, A Bird's Eye View of the Organon, A Dictionary of Domestic Medicine and Homeopathic Treatment, Catarrh, Colds and Grippe, Cholera, Diarrhea and Dysentery, Clinical Repertory, Constitutional Medicine, Diseases of Heart and Arteries, Grand Characteristics of Materia Medica, Gunpowder As A War Remedy, Hahnemann and Pracelsus, Homeopathy Explained, Indigestion-Its Causes and Cure, Non-Surgical Treatment of Diseases of Glands and Bones, Prescriber, Radium As An Internal Remedy, The Revolution in Medicine, The Therapeutics of Cancer, Therapeutics of the Serpent Poisons, Tumours, Whooping Cough. Also, Call of the Sword, England Under the Heel of the Jew. (Winston 1999, www.en.wikipedia.org/wiki/John_Henery_Clarke).

Clarke (1927) in his subsequent book, *Constitutional Medicine With Especial Reference to the Three Constitutions of Von Grauvogl*, wrote,

> It was through Hahnemann's insistence on the necessity of observing Concomitant Circumstances in relation to symptoms that Grauvogl was led to make his great generalisation. The homeopath abstracts first from the symptoms of the individuality of the patients in connection with the state of the outer world in which they have existed from their birth and out of which the bodily constitution is developed. The bodily constitution is hence the general cause. If a patient who has been for a long time annoyed by this circumstance that every draught of air affects him unpleasantly, he is not cured. Such constitutional conditions which make themselves known by such accompanying circumstances, give us, hence, the only right indications.

1. The Hydrogenoid Constitution is characterised by an excess of Hydrogen and consequently of water in the blood and tissues (corresponds closely with Hahnemann's sycosis).

2. The Oxygenoid is characterised by an excess of oxygen, or, at lest, by an exaggerated influence of oxygen on the organism (Hahnemann's syphilis).

3. The Carbo-nitrogenoid Constitution is characterised by an excess of carbon and nitrogen (Hahnemann's Psora) (Clarke 1927).

His case taking pursued this constitutional line as a consequence. For Clarke there are many different kinds of similarity, as well as of degrees, and every kind should be available for the prescriber's use. In *The Prescriber* he says,

> There is similarity between drug and disease in organ-affinity; in tissue-affinity; there is similarity of diathesis; similarity of sensations and conditions-all these and other kinds of likeness

are available for the prescriber to find his correspondence in; and he is no friend of Hahnemann, or of Hahnemann's system who would tie up practitioners to any one of them (Clarke 1885).

His colleague Burnett had a different stance and therefore a different approach to taking the case. In his book,

> Diseases of the Veins Burnett says, If we follow Hahnemann's method of historical case-taking we see strange things, as to the really primitive causes of diseases. In my own practical experience I trace cases of diabetes and cataract to the surgical traumatism inflicted in operating for piles (Burnett 1881).

His fame and reputation grew for his ability to cure cancer. Burnett in his book,

> Curability of Tumours says, A case of large abdominal tumor: The tumour presumably had its origin in a fall, eight years ago, on the left side, which fractured the ribs. This was cured by two remedies Bellis perennis and Ceanothus americanus. Two factors were helpful, traumatism and specificity of seat, or organopathy. A tumour may be cured purely on symptoms; indeed this has been done time and again (Burnett 1898).

Burnett maintained that in the majority of cases of tumour the finer symptoms available for basing a homeopathic prescription upon were often lacking. It was necessary therefore to find the indications elsewhere. There were two sources from which he obtained his tumour curing remedies, organ specific remedies. He argued that with these remedies the similarity lay chiefly in the locality and direction of action. The other source of curative remedies he found were nosodes (Clarke 1908).

James Compton Burnett was born in 1840 and died in 1901. He attended medical school in Vienna, Austria in 1865. He had his first lesson in homeopathy from reading Dr Hughes's two books, Manual of Pharmacodynamics and Manual of Therapeutics. Burnett was one of the first to speak about vaccination triggering illness. This was discussed in his

> book, Vaccinosis, published in 1884. Along with other nosodes, he introduced the remedy Baccillinum. A prodigious writer he published over twenty books in his lifetime. Clarke, Cooper, and Compton Burnett together formed the 'Cooper Club'. This regular meeting of leading British homeopaths was the source of many of the symptoms in Clarke's Dictionary of Materia Medica. Burnett's writings: Gold as a remedy; Gout; Curability of Cataract with Medicines; Vacinosis and its Cure by Thuja; On fistula and its Radical cure; Ringworm; Natrum Muriaticum; On Neuralgia, Diseases of veins; Diseases of Spleen & their remedies; Organ diseases of Woman & Sterility; New cure for Consumption; Change of life in Women; The diseases of Liver & Skin; Curability of Tumors; Fevers & Blood poisoning; 50 Reasons for being a Homoeopath; Valvular disease of the heart; Enlarged Tonsils cured by Medicine; Delicate, Backward, Punny & stunted Children; Tumours of the Breast; On the Prevention of Hare- Lip, Cleft- Palate (Chitkara 1921)

Boger

Boger was born in 1861 in western Pennsylvania. He graduated in pharmacy from the Philadelphia College of Pharmacy and later in medicine from Hahnemann Medical College of Philadelphia. There is some debate on the accuracy of his translation work. Nevertheless he brought *Böenninghausen's Characteristics and Repertory* into English in 1905. He says in Studies in the Philosophy of Healing, *The gist of the case my be featured in any one of the three parts* (Constitutional, General and Peculiar). In the Boger method fewer symptoms were used and special stress was put on pathological generals,

> Boger's Books; Böenninghausen's Characteristics and Repertory
>
> Studies in the Philosophy of Healing
>
> Boger's Diptheria
>
> A Synoptic Key of the Materia Medica, General Analysis with Card Index, Samarskite; A Proving, Study of Materia Medica and Case Taking
>
> The Times which Characterize the Appearance and Aggravation of the Symptoms and their Remedies (Winston 1999, www.hpathy.com, www.wholehealthnow.com.

for instance if the *case presented several excoriating discharges the rubric Acridity, in Boger's General Analysis, would be taken, if the patient complains of marked dryness of mouth, rectum, skin, the general rubric Dryness would be used. In this method the mentals are prominent and take first place, as in the Kent method* (Wright-Hubbard 1977).

Boger's (1939) opinions and guidelines for taking cases:

1)	The common way of eliciting well-known key-notes and prescribing accordingly is a most pernicious practice, which has earned a deserved odium and is no improvement upon the theoretical methods of the old school.
2)	To be ruled by clinical observations and pathological guesses is most disastrous. Such reports mostly lack individuality and at best describe only end products; standing in strong contrast to those expressions which reveal the real mind, whether in actions, words or speech.
3)	The past history and the way each sickness developed is both useful and interesting, for most persons develop symptoms in a distinctive way through the most diverse affections. Such constancies are truly antipsoric and it should be your pleasure to search out the differentiating indications from among them.
4)	Generally best to allow a free statement of the case in the patient's own way while we take pencil memoranda of the salient points, gradually filling in the deficiencies by such questions as the notes suggest.
5)	As every sickness, whether natural or induced, is the child of a combination of events which never again produces its exact self, it follows that the best indicated remedy is the one holding the closest similitude thereto in location, origin, modality, mental condition, concomitants, peculiarities and time.
6)	Objective phenomena, being exempt from self-interpretation and allowing the largest scope to the acumen of the examiner are withal the least deceptive and should receive our first and best attention. This is particularly helpful in the examination of children.

7)	The facial expression, the involuntary posture, the temperature both localized and general, alterations of colour or consistence, the state of the reflexes including sensibility, the odour of the patient, etc., are but a few of the points to be noted.
8)	It is only when an ordinary symptom appears in an extraordinary place or way that it becomes of much value.
9)	Sensations are expressed according to the mentality of the subject and vary from the simple indefiniteness of those of childhood to the hysterical loquacity which takes on every symptom thought of: it therefore follows that the attributes of the symptoms are of far greater importance than the sensations themselves.
10)	In certain cases by paying more attention to the time, manner and circumstances under which a given symptom occurs we succeed in not only diverting the mind of the patient, but in gaining a great deal of very valuable information.
11)	It is far better to be able to see the general picture and use the key-note as a differentiating point, just as we would use a modality.
12)	The final analysis of every case, therefore, resolves itself into the assembling of the individualistic symptoms into one group and collecting the disease manifestations into another, then finding the remedy which runs through both, while placing the greater emphasis on the former.
13)	Each case presents a slightly different alignment of symptoms, particularly in the latest and most significant development which is usually but an outcropping of another link in the chain of individualistic symptoms belonging to the life history of the patient. This way of looking at the matter presupposes the taking of a pretty thorough case history, but furnishes a therapeutics key to almost every sickness for a long period of time

Nash

Eugene Beauharnais Nash in the preface *Leaders in Homoeopathic Therapeutics* (1913) focused on characteristic symptoms.

> The elder Lippe was remarkable for such ability...Every symptom has its pathological significance, but we cannot always give it in words; but the fact that it has such meaning is sufficient reason for prescribing on the symptom or symptoms without insisting on, or trying to give, the explanation...The majority of the cases, however, do have, standing out like beacon lights,

some characteristic or keynote symptoms which guide to the study of the remedy that has the whole case in its pathogenesis.

T. F. Allen

Further advice came from TF Allen. He received his undergraduate education at Amherst College and his medical degree from New York University. After serving as a surgeon during the Civil War he returned to New York where he partnered with Carroll Dunham. He also studied homeopathy with Wells in Brooklyn. In 1871 Allen was appointed Professor of Materia Medica at the New York Homoeopathic Medical College. Later he served as president from 1882-1893. Allen compiled the Encyclopedia of Pure Materia Medica over the course of 10 years. It was a comprehensive record of all the provings of homeopathic medicines recorded up to that point. Hering, Dunham, Adolph Lippe, and Richard Hughes all contributed to it.

> Allen's other publications were Ophthalmic Therapeutics (1874)
>
> The Symptom Register (1880)
>
> Handbook of Materia Medica and Homeopathic Therapeutics (1889)
>
> Böenninghausen's Therapeutic Pocket Book (1891)
>
> A Primer of Materia Medica (1892)
>
> Pocket Characteristics (1894)

He focused on the results of case taking and divided symptoms into determining and resulting categories.

> Determining symptoms are those which precede and determine the development of a lesion, which, when established, becomes the fountain of new and resulting symptoms. Resulting are those which are not of prime importance to the therapeutist who seeks to arrest the progress of the real malady.

He concludes:

1. Some symptoms are of more value than others.
2. The most valuable to the therapeutist are the determining symptoms, both in acute and chronic diseases.

Drysdale and Allen both emphasised that a characteristic symptom was not to be found in every case. Success was to be determined by acuteness of observation in recognizing the peculiarities of the patient.

When it came to the specifics of case taking he wrote (T.F. Allen 1889):

1)	Note carefully and completely the various complaints of his patient and add thereto his own observations concerning his condition, that is to say, he must get all of the subjective and objective symptoms.
2)	Most symptom lists are extremely complicated; in chronic complaints the observation that one organ after another has become involved finishes series of symptoms from new foci, as it were, the lately developed symptoms often overpower and obscure previous affections; in acute diseases the immediate symptoms are complicated by a series of old chronic troubles which, likely as not, have so affected the vitality of the individual that the acute disease has become possible. In the latter case (frequently in scarlatina and the other so-called zymotic diseases), we find our patient unresponsive to the remedy selected for the most numerous and apparently important symptoms, and are compelled to fall back upon a careful analysis of a few chronic troubles. Still we must prescribe very frequently for a few severe and distressing symptoms, and postpone for a time the investigation of the past history and present complications of the malady.
3)	In these acute diseases a knowledge of the nature of the morbid process enables the expert to separate the symptoms due to the recent malady from those which are contingent and individual and which must be considered most seriously.

> 4) In chronic diseases the conditions are somewhat different, and as a rule the symptoms are less complicated, but it frequently becomes necessary to exercise great partiality toward a few symptoms to the exclusion of the many. In most of the chronic maladies which show no tendency to recover, but rather to involve one organ after another, the original symptoms become obscured. For example, in cancer, the tumor, with its destructive metamorphoses, has developed from the underlying cachexia which has determined its manifestations. This secondary development gives rise to new and obtrusive symptoms which may entirely mask the real disease. Consumption develops from the scrofulous habit. The Lithaemic diathesis gives rise to a host of degenerative changes in various organs and tissues which develop new sets of symptoms. In all of these and other similar diseases it becomes our duty to investigate thoroughly the nature of the morbid processes, to study the evolution of the malady and separate the symptoms into groups. While it may be true that the absolute totality of all the symptoms would include the original, determining and essential symptoms of the case, yet he who fails to grasp the full significance of all the symptoms will fail to appreciate the overpowering value of the few. It is then necessary to get at what is characteristic in the patient in all forms of sickness

H. C. Allen

Henry C. Allen (1836 - 1909) is mentioned in this context because it was he who provided a handbrake to the Kentian enthusiasm that led homeopathy in America into the 20th century. A descendant of the Revolutionary War hero, Ethan Allen, he studied medicine at the College of Physicians and Surgeons in Ontario, Canada and received his homeopathic training at Western Homeopathic College (Cleveland Homeopathic

> Besides writing many articles in homeopathic journals he wrote numerous books. Some of Henry Allen's well-known works include:
>
> Keynotes of the Materia Medica with Nosodes.
>
> The Materia Medica of the Nosodes.
>
> The Homeopathic Therapeutics of Intermittent Fever.
>
> The Homeopathic Therapeutics of Fever.
>
> Therapeutics of Tuberculous Affections.
>
> He also revised Böenninghausen's Slip Repertory, which he updated and arranged for rapid and practical homeopathic work.

College) in Cleveland, Ohio where he graduated in 1861. After his graduation, he entered the Union Army, serving as a surgeon under General Grant. After the Civil War Allen accepted the professorship of Anatomy at Cleveland and first started the practice of medicine. He later resigned this post to accept the same chair at the Hahnemann Medical College of Chicago. In 1875 he moved to Detroit and was appointed Professor of Materia Medica at the University of Michigan, Ann Arbor in 1880.

> One of the stumbling blocks to progress in the study of homeopathy is the way we take our cases. We do not go back to Hahnemann's system of therapeutics. There is a broad distinction between symptoms of diagnosis and symptoms of therapeutics. Diagnostic symptoms are those of the disease, and the therapeutic symptoms go down to the patient himself. Now, the more valuable symptoms are for diagnosis the less valuable they are for the selection of the remedy. The practice of homeopathy is just as simple as 'rolling off a log.' Read §152 of the Organon. Take the individual symptoms, and select those peculiar as your guide, and it will be astonishing how easy it is to prescribe for a case after you have taken it. That is where the trouble lies. Hahnemann has told us that anybody can prescribe for a patient after the anamnesis is well taken (www.wholehealthnow.com).

Allen actively worked for reinstatement of the *Organon* in college curricula and was largely responsible for its wide-scale use during the turn of the 20th century. Like Hahnemann and Hering before him, Allen passionately defended the inductive method described in the *Organon*. He was vocal in his disagreements with Kent over the publication of unproven remedies who at one stage was describing remedies for which there were no provings or clinical experience. For example, Kent would combine the qualities of *Alumina and Silica* and speculate on the symptoms that would exist in Alumina silicata. At the Homeopathic Congress of June 1908, Allen accused Kent of publishing unreliable materia medica. Kent retracted his position and never published a 'synthetic' remedy again and later removed them from the 2nd edition of his *Lectures on Homeopathic Materia Medica*.

While there is an undoubted richness that emerges from the homeopaths that contributed to the literature in the 50 years after Hahnemann's death, nevertheless it was a disperate body of work and has contributed to much of the confusion, and questions that we are faced with today when it comes to best practice in homeopathy.

Summary of Best Practice Post-Hahnemann

Böenninghausen

Condition/Sensation, Location/Modality

Dunham

To take the case requires great knowledge of human nature, of the history of disease and of the materia medica

Bidwell

The physician should not be in a hurry

Hering

The symptoms of a case and the symptoms of a medicine must not only be alike, one by one, but in both, the same symptoms must be of a like rank

Hughes

The remedy should not only match the symptoms but also the sequence

Burnett

If we follow Hahnemann's method of historical case taking we see strange things, as to the really primitive causes of diseases. In my own practical experience I trace the cause of diabetes and cataract to the surgical traumatisation inflicted in operating for piles

What the Case Taker Needs

Patience

Chapter 4

Kent

- Classical
- Repertory, Types, The Person not the Disease
- Swedenborg
- Mind
- Kent's Instructions on Case Taking
- The Science of Case Taking for the Lower Plane of Homeopathy
- The Art of Case Taking for the Higher Plane of Homeopathy
- What the Homeopath Needs
    Tact and Timing
- Kent and Peculiarity
- Hysteria, Exaggeration and the Irish

In this chapter you will
1. Learn about the incalculable impact of Kent on the development of Homeopathy.
2. Identify the crucial features of his philosophy and its relationship to case taking.
3. Consider the influence of Swedenborg and Kent on modern contemporary homeopathic practice.

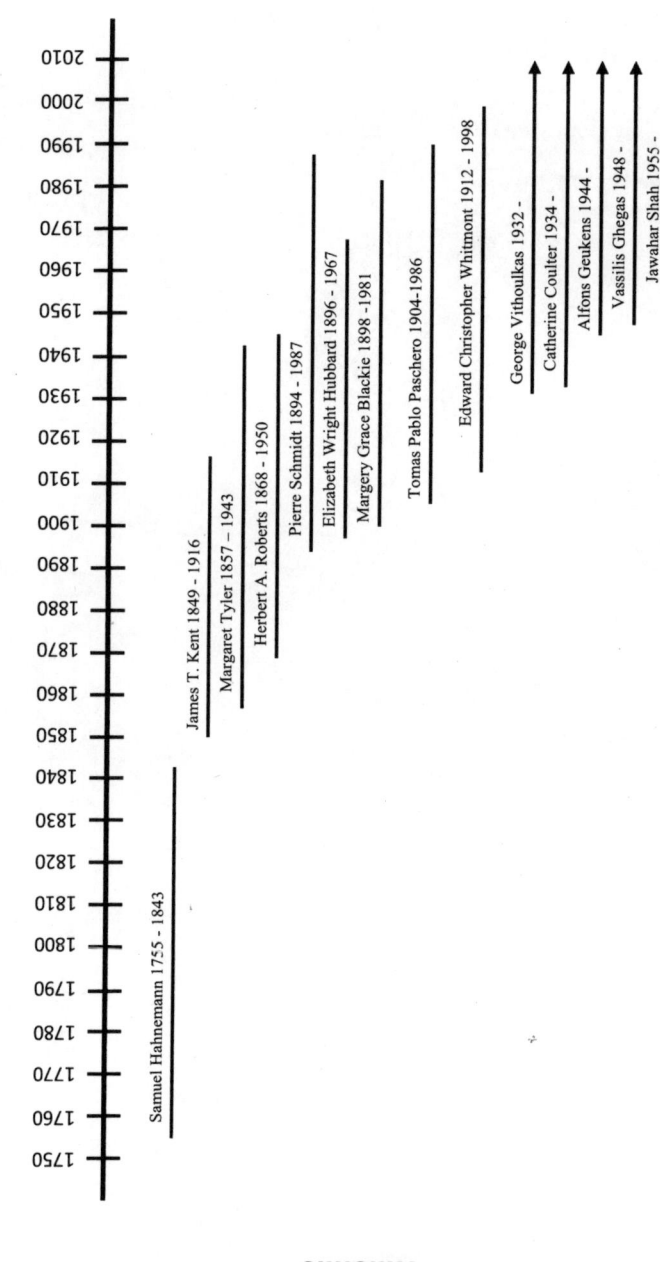

Timeline

- Samuel Hahnemann 1755 - 1843
- James T. Kent 1849 - 1916
- Margaret Tyler 1857 – 1943
- Herbert A. Roberts 1868 - 1950
- Pierre Schmidt 1894 - 1987
- Elizabeth Wright Hubbard 1896 - 1967
- Margery Grace Blackie 1898 -1981
- Tomas Pablo Paschero 1904-1986
- Edward Christopher Whitmont 1912 - 1998
- George Vithoulkas 1932 -
- Catherine Coulter 1934 -
- Alfons Geukens 1944 -
- Vassilis Ghegas 1948 -
- Jawahar Shah 1955 -
- Rajan Sankaran 1960 -

Chapter 4
Kent

If the patients answer was yes or no the question was badly formed. (Kent 1900)

Symptoms are but the language of nature, talking out as it were and showing as clearly as the daylight the internal nature of the sick man or woman...It is nonsense to say that prior to the localization of the disease; the patient was not sick. (Kent 1900)

The physician spoils his case when he prescribes for the local symptoms and neglects the patient. (Kent 1921)

For a century James Tyler Kent has held a special place as one of the most influential homeopaths. His significance has been incalculable molding a generation of homeopaths. His impact on George Vithoulkas in particular has shaped contemporary homeopathy. Others include Herbert Roberts, Margaret Tyler, Marjorie Blackie, Elizabeth Wright-Hubbard, Pierre Schmidt, Pablo Paschero and Vassilis Ghegas, the leaders, authors and influencers of their generation. Others influenced by Kent, and thus the direction of 21st century homeopathy have been Edward Whitmont and Catherine Coulter who added their own experience and insight to the psychological profiles of the polychrest remedies. Furthermore, currently active contributors include Rajan Sankaran, Jayesh Shah and Alfons Geukens each of whom owe their variations of method and practice to Kentian roots.

Classical

Every homeopath in the western world has had that phone call asking, 'Are you a classical homeopath?' The answer is of course 'Yes,' but then again it may as well be, 'What do you think classical is?' Invariably the questioner says that a classical homeopath is one who uses one remedy, a high potency and just once. It seems astonishing that this 'classical' or 'pure' homeopathy is so far from the homeopathy that Hahnemann practiced. Kaplan has an elegant definition of classical homeopathy (Kaplan 2001:46) emphasizing the way Hahnemann practiced, with multiple anti-psoric medicines being needed to cure the patient and repeated visits necessary over time. It depends on your point of view.

Classical is such an interesting term. It's used in relationship to music, jazz, homeopathy, and cricket. Ask any Indian cricket fanatic who the best batsman is and of course the answer would be Tendulkar. His batting has defined a generation and his skills and mastery have been observed with wonderment from the beginning of the 1990s to the present. He is the classical batsmen of this generation with Dravid a close second. In this context his style is defined as upright, correct, elegant, pure. In cricket anyway this is what the term *classical* tends to mean.

But in homeopathy the word has often been misused and unfortunately to many, the term 'classical' means 'constitutional'. This is the source of much confusion. Simply stated, constitutional prescribing involves taking the whole person into account as far as possible, and treating the person simultaneously on all levels-physical, mental and emotional. The expression 'treat the person, not the disease' may be accurately applied to this method (Master 2001c). That said, debates about constitutional and classical inevitably lead back to Kent.

Repertory, Types, The Person not the Disease

One of his greatest contributions to the profession of homeopathy, and its teachings, was his completely unique style of repertory. Although others exist, Kent's *Repertory*, is still the popular choice, and has been described as more complete, systematic and precise. Kent is also known for developing 'pictures' of constitutional types of patients. A well-known example would be his description of Sulphur as 'the ragged philosopher.' There are many works based on the principles and ideas of Kent, Margaret Tyler's *Homeopathic Drug Pictures* being a notable example.

Kent was born on 31 March 1849 at Woodhull, New York and in 1873 he completed medical studies in allopathic, homeopathic, naturopathic and chiropractic at the Institute of Eclectic Medicine in Cincinnati, Ohio at the age of 25. But he had little regard for homeopathy. In 1874 he married a Baptist like himself, settled in St. Louis and began practice. In 1876 he became the Professor of Anatomy at American College of St. Louis. During the same year, his wife became seriously ill and was cured by a homeopath resulting in his complete and enthusiastic conversion. In 1881 he accepted the chair of Professor of Anatomy of the Homeopathic College of Missouri and then the Chair of Surgery and later Professor of Materia Medica. In 1890 he became the Dean of Professors at the Post-Graduate Homeopathic Medical School of Philadelphia and held that post until 1899. Around this time Kent began to study the works of Swedenborg and adopted his philosophy.

Swedenborg

Kent's philosophy, on which he based his approach to case taking and the grading of symptoms, was deeply influenced by teachings of Emanuel Swedenborg. *'All my teaching is founded on that of Hahnemann and of Swedenborg; their teachings correspond perfectly.'* (Kent 1900). His second marriage to Clara Louise was reported in the New Church News, and his major writings started to reflect the teachings of Swedenborg. Kent, in delivering his lectures at the Post Graduate School infused his teaching with the 'New Church' doctrine to an extent that it developed a reputation as a Swedenborgian institution. Swedenborg's ideas ranged over wide fields in science, philosophy, theology, and religion (Carlston 2003). For Kent, Swedenborg's thought was completely congruent with Hahnemann's, only more far-

---

Kent's Books and Contributions

Repertory of the Homeopathic Materia Medica, 1897

Lectures on Homoeopathic Philosophy, 1900

Lectures on Homoeopathic Materia Medica, 1905

New Remedies

Lesser Writings

Clinical Cases

What the Doctor Needs to Know

Kent's Aphorisms and Precepts from extemporaneous lectures

Kent's Final General Repertory, Schmidt and Chand, 1980

Kent's Repertorium Generale, Jost Künzli von Fimmelsberg, 1987

(http://www.hpathy.com/biography/james-tyler-kent.asp)

reaching. 'The principle of likes extends throughout existence,' wrote Swedenborg, 'and, in fact, is the means by which the world is manifest.' In the words of Kent, *Through familiarity with Swedenborg, I have found the correspondences wrought out from the Word of God harmonious with all I have learnt.*

Swedenborg's philosophy centered on love. He saw love as the essence of all human beings. He argued, *'love is what we are and the basis of our existence. Love is life. Feeling, not thought, is the substantive element in life.'* Swedenborg himself believed intelligence was far less important than love. He also believed that love was more important than faith. Kent's *Lectures on Homeopathic Philosophy* was liberally pasted with Swedenborgian terms and concepts. 'Will' and 'Understanding', for example, were terms that Kent used often in his lectures. Swedenborg considered Will and Understanding to be the two fundamental elements of a human being. According to him, Will is the volitional quality, intentionality in another word. Understanding meant discrimination, the capability of discernment. Will was the engine, while Understanding the captain or rudder (Winston 1995, Kaplan 2001).

Mind

For Kent the Mind came first. Disease originated there. Nevertheless homeopaths erroneously think that because this was the corner stone of Kent's philosophy that this was all he prescribed on, asked about or cared about. While rightfully seen as the first to discuss psychosomatic prescribing he is often wrongfully tarred with doing nothing else, or being responsible for the failings and inadequacies of those homeopaths who use his name or follow his ideas. There is an often forgotten pragmatism and practicality in his homeopathy.

Gypser and Dimitriadis

Significant change of emphasis in homeopathic education has taken place in this generation. Teachers in the UK in the 1980's and 90's said, 'Read Kent, understand his philosophy', and they pushed his books as seminal texts in understanding how to practice. It is extraordinary that virtually no student these days has his *Philosophy*, his *Materia Medica* is rare and *Lesser Writings* is unheard of. Gypser in Germany and Dimitriadis in Australia have argued that an imbalance in our emphasis as case takers and homeopaths has been too long in being righted. They have argued that it is necessary to look at Kent's work critically and compare it to the ease of the approach of others. 'Kent is just so spiritualist,'

Hierarchy of symptoms: When the case has been fully taken, those symptoms which are considered to be characteristic are graded in importance in the following hierarchical order:

First	Mental and emotional symptoms (Kent considered the symptoms pertaining to the will, to be most important; those of the emotions and understanding or intellect to be next most important and those pertaining to the subconscious to be of lesser importance).
Second	Physical general symptoms (those pertaining to the whole person, e.g. chilliness, fever, sweat, sleep, sexual functions, menses, cravings and aversion, etc)
Third	Physical particulars and disease symptoms (those pertaining to certain parts of the organisms or to the disease state itself, e.g. headache, arthritis, chilblains, coryza etc). Wherever possible the remedy prescribed must bear similarity with the mental/emotional state, as this is perceived as being originally affected. In the absence of clear mental/emotional symptoms, the physical general symptoms take precedence. Disease symptoms and local symptoms are considered the end results of a disorder at the higher level and are, therefore, given the lowest hierarchical importance.

a French homeopath said to me once. 'These high potencies are ridiculous.'

Without doubt his emphasis on suppression seems out of step with modern city patients and his references to contraception and to negroes with slashing blades lose him votes with modern students. Even the mustache puts people off. Compared to Hahnemann's broad forehead and gentle eyes, his Aries pioneering intensity, Kent seems austere and unapproachable, moral and very judgmental behind those whiskers. All superficialities aside what we know for sure is that his case books demonstrate a very different type of homeopathic prescribing to his philosophy book. Moreover his advice on case taking is remarkably practical.

Kent's Instructions on Case Taking

1.	Patient's own words.
2.	Fresh line for each new symptom.
3.	Bystanders, if anxious, do not give correct information.
4.	Collateral questions and no direct questioning.
5.	Aim of symptom collection to find pathological diagnosis, prognosis and materia medica. Symptoms with respect to materia medica are the key to the prescriptions.
6.	The physician should work instantly to ascertain the condition of the patient and what relation they maintain to materia medica.
7.	Get the original form of the malady.
8.	The circumstances of life, habit and also slightest particulars must be studied.
9.	The question of modesty should be laid aside.
10.	Exaggerators and too lazy patients do not present the true picture of sickness.
11.	A physician should never prescribe for an acute and chronic trouble together.
13.	Not to be prejudiced.

It is argued by many that Kent took homeopathy to a different level. He differentiated two planes of practice, the lower plane of homeopathy pertaining to the science of homeopathy and the higher plane of homeopathy pertaining to the art of practice. He gave separate instructions for case taking for both states.

The Science of Case Taking for the Lower Plane of Homeopathy

Examination of the Patient

1. The record can be arranged by dividing the page into three columns. The first contains the dates and prescriptions, the second is for emphatic symptoms, while the third one is for modalities.
2. Always leave the patient in freedom. Do not put words in his mouth. Say as little as you can, but keep the patient talking and keep him close to line.
3. Get into a fixed habit of examination then it will stay with you.
4. After the patient has detailed his sufferings, then proceed to make enquiries. Question the patient, then his friends, and observe for yourself if you do not obtain enough to prescribe then go back to the particulars.
5. After much experience you will become an expert in questioning patients so as to bring out the truth.
6. If you neglect making a careful physical examination the patient will be the first sufferer, but in the end both you and the system will suffer from it.

7. No homeopath ever discouraged the true study of anatomy and physiology. It is important not only to know the superficial but the study of real and profound character, to be able to recognize one symptom image from another.

Other Hints and Suggestions

1. Mental symptoms are more important.
2. Sleep symptoms are important.
3. Menstrual symptoms are important.
4. The flash of the eye is important, it will tell things that can not be told by the nurse.
5. It is important for the physician to know the value of the expression.
6. The symptoms that arise after the administration of powerful medicine are not indicative of a remedy. (Drugging is only a master of changing the symptoms and masking the case.)
7. Remember circumstances of a man's life govern his actions and reactions, symptoms and the development of symptoms. All such circumstances ought to be examined, which sustain or give rise to disease so by their removal cure may be facilitated.
8. A great deal depends upon the physician's ability to perceive miasma and what symptoms constitute it.
9. Get all the symptoms first and then commence your analysis in relation to remedies. Keep out of the mind while examining a case, some other case that appears to be similar and the remedies that have treated it in past.

10. The physician must be possessed of an uncommon share of circumspection and tact, knowledge of human heart, prudence and patience, to be able to form a true and complete image of the disease in all its detail and to put patients at ease. Remember the most impatient hypochondriac never invents sufferings and symptoms that are void of foundation. Truth can be known by giving such a patient only placebo and see whether the symptom are consistent or not (if symptoms are not consistent then think hysteria).

11. The homeopathic physician must be acquainted with the signs and symptoms of human diseases. Different diseases are only a change in combination of those symptoms in manner and representation. There is order, perfect order, in every sickness that presents itself. It rests with the physician to find that order.

The Art of Case Taking for the Higher Plane of Homeopathy

So while emphasizing gathering information he also argued that the quiet, silent manner of perception is to be cultivated (Kent 1921:658). With the true physician, discrimination is not with the eye alone; the consciousness of discrimination seems to occupy his entire economy (Kent 1921:658). Observation is the key.

> If prescribing is to be made easy, it is to be done by securing such a perfect view of the whole case as would be expressed by saying that. 'The sole basis of the homoeopathic prescription is the totality of morbid signs and symptoms'. as Hahnemann taught so many years ago. It will be seen, therefore, that carelessness in taking the symptoms, as well as in viewing the symptoms

after they are noted, must lead to indifferent results. Remember that it is not the totality of the symptoms taken by a careless or ignorant physician that constitutes the basis of a homeopathic prescription, but the totality of all the symptoms the patient has (Kent 1921:477).

Let me say that a part of the study of materia medica consists in the observation of sick people. A busy physician learns without books, though of course he should familiarize himself with the literature, so that from reading, as well as observation, he may acquire knowledge of the general nature of sickness. When he listens to the patient's story or makes a physical examination, he knows how such cases usually conduct themselves. He knows what to expect. He knows the natural trend of sickness and instantly recognizes what is strange and unusual unless he knows what is natural. So your books on symptomatology and pathology, diagnosis, etc., will tell you much of this, but as you gain experience in homoeopathic practice you will get a much finer idea of this because your materia medica teaches you to observe more closely. The materia medica man learns to single out and trace every little thing in order to individualize. So it may be said that years of observation in studying disease, studying the sick man along with the materia medica, will open to the mind a much grander knowledge of the sickness of humanity than can be had by practicing traditional medicine. Traditional medicine benumbs the ability to observe (Kent 1905:414).

In the Aethusa patient there is much in the face and aspect to indicate the remedy; so much can be seen and comes within the observation, and so little questioning is necessary, that a sort of snap-shot prescribing can be done, but it is not to be recommended. A busy physician, one who really and truly studies his materia medica, and has learned the principles, will in time do a great deal of what seems to be snap-shot prescribing, but he really does not do so, because he puts together many things that outsiders would not think of Aethusa then shows itself upon the surface, whereas in many remedies there is nothing seen upon the surface, because they manifest themselves in inner or deeper sensations. Let me lay a case before you to illustrate this. For instance, take a robust looking fellow, who declares himself fairly well, out to lunch with you. You have noticed for some time that his nose is all the time peeling off; at once there is a star. He never talks about his health. Pretty soon, while lunching, the door slams and he jumps. That is the second point. Then he tells you how much he eats, how well it affects him, how good he feels after eating, and you have noticed yourself that he eats a good deal. You have not asked him to tell you any symptoms. Finally you shove the pitcher of milk over to him, and he says, 'Oh, I can't drink milk; if I take milk it give me diarrhea; I never think of taking it.' Who could not prescribe for that fellow without taking him into the office? Who would think of anything but Natrum carb for such a case? Sometimes you can find out the whole story by getting a stubborn patient to go and dine with you (Kent 1905:27).

The study of the face is a delightful and profitable one. It is profitable to study the faces of healthy people that you may be able to judge their intentions from their facial expressions. A man shows his business of life in his face; he shows his method of thinking, his hatreds, his longings, and his loves. How easy it is to pick out a man who has never loved to do anything but to eat - the epicurean face. How easy it is to pick out a man who has never loved anything but money - the miserly face. You can see the love in many of the professional faces; you can single out the student's face. These are only manifestation of the love of the life, which they live. Some manifest hatred; hatred of the life in which they have been forced to live; hatred of mankind; hatred of life. In those who have been disappointed in everything they have undertaken to do we see hatred stamped upon the face. We see these things in remedies just as we see them in people. The study of the face is a most delightful one. A busy, thoughtful and observing physician has a head full of things that he can never tell things he knows about the face. So the face expresses the remedy (Kent 1905:333).

What the Homeopath Needs

Reading any of Kent's work confirms that he was never shy in giving his opinions (Kent 1900 Lecture 22).

An unprejudiced mind! At the present day there is almost no such thing as an unprejudiced mind.
Go out among the doctors who profess to practice Homeopathy and you will find they are all full of prejudice. They will at once commence to tell you what they believe; one believes one thing and another thing; they all have varying kinds of belief.
Go into anything that you have a mind to and you will find man full of prejudice.
This state of prejudice exists in the examination of a patient.
The physician goes to the patient prejudiced as to his own theories.
He has his own ideas as to what constitutes the correct method of examination, and so he does not examine the patient for the purpose of bringing out the truth, the whole truth and nothing but the truth.
His prejudices lead him to snap the patient up as soon as he begins to tell his story.
It is certain that the true man is one freest from prejudices, one who can listen, who can examine evidence and who can meditate.
If a physician goes in with a prejudice for a certain potency or a certain disease, or a prejudice against certain principles, he is not in a rational state, he is not in freedom with the patient and he goes into the examination in ignorance, and if he cannot free himself from prejudice he cannot prescribe.
Listens to the friends of the patient and observe without prejudice, with wisdom and with judgment.
That is doing it without prejudice and for this a sound understanding is necessary, with a clear knowledge of all the things relating to the subject and to all of his duties.
Fidelity is necessary. This faithfulness would never be shown by one who had not removed all his prejudices by opening his mind to the principles and doctrines.

Further more he gave very practical advice on maintaining records (Kent 1900 Lecture 23):

> One of the most important things in securing the image of a sickness is to preserve in simplicity what the patient tells us in his own way unless he digresses from the important things and talks about things that are foolish and not to the point; but as long as he confines his information to his own sufferings, let him tell it in his own way without interruption and in the record use his own language, only correcting his grammatical errors for the purpose of procuring the record as perfect as possible.
>
> - If you use synonyms be sure that they are synonyms and cannot be perverted.
> - Of course, when the woman speaks of her menstrual period as 'monthlies' or as her 'show', the more suitable medical term is 'menses', which is a synonym for those expressions, and is more expressive than her own way of calling it 'a show'.
> - So in general terms you can substitute terms of expression so long as you do not change the idea.
> - Of course, the changing of 'legs' into 'limbs' if you feel like making such a change is not a change of thought, but be sure in making a change it is not a change of thought.
> - It is one of the most important things in forming the record of a patient to be able to read it at a subsequent examination, without being disturbed by the repeated statements of the patient.
> - If you write a record in consecutive sentences, you will be so confused when hunting out the symptoms of the patient that you will be unable to form an image of that sickness in the mind.
> - It is truly impossible when the mind is full with the effort at hunting out something to listen with proper and concentrated attention.
> - You should divide your page in such a manner that when the patient is talking to you about this thing and that thing and the other thing of her symptoms, you can with one glance of the eye look down over the page of the record and see everything there is in that page.
> - If your record is not so arranged, it is defective.
> - Now, a record can be so arranged by dividing the page into three columns, the first of which contains the dates and prescriptions, the second the emphatic symptom or headings and the third things predicated of the symptoms.

Kent had some strong opinions,

- *Among pupils who have been taught here, I know some who have merely memorized and some have not even memorized but have fallen away.*
- *These students are violating everything they have been taught; they have gone to low potencies, making greater and greater failures, to the shame of the tutor and the science they profess to follow.*
- *I expect some in the sound of my voice will be doing this five years from now; this is a warning, stop before you go too far, or you will not feel the fault is your own.*
- *You will think you were hypnotized and led into false ways.*
- *If you neglect making a careful examination the patient will be the first sufferer, but in the end you yourself will suffer from it, and homeopathy also.*
- *The questions themselves that Hahnemann gives are not important, but they are suggestive and will lead you in a certain direction.*
- *Question the patient, then the friends, and observe for yourself; if you do not obtain enough to prescribe on, go back to particulars. After much experience you will become expert in questioning patients so as to bring out the truth.*
- *Store up materia medica so as to use it and it will flow out as your language flows.*
- *You must put yourself on a level with the form of speech your patients use.*
- *Be sure you have not put any words into your patient's mouth or biased his expression.*
- *You want to know all the particulars but without asking about it directly.*
- *If you ask a direct question, you must not put the symptom in the record, for ninety-nine times out of a hundred the patient will answer by 'Yes' or 'No'.*
- *If the patient's answer is 'Yes' or 'No', your question was badly formed.*
- *If a question brings no answer let it alone, for he does not know or has not noticed.*
- *Questions giving a choice of answers are defective.*
- *Ascertain the precise part of the body the pain was in and the character of the pain, etc.*
- *In investigating a case there are many things to learn, the length of the attack, appearance of the discharge if it be a case of vomiting, its character, the time of day, etc.*
- *Every student should go over these questions framing collateral questions, and practicing case-taking.*

Tact and Timing

Kent too emphasized the necessity of tact, timing and remaining silent.

- Leave the patient in freedom always.
- Do not put any words into his mouth.
- Never allow yourself to hurry a patient; get into a fixed habit of examination, then it will stay with you.
- It is only when you sustain the sharpest kind of work that you can keep up your reputation and fulfil your highest use.
- Say as little as you can, but keep the patient talking and keep him talking close to the line.
- If he will only talk, you can find out symptoms in general and particular.
- If he goes off, bring him back to the line quietly and without disturbing him.
- There is not much trouble in private practice.
- There you will do a better average of work.
- All sleep symptoms are important, they are so closely related to the mind, the transfer from sleep to waking, from cerebrum to cerebellum, is important.
- Old pathologists were unable to account for difficult breathing during sleep.
- The cerebrum rules respiration during sleep.
- To know the functions of the brain, the functions of the white matter and gray matter, is important.
- A rational knowledge of anatomy is important.
- No homoeopath ever discouraged the true study of anatomy and physiology.
- It is important not only to know the superficial but the real, profound character, to enable you to recognize one symptom-image from another.
- Study this paragraph carefully and meditate upon it.
- If you do not form habits now, you will not form practice hereafter.
- You have no regular course and will get into habits you cannot break up.

It should be remembered that Kent's practice was unlike anything we would recognize today. For him the civil war was a short decade ago and the developments in orthodox drugs not widespread. It is a hard perspective to grasp for the student in Galway, Boulder or Sydney in the 21st century.

- *The flash of the eye is important; it will tell things that cannot be told by the nurse.*
- *It is important for the physician to know the value of expression.*
- *When the patient stares with glassy eye, is he injured about the head, is he suffering from shock, intoxication or typhoid fever, or some disease in which the mind is stunned?*
- *The physician immediately proceeds to ask, 'How long has the patient been in bed?'*
- *If the character is above reproach, he will not suspect intoxication; if the patient has been sick for many days with fever, tongue coated, abdomen sensitive, etc., he is fully entered upon the course of typhoid fever.*
- *The physician must know immediately upon entering the room what the state of the patient resembles; apoplexy, coma, opium poisoning, etc.*
- *A physician is supposed to set his mind to work instantly, to ascertain the condition of the patient and what relation the symptoms maintain to the materia medica.*

But there is no doubt that some of his opinions go against the contemporary grain. His opinions on other treatments are well out of step with modern western patients,

> The whole aim of the physician is to secure the language of nature. If it has been masked by medicines, it cannot be secured. Any meddling will so affect the aspect of the case that the physician cannot prescribe, and the physician who does this meddling must inevitably be driven into bad methods or into allopathy. I have looked over the work of bad prescribers and have wondered what on earth they could see in homeopathy to attract them, they do not cure folks. They have no cures to present. The patients cannot well be satisfied by these things. It is true that once in a while a strong, vigorous, robust patient, when he gets a homeopathic remedy, will go on getting well through

a mess of symptom changing and drugging, so that in spite of this meddlesome practice he will recover. The physician in that case, knows not what remedy to attribute it to, for he has given a great many. But only the most vigorous constitution will stand such homeopathic villainy. Some vigorous patients, after getting the homeopathic remedy, go on and get well in spite of their indulgences in wine, in eating, etc. it is wonderful what their own powers will do in throwing off disease. In ordinary cases, however, we see so many things; confusion is brought about at once if the physician administer another medicine in place of administering placebo.

He often rubs the modern reader up the wrong way.

To illustrate that more particularly, and to bring it down to a practical basis, we may say that the examination of every woman relates to her eating, her stool, her menstruation, her bathing, her dress, because these are the things natural to her. These are the circumstances in which her symptoms may come or may not come. Until the woman is educated to it she does not understand. 'What do you mean, Doctor?' she says. Then I may say, 'You have given me these symptoms; you say you have headache, stomachache, etc. Now will you proceed to relate to me under what circumstance this headache appears, how it is affected by your changes in dress, by the changes in weather, how it is affected before, during or after your monthly indisposition and so on.' Now, these are the natural circumstances. In addition to these another group of circumstances comes up, a group of circumstances somewhat different, in relation to ordinary occupation. Every person will have circumstances more particular than those in general. Occupation will make changes in the circumstances of young women. She may be standing upon the floor of Wanamaker's store all day, and this has produced a condition of prolapsus; or she may lead a sedentary life at her work as seamstress, or she may be at some other occupation, the circumstance of which will develop her psoric manifestations. Modes of life mean a great many different things. They come in as supernumeraries over and above the natural conditions and circumstances of life. The natural functions and circumstances of life have to be considered in relation to the mode of life.

Kent and Peculiarity

He was clearly a man of his time. But by stripping away the Victorian in him reveals a solid strategy and ethos of sound observation.

- The patients generally call attention to the commonest things, while it is the strange and peculiar things that guide to a remedy.
- The symptoms most covered up from the observation of the physician are often the things guiding to the remedy, but finally they leak out in some way.
- The symptom is of such a character that the patient says of it, 'I have always had it and I did not suppose that had anything to do with my disease'.
- When asked, 'Why did you not tell me that before?' he says, 'I did not suppose that amounted to anything, it is so trivial.'

An Anecdote from Kent

Let me illustrate it. A patient comes along with a pallid face, a rather sickly countenance, tired and weary, subject to headaches, disorders of the bladder and disturbances of digestion; and in spite of all your questioning, you fail to get anything that is peculiar. You set the patient to thinking and to writing down symptoms, and she comes back month after month and you give her Sulphur, Lycopodium and a good many medicines. You can sometimes find out whether she is a chilly or hot-blooded patient, and thus you can get a little closer among the common remedies; but the patient says one day, 'Doctor, it seems strange that my urine smells so queer, it smells like that of a horse.' Now at once you know that is Nitric acid. 'How long have you had this? 'Oh, I have always had it, I did not think it amounted to anything.' If you examine the common things belonging to Nitric acid you will find that it possesses all the features of the case.

Hysteria, Exaggeration and the Irish

While we all prefer to see ourselves as unprejudiced Kent's lack of neutrality often slipped through the cracks.

> There is another kind of patient spoken of here, those that 'depict their sufferings in lively colors, and make use of exaggerated terms to induce the physician to relieve them promptly.' This is especially characteristic of the native Irish as a class. You will find that they will exaggerate their symptoms, really and sincerely believing that the doctor will give them stronger medicine if they are very sick and will pay more attention to them; and if they do not exaggerate violently, probably he will turn them off with a simple remedy. Then we have the exaggeration of symptoms by sensitive people. It is an insane habit, such as belongs to hysteria. The physician will be helpless in the hands of these exaggerators, because homeopathy consists in securing the whole truth and nothing but the truth; it is just as detrimental to get too much as to get too little. Any coloring which is expressed, whether by the patient or by the physician, will result in failure; It is true that this tendency to exaggeration must be considered as a symptom. When you have found a patient to exaggerate a few symptoms into a large number, you can simply mention in your note 'tendency to exaggerate symptoms', which is covered by some of our remedies. Such a state is misleading, for you do not

know what symptoms the patient has and what the patient has not (Kent 1990).

Both Hahnemann and Kent used placebo in such situations. It's an option not available to homeopaths in the west nowadays.

> You may rest assured that no patient without symptoms would consult a physician; the patient would not be likely to manufacture the entire sickness; the fact that she has a desire to present herself to the physician and has a desire to exaggerate her symptoms and sufferings is in itself a disease, because no well person would do that. Hence this must be considered; perhaps it is the first and only element that can be considered of that which such patients give out. This exaggeration must be measured with discretion and wisdom. 'Even the most impatient hypochondriac never invents sufferings and symptoms that are void of foundation, and the truth of this is easily ascertained by comparing the complaints he utters at different intervals while the physician gives him nothing at least that is medicinal'. Hahnemann's plan would be to give no medicine and to compare the symptoms that the patient gives from time to time.

The physician must be possessed of an uncommon share of circumspection and tact, a knowledge of the human heart, prudence and patience, to be enabled to form to himself a true and complete image of the disease in all its details.

He must live the life of the neighbor, and be known as a man of honor, as a man who may be believed and respected, as a candid man.

He was an upright kind of bloke,

If a man has carried out his heart's desires without any self-control he is a man unworthy of respect. If he has on the other hand controlled those impulses, he has become a man worthy of respect. In time the physician who does this will become so well acquainted with the human heart that he has apathy and knows what constitutes the language of the affections.

Best Practice Kent

Chapter 23

Set up your page well to start
Ask the relatives
No direct questions
Be Silent
You are like an interrogator of a witness

Chapter 24

Look to the expression
Look for the cause
Look to when the patient was last healthy
Look to the circumstances the patient is in

Chapter 25

Focus on the peculiar
Spot those people who colour their symptoms
Deal with lazy people
Be candid and upfront with delicate matters

From other works

Have a knowledge of human nature
Be quiet and cultivate silence and perception
Have a knowledge of the human heart
Be circumspect
Have honour
Be a neighbour
Be candid

Chapter 5

Post Kentian Approaches

- Schmidt
- Tyler
- Wright-Hubbard
- Roberts
- Close
- Getting Mental Symptoms
- Best Practice Post Kentian

In this chapter you will

1. Learn the case taking opinions and directives of the major writers in homeopathy after Kent's time.
2. Understand the profound influence of Kent's pupils and colleagues in the development of 20th century homeopathy.
3. Identify the continued historical development of case taking.

Timeline

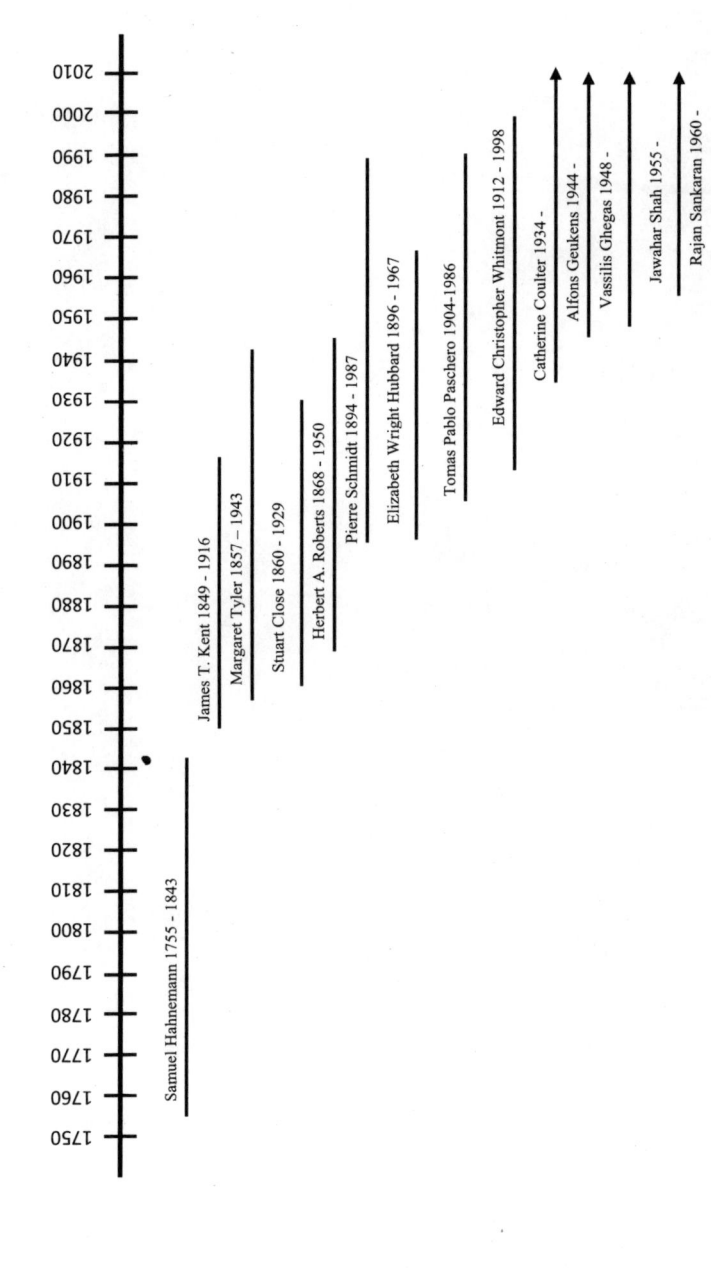

- Samuel Hahnemann 1755 - 1843
- James T. Kent 1849 - 1916
- Margaret Tyler 1857 – 1943
- Stuart Close 1860 - 1929
- Herbert A. Roberts 1868 - 1950
- Pierre Schmidt 1894 - 1987
- Elizabeth Wright Hubbard 1896 - 1967
- Tomas Pablo Paschero 1904-1986
- Edward Christopher Whitmont 1912 - 1998
- Catherine Coulter 1934 -
- Alfons Geukens 1944 -
- Vassilis Ghegas 1948 -
- Jawahar Shah 1955 -
- Rajan Sankaran 1960 -

Chapter 5
Post Kentian Approaches

The interrogation above all must be methodical. (Schmidt)

Symptoms are the outward and visible signs of the inward disturbance of the vital force which will ultimately produce morbid states, and when these symptoms are removed the disease ceases to exist. (Roberts)

Built upon Kent's instructions and emphasis, the giants of twentieth century homeopathy formed and molded the case taking styles for generations of subsequent western homeopaths. They encouraged questionnaires, and we see in most of the casework and the questions of modern homeopathic students the influence and shadow of these writers. The rift that developed between American and British homeopathy in the late 19th century was more about the method and emphasis rather than case taking styles. The high potency emphasis of Kent and his followers prevailed at that time and deeper into the 20th century as well. Böenninghausen, Hughes and Dudgeon's approaches were relegated to a few homeopaths prescribing in corners of the homeopathic world. The emphasis was on types, personality, essences, and drug pictures rather than the simple application of the similar principle from the words of the prover embedded in Allen's *Encyclopedia* or Hahnemann's *Chronic Diseases* to the case (Kaplan 2001). After all, who wants to read dry proving documents and proving symptoms when a great lecturer could stand and perform a song and dance that was far more interesting and captivating. These days the balance is one back towards the centre and good modern homeopathic education emphasizes both the original source material and the value of the synthesized approach to materia medica.

Schmidt

Pierre Schmidt is deserving of a chapter of all on his own. Just as there is tremendous benefit in reading all of Kent (1900) Chapters 23-26 in his *Philosophy*, I would advocate that all read the *Art of Interrogation*. It's not the easiest title to digest. In fact when I saw it on a book list when I was a student and began to read it I hated it. The idea of me as an interrogator didn't fit with the perception I have of myself as a kind, healing, openhearted good person healing all and sundry. But then the more I practice the less I seem to need to be liked. These days when I take the case I notice that I often do act like a policeman or investigator. In my own postgraduate course all of the students who participate watch Sherlock Holmes movies or *Insomnia* with Al Pacino, a perfect example of an investigator who arrives at a crime scene.

Schmidt's posture is similar to Hahnemann yet with a Kentian twist. He was both conservative and medical, yet at times surprisingly esoteric with references to astrology and graphology. Nevertheless his work is full of gems, and his questionnaire, while still a questionnaire, has enough flexibility in it to be useful especially for the beginner.

A legitimate question is, why did he write and speak of interrogation? Just as I've been arguing in the case of Hahnemann or Kent, it is important to remember what was happening historically. While the modern student starting their homeopathic diploma, degree or medical qualification will shrug their shoulders and ask, 'Why do I need to bother to read this book?' it is important to remember that not all modern students in all countries and not all students in the past had the benefit of such training. For example in the case of Schmidt,

> To finish with this introduction, I cannot sufficiently criticize the method quoted in the book recently published, 'La doctrine de l'Homoeopathic francaise' where the physician, after a short physical examination, asks the patient about the symptoms of Sepia suggested by a yellow saddle he has observed on her nose, or those of Lycopodium on an irritable man complaining of his liver. This we may call the 'torpedo method,' in French 'le torpillage'. Because a patient has red lips you would ask him: 'Have you not an empty, all-gone sensation in the stomach before noon?' 'Do you not find it disagreeable to be in a standing position quite a while?' 'Are you not obliged to put your feet out of the bed at night because they are burning'. 'You probably drink much and eat little, and...'

Appropriately, Schmidt acknowledges all of his influences:

> Hahnemann, in his Organon, devotes more than sixty three paragraphs where he speaks about the examination of the patient. Von Böenninghausen gives us excellent advice on how to take the case. Jahr furnishes also a questionnaire, as well as others like Mure, Perussel, Molinari, Landry, Claude, then, more recently, Close and Kent, this last the only one who gives us a full

questionnaire comprising more than thirty-two pages, entitled What the Doctor Needs to Know in order to Make a Successful Prescription. Finally, there is that of Dr. Margaret Tyler. But I bear in mind also the famous lecture of Constantine Hering, published in 1833 in the 'Bibliothéque Homoeopathique de Genève,' in which he sets forth the theme how to trace the picture of the disease, his rules being summed up in four words; to listen, to write, to question, to co-ordinate.

Schmidt while a doctor, does not appear to have been an allopath. Throughout the *Art of Interrogation* and his other works he encouraged homeopaths to desist in attempting to label disease. This even while he was treating physical pathology, such as diphtheria himself. This was dismissed as hunting after end-products, after the results of disease. He followed Hahnemann's line and clearly saw Kent's contribution as an addition to that.

If a patient presents herself to you with varicose veins and pain in the lower limbs and you give her Fluoric acid, Calcarea fluorica or Hamamelis, you will have treated only the vascular walls, but not all the varicose patient. This is only a travesty of homoeopathy. It is the application of a remedy to a diagnosis, it is allopathic prescribing with homoeopathic remedies.

He gave solid and clear advice;

1) The minimum of the best questions to be asked a patient when the time is limited.

2) Most important and most necessary those questions to discover, not the pathological diagnosis but the therapeutic diagnosis, the general remedy corresponding to the patient.

3) The questions to be asked, those for which we are sure to find a correspondence in our repertories and materia medica.

Of course, it goes without saying that the questions asked must be according to the purest principles of homoeopathy:

a) To avoid direct questions, for we know, if the patient answers with yes or no, the question is badly formed.

b) Never to ask a question putting an answer, so to say, into the patient's mouth, thus making sure not to bias his answer.

c) To avoid all questions where the patient is obliged to choose between two different alternatives, and respect the sacred rule to leave the patient always his own choice.

Of course, the physician must put himself, as Dr. Kent says, on the level of language comprehended by his patient. His attitude of seriousness and benevolence must help to stimulate the confidence of his patient. On the other hand, he must know sufficiently his materia medica, so that his questions will be adapted to the comparison he will have to make further on. 'Store up your materia medica so as to use it, and it will flow out as your language flows', in the well-known words of Kent. The physician, by his manner of interrogation and general questions, must do everything not to determine, but to let the patient himself characterize the particular facts. 'Say as little as you can, but keep the patient talking and help him to come close to the line and keep to the point' (Schmidt 1996).

We can never sufficiently bear in mind how difficult is the art of interrogation, and all the importance that should be given to it. 'One can learn very much from Socrates', observes Hering, 'and the study of Plato is as important for us as Hippocrates'.

To avoid all ambiguity, I will first give you some questions that in the course of your own practice you also will have frequently heard, demonstrating that many physicians show by the questions they ask that they have not grasped the thought of individualization; for example:

1) Direct questions (a) Are you thirsty? (b) Are you irritable? (c) Have you pain in the stomach?
2) Suggestive questions (a) You do not stand the cold very well, do you? (b) You surely prefer to be consoled? (c) I suppose that you don't like too greasy and too rich food?
3) Questions where the patient must choose (a) Do you prefer dry or wet weather? (b) Do you dream about sad or cheerful things? (c) Are your menses dark or light?

Schmidt considered that the cause of the condition needed to be determined. And he also wrestled with emphasis of the different types of symptoms he was receiving.

What classification is to be adopted? On one side, we have the counsel given by Hahnemann in his Organon, then the remarkable study of Kent in his 32-33 chapters concerning the value of symptoms, then the numerous classifications established by Grimmer, Gladwin, Green, Loos, Margaret Tyler, Del Mas, Stearns, to quote only those worthy of notice. It is impossible to discuss here every one of the proposed classifications, the broad lines of which, nevertheless, converge in the same direction: First mental symptoms, then general symptoms, then cravings and aversions, then sexual symptoms, and finally sleep and dreams. After this list come the local symptoms related to the organs. But if, theoretically, this classification seems the most acceptable, practically, it is not so; and about this experience has proved to me precious teachings. In my early days of practice, I used always first to ask the mental symptoms, but very soon I came to see I was mistaken. In fact, an unknown patient, knowing nothing whatever about homoeopathy, feels hurt or resents this interrogation about his character when he comes to see you for a headache, a stye or an enlargement of his prostate. Very often too, he imagines that you are mistaking him for a mental case, and that you are making a disguised psychoanalysis. Very shortly, the physician sees by the patient's way of answering, his attitude and his look, the error the himself is committing. On the other hand, to make the interrogation of the mental symptoms at the end of the questionnaire is also a mistake. Because then the patient is tired and has his mind on the fact that those questions have nothing to do with his disease, and have no relation whatever to it. Thus he answers shortly, curtly, badly, manifesting very soon his impatience and his desire to get rid of the inquiry.

While having a Kentian slant, it seems that his philosophical emphasis on the value of mental and emotional symptoms didn't mean that he pursued these doggedly and inappropriately. Overall it seems a very balanced approach.

This is why experience has taught us that it is preferable to begin with the general symptoms, then to ask the questions related to the mentality, explaining rapidly to the patient the difference here between homoeopathy and allopathy, the former being able to compare these symptoms with those obtained on the man in health, because of homoeopathic experimentation only supposed to be made on the healthy man, and not, as the ordinary school does, on animals. Then come the aversions and alimentary cravings, then the symptoms related to the sleep and dreams, and finally, for ladies, those concerning the menses if it is possible to do so. The questions related to the sexual sphere can almost never be asked in the first consultation, especially in a short one. Sometimes it can be touched on when one is asking about heredity or personal history. To close with, it is good to reconsider some of the symptoms predicated by the patient, especially those considered as rare, peculiar and striking, strange or uncommon, and to examine their modalities in order to see if really they deserve important consideration (Schmidt 1996).

Here is the list of symptoms to be taken into consideration:

1) General Symptoms
Hour of aggravation, periodical season aggravation; by the weather: dry, wet, cold, hot, fog, sun, wind. Changes of weather: snow, storms; aggravation of temperature, draughts of air; tendency to take cold, desire or aggravation by the air: aggravation of position, by motion or by repose, riding in cars, sailing, prandial aggravation, appetite and thirst, aggravation by certain foods, wine, tobacco, drugs, vaccinations, cold or hot baths, seashore or mountain, clothing, wounds slow to heal, haemorrhages, fainting in rooms full of people, laterality (side affected).

2) Mental Symptoms
The mental state of a human being can, on the whole, be resolved into four or five essential points: life or death, emotions, fears, irritability and sadness; and all these under hyper or hypo-manifestations.
The theoretical classification would be thus:
a) Symptoms relating to the instinct of self-preservation (death, suicide).
b) Ailments from grief, vexation, mortification, indignation, anger, bad news, disappointed love, and c.
c) Fear, anguish, anxiety.
d) Irritability, anger, violence, impatience, hastiness.
e) Sadness, weeping, despair, effect of consolation.
Then, certain symptoms having no relation to these categories as, for example, jealousy, absent-mindedness, concentration, mania of scruples and as to trifles; modifications of the character before, during and after menses.
Instead of following this questionnaire in the above-given order, it would be better to follow it in the reverse order; because one must begin with symptoms rather superficial and which do not go too deep into the mind of the patient, which latter is ultimately to be discovered.

For the practitioner who has his eyes open as well as his understanding, there are numerous mental symptoms that can be observed without saying one single word, as for example, timidity, loquacity, egotism, easily offended, embarrassed, exhilarated, easily startled, haughty, needless, suspicious, laughing immoderately, even some memory troubles, quiet or hurrying disposition, sighing patients, restless, weeping when speaking about certain symptoms, also, there are certain symptoms of which there is no need to ask the patient because he will tell them himself, either because he came for this purpose, or suffers really very much on account of it. Very often, also, friends or relatives may have written of those symptoms to you before the consultation, if they are sufficiently striking, as, for example, the refusal to eat, the desire to escape, sometimes even fear of suicide (Schmidt 1997).

3. Aversions and Alimentary Cravings	
a) Sweets, pastry, delicacies	e) bread, fruits, fish, meat
b) salty things	f) milk, coffee, wine, beer
c) sour, strong and spiced food	g) state of thirst and appetite
d) greasy and rich foods, butter	

4. Sleep and Dreams
a) Position of the body, head and extremities during sleep
b) What the patient is doing during sleep: laughs, starts, talks, shrieks, weeps, is afraid, grinds his teeth, keeps eyes or mouth open
c) Quality of the sleep: hours and causes of wakings, of sleeplessness and sleepiness;
d) All about dreams.

5. Symptoms Concerning the Menses and the Sexual Sphere
a) Menses too late, duration, abundance, colour, quality, consistence, more day or night, influence of the character or other particular symptoms before, during and after the menses shortly all about what we call the 'Molimen.'

6. Rare, strange and peculiar symptoms indicated by the patient, with their modalities and related phenomena and the making more precise the main symptoms for which the consultation was made.

How to formulate the questions

Schmidt's advice was so comprehensive that it has been replicated here almost in its entirety (Schmidt 1997).

> It is not a bad procedure to say to the patient at this time: 'I have listened to you until now without interrupting you, now we will change the role, and please don't be astonished if I seemingly stop you while answering, to ask you the next question, because this will mean that the answer I was waiting for is obtained. Do not believe that by so doing, I underestimate your answer, but this only signifies that a longer explanation will bring neither useful nor new details in the case.'

General symptoms
1) At what time in the twenty-four hours do you feel worst?
2) In which season do you feel less well?
3) How do you stand the cold, hot, dry, wet weather?
4) How does fog affect you?
5) What do you feel when exposed to the sun?
6) How does change of weather affect you?
7) What about snow?
8) What kind of climate is objectionable to you, and where would you choose to spend your vacation?
9) How do you feel before, during and after a storm?
10) What are your reactions to north wind, south wind, to the wind in general?
11) What about draughts of air and changes of temperature?
12) What about warmth in general, warmth of the bed, of the room, of the stove?
13) How do you react to extremes of temperature?
14) What difference do you make in your clothing in winter?
15) What about taking colds in winter and in other seasons?
16) How do you keep your window at night?
17) What position do you like best-sitting, standing, lying?

Post Kentian Approaches

18)	How do you feel standing a while, or kneeling in church? You remark that this question of the standing position comes again. You will find this way of repeating it is intentional here and there in the questionnaire. It is a very useful and necessary procedure for verification.
19)	What sports do you engage in?
20)	What about riding in cars or sailing?
21)	How do you feel before, during and after meals?
22)	What about your appetite, how do you feel if you go without a meal? It will be often answered to you: 'I can easily go without a meal but I never can stand a big dinner or banquet.' A question that you did not ask, but which demonstrates that the question was well formulated as it made the patient talk and left him his own choice.
23)	What quantity and what do you drink? What about thirst?
24)	What are the foods that make you sick, and why? (If the patient does not answer after a while, just ask looking closely at him: sweets, salty things, sour, greasy food, eggs, meat, pork, bread, butter, vegetables, cabbages, onions, fruits?
25)	What about wine, beer, coffee, tea, milk, vinegar?
26)	How much do you smoke in a day, and how do you feel after smoking?
27)	What are the drugs to which you are very sensitive or which make you sick?
28)	What are the vaccinations you have had, and the results from them?
29)	What about cold or warm baths, sea baths?
30)	How do you feel at the the seaside, or on high mountains?
31)	How do collars, belts and tight clothing affect you?
32)	How long are your wounds in healing, how long in bleeding?
33)	In what circumstances have you felt like fainting?

Mental symptoms	
34)	What are the greatest griefs that you have gone through in your life? (Quite often the the patient will lower the head and look quite moved, and a kind word of the doctor will be needed. It is why, as soon as the extra-version or self-expression has been made, this following question will make the patient look at you again in an astonished way, and sometimes with a happy smile)
35)	What are the greatest joys you have had in life? These two questions are very important and, when asked at the right moment, will pave the way for the coming questions.
36)	At what time in the twenty-four hours do you feel in the blues, depressed, sad, pessimistic?

37)	How do you stand worries?
38)	On what occasions do you weep? (If the patient cannot answer, we will just ask-not losing for one second his expression-music, at reproaches, at which time of the day? Certain people can refrain from weeping, some others cannot).
39)	What effect has consolation on you? If the answer is, 'It depends by whom', you may say 'Just by people you like', because very often people say they do not like to be comforted because they think of members of their family they hate.
40)	On what occasions do you feel despair?
41)	In what circumstances have you ever felt jealous?
42)	When and on what occasions do you feel frightened or anxious? (If the patient does not answer, ask: Some people are afraid of the night, of darkness, to be alone, of robbers, of certain animals, of death, of certain diseases, of ghosts, to lose their reason, of noises at night, of poverty, of storm, of water. According to the way of answering, you will at once see the real fears, and be able to discriminate those which are not to be taken into consideration.
43)	How do you feel in a room full of people, at church, at a lecture?
44)	Do you go red or white when you are angry, and how do you feel afterwards?
45)	How do you stand waiting? (If he does not answer, just question him about impatience.)
46)	How rapidly do you walk, eat, talk, write?
47)	What have been the complaints or effects following chagrin, grief, disappointed love, vexation, mortification, indignation, bad news, fright?
48)	In time of depression, how do you look at death? Certain patients have presentiments of death, thoughts of death, even desire to die; others have tendencies or desires of suicide, some would be courageous enough to do it, others are afraid, in spite of desiring it.
49)	Tell me all about over-conscientiousness and overscrupulousness, about trifles; some people do not care about too much details and too much order.
50)	What about your character before, during and after menses?

During all these questions, the physician must by kind words put his patient at ease, but must watch him very closely, without the patient's noticing it.

Food cravings and aversions	
a)	What is the kind of food for which you have a marked craving or aversion, or what are those that make you sick or you cannot eat? Here also, it is very important to watch very carefully the expression of the patient, because it is very easy to read on the face by observing the corners of the mouth coming down if the patient is disgusted, or on the contrary coming up with big shining eyes if the craving or a strong alimentary attraction is felt. Then, one can add, for example:
b)	What about pastry and sweets?
c)	What about sour or spiced food?
d)	What about rich or greasy food?
e)	How much salt do you need for you taste?
f)	What about thirst and what do you drink? Coffee, wine, beer.

Of course, all those questions have been already asked in the beginning of the questionnaire, but by asking them again, you are able, by doing some cross questioning, to determine if they have been answered well the first time or not.

Sleep	
a)	In which position do you sleep, and since when that position? Where do you put your arms, and how do you like to have your head?
b)	What are you doing during sleep? (If the patient does not answer, you add, Some people speak, laugh, shriek, weep, are restless, are afraid, grind their teeth, have their mouth or their eyes open.)
c)	At what time do you wake up, or when are you sleepy? What makes you restless or sleepy?
d)	What about dreams?

For ladies, menses	
a)	At what age did they begin?
b)	How frequently do they come?
c)	What about their duration, abundance, colour, odour, what about clots?
d)	At what time in the twenty-four hours do they flow most?
e)	How do you feel before, during and after menses?

Schmidt's Idiosyncrasies

...A good physician should be able in the first consultation to make his patient laugh or cry, and so doing, he was assured that the contact was made, as he was able to put in vibration the living human being who was asking for help.

Pierre Schmidt as a physician insisted on the necessity of medical knowledge, including not only classical medicine, homeopathy but also elements of acupuncture, manual medicine, knowledge about semiology, morpho-psychology, iridology, graphology and numerology. Some other points from *The Art of Case Taking* and *The Art of Interrogation* (Schmidt, 1996, 1997) may surprise.

1) The main thing is first to take note of all your observations absolutely neutrally.

2) Divide the page into two parts. To the left, you write all the pathological symptoms, the pathognomonic symptoms of the disease (Cough, fever, sweat in tuberculosis). On the right side which are the non-pathognomonic symptoms - the symptoms that are not habitually occurring in this disease (Desire for vinegar in tuberculosis).

3) In cases at the end and in many chronic diseases e.g. multiple sclerosis, there are almost no symptoms of the patient. You have only symptoms of the disease. All those individualising symptoms fade away. These cases then become difficult to cure.

4) The first thing after having heard the patient is to allow him to tell all about the disease.

5) Hahnemann has described 22 very interesting different diagnoses and diseases or troubles that the patient hides.

6) A good homoeopath should know graphology because it helps very much.

7) Now nominology may help through the name of the patient. Every name is a vibration. The name that you are given when you are born is not something in the air. This name has a science about it.

8) Besides this, there is numerology. By the name and birth-date of the patient you can tell his character. At once, you know his tendency. You know if he is stubborn, very sensitive to beauty or form, or if he is a businessman, etc.

9) You can look into his eyes and see by the form of his pupil what he is hiding. I looked into the patient's eyes and the pupil which was supposed to be round was not round at all. In the 12 o'clock position was a sign of grief. So I said to the girl, 'I think you have a grief connected with your sweetheart.' She began to cry and the mother said, 'Yes, that is so but she would not tell me earlier'.

10) If it is in the left eye, it is not all grief. Every body is divided into two parts or two poles, the right one is the father's side, the left one is the mother's side. If it is in the left eye, it is a revengeful feeling, or rage inside, an angry feeling against somebody e.g. it could be a secretary whom the boss is criticising and fault-finding, so she comes every day already trembling and says all day she is constipated, because she is always under fear.

11) If you have a flattening of left eye at 6 o'clock (position) instead of at 12, it is something else, it means that the patient has flat feet. So you must give her something to put in her shoe.

12) Now, when you put a light into the pupil from sideways or so, the pupil at once contracts and a normal pupil contracts and remains contracted as long as there is light. Instead of this if you see the

pupil always contracting and dilating, what is this? This is found in a vagosympathetic patient. Such patients have alternating troubles. They have alternated constipation and diarrhoea and their characteristic moods are always either up or down, like the pupil, always up and down, never at the centre.

13) There are at least 10-12 diseases which can be diagnosed only by looking into the pupil

14) We must know how to ask for mental symptoms. If you are not able at the first consultation to make a patient cry or laugh, if you do not touch the heart of the patient you will not find the remedy.

15) Big bulging lips express people who are very greedy for eating, good eating; also for love, because you kiss with the lips. This corresponds to the genital parts.

16) Only by looking at the face, you may know everything in the body.

17) There are people who by looking at the hand or at the nails can tell you everything and some of them by the form of teeth. They can tell you everything from the skull.

18) One of my pupils had discovered that the ear is the inverse of the fœtus and that there you have the vertebral column above, and below that the eyes and the nose, then you have skin. There you have the geographical map of the whole body in the ear, and by touching certain points with the needle, sometimes you can cure things at once.

19) Fifth, the sexual symptoms. Of course, this requires the tact and the delicacy of thought of the physician to talk of this question with the patient.

20) You will never begin with this. If you know how to handle

human hearts and human beings, they will tell you very easily their troubles, especially their sexual troubles.

21) The more an allopath grows old, the more he is pessimistic; the more the homoeopath grows old, the more he is enthusiastic and optimistic

Tyler

Somebody said the other day, 'If the case is well taken, any fool can find the remedy'. Certainly, if the case is not well taken, it is impossible to find it. Tyler.

While Tyler is not necessarily to the taste of the genY student of 2010 she gives solid guidelines in her book *Different Ways of Finding the Remedy* (Tyler 1928). Predominantly she encourages homeopaths not to pursue a pathological case-taking approach.

> After writing the patient's story start on the quest of the 'strange, rare and peculiar'. That is to say, you take him through it again, and make him amplify and qualify his statements.
>
> An asthma patient can only breathe when lying flat, or in the knee-elbow position, may be peculiar to this case, and highly diagnostic of one, or of two or three remedies. You will underline that. If you are so skilful, or lucky, as to get two or three invaluable symptoms, your work may end here. For turning up the drugs that have caused these symptoms, you may find in one of them a complete picture of the patient's case, disease and all.
>
> This seems to have been a common method of finding the remedy with Dr. Erastus Case, and it led him to brilliant results with many rare remedies that would not 'work out' by more tedious repertory methods. Next, you try to extract anything definite and well-marked in the general symptoms of the patient:

his (especially) altered reactions to environment, mental and physical. The effect on him of temperature, humidity, thunder, foods, light, noise, smells; his cravings and aversions, with delicate probings for mental symptoms, especially where these denote change from his normal. You may get help from nurse, from friends or relations (who will often lie, by the way, if the patient is present). And all the time you are using your own observation to check, to confirm, and to note the things that you are not told.

She is certainly candid.

Dr. Burnett used to say, 'With children, lunatics and liars, you have to use your own observation'.

Remember, 'leading questions evoke misleading answers'. Make the patient consider. Never ask a question that can be answered by yes or no. Only record what is considered and definite.

She is firmly Kentian in approach.

Mental symptoms, most precious of all, if marked and true, have been angled for, and, where definite and reliable, recorded. Where these deviate from the patient's normal, they are of the highest importance. They may be used as eliminating symptoms. And now THE CASE HAS BEEN TAKEN.

Moreover she reminds us of the central yet controversial role of placebo.

Another way not to do it is to be too ready with your prescription. If you take a lot of trouble with a case (when you know how!) it will give you very little trouble afterwards. (Conversely, if you take very little trouble to begin with, it will give you endless trouble, many times repeated. If you are not sure, give a placebo, and wait. Hahnemann says a week's placebo to start with, anyway! (Tyler 1927).

Wright-Hubbard

A case well taken is half cured, one of the masters said. (Wright-Hubbard)

Elizabeth Wright-Hubbard, Tyler, Close and Roberts are in the same tradition and her book, *A Brief Study Course in Homoeopathy* (1977) is a gem. Again the amount of placebo advocated is surprising.

> He must not prescribe anything but placebo, in a chronic case, until he has complete case taking.

> The physician must be receptive, like a photographic plate ready to receive the image of the patient. He must clear his mind of other preoccupations and of previous opinions about the patient. He must be tranquil, cordial, and after the first greeting and question, 'What brings you to see me?' or 'Tell me what it is that troubles you'. He must be silent.

This was the advice given to students in the UK in the 1980's and 90's. The emphasis was on mental symptoms, sometimes slipping into personality traits. While this slanted the case taking towards the psychological it was nevertheless thorough.

> The physician must allow the patient to tell his own story in his own way. Questions or interruptions of any sort derail the patient at this stage, and may cause the doctor to lose essential information.

> The physician must observe from the moment the patient enters. The office should be so arranged that the light falls on the patient.

> The main points to be noted are: (a) Personality of the patient. (b) His apparent state of mind both in himself and in relation to

the doctor (whether depressed, shy, suspicious, secretive, afraid, ashamed, etc.). (c) His apparent physical status (signs of disease in gait, complexion, difficulty in breathing etc.). (d) Traits of character as shown in dress, cleanliness, neatness, pride, etc.

The physician must record every item which seems to him important, in the words of the patient, both in what the patient says and in what he himself observed, in a column at the left of his paper, leaving at least an inch blank between the items to be subsequently filled in as the patient reverts to that subject or, later, when the physician questions about it. He may prefer to put facts pertaining to history on one sheet or in one column, those pertaining to actual physical symptoms in another, and mentals in a third, but this requires experience and adeptness. It is safer for the beginner to list them all as they come and sort them later in the working out of the case.

When the patient has come to a full stop the physician may say, 'What else?' The object is to drain the patient dry of what he knows of himself.

If the patient is loquacious, time may necessitate the prevention of irrelevancies and the utmost tact is needed to keep him on the main track and yet not lose important side lights.

Give a few remarks on the need of knowing patient as a whole. This pleases the patient and ensures cooperation in answering the often rather intimate questions which must follow.

The patient should be definitely told that the physician must do a complete physical examination and the necessary routine laboratory tests at the next visit. Instructions for bringing a 24-hour urine specimen should then be given. This makes the patient realise that in addition to the interest in all details of the case the physician is going to be thoroughly scientific.

The mental symptoms and characteristics of the patient are the most important if strongly marked. These should usually be elicited last when the patient's confidence has been more fully gained.

Especial tact and insight on the part of the physician are needed to evaluate the emotional causes of disease, for instance, few patients would know that ailments from mortification might be the most important symptom in their case, or that suppression of sex needs or anger might rank as a leading cause in their illness.

At the close of the interview **the patient must be made to feel that the physician is deeply interested in his case**, that he will take the hours needed to thoroughly study up (to repertorize) the case, and that the special method of homeopathy can bring not only relief but also a fundamental improvement in the whole constitution which will tend to ward off subsequent illness and increase the powers and well being of the patient. A thorough physical examination and the routine laboratory work, or any extra tests suggested by the history, must be done on every new patient and at least yearly on old patients, and the patients instructed as to why they should not use other drugs during homeopathic treatment what the dangers of suppression are, when they should report back, and what they may expect as the immediate results of the treatment. One other point may be valuable in knowing the patient and that is to get the version of the immediate family or close friends. This is sometimes dangerous, as nervous patients hate to know that they are being talked over, but the wise physician can take much contradictory evidence and arrive at a more just and sympathetic evaluation of the case. By this time the physician should have a remarkably accurate picture of the patient in all his phases subjective, objective, pathological. From this totality of symptoms he can, by correctly evaluating the symptoms as we will show in a subsequent lecture, derive a true image of the patient and the remedy (Wright-Hubbard 1977).

Other advice she gave was immensely practical encouraging the student to use the questionnaire until it was memorized and second nature. The emphasis on searching for mental symptoms at the end of the process is also of value to gain confidence and better details. Moreover her verifying symptoms with cross-questions when the patient did not understand or answer the question well is of great use. *Accept no diagnostic suggestions or pathological theories or former opinion of other physicians as these are deceptive guides for the selection of a drug* (Wright-Hubbard 1977).

Roberts

H.A. Robert in his book, *The Principles and Art of Cure by Homoeopathy* (1936) advocated a different order for the process but essentially the same ethos.

> The attitude of the physician should be one of absolute rest and poise, with no preconceived ideas nor prejudices. He should be in a quiet, listening attitude, and as the case is presented to him he should have no previous impressions as to what remedy the patient will require.
>
> The first thing to note is the patient's name, age, sex, vocation and, if possible, avocation.
>
> Then a record of the family; that is, the age of the parents, their

general health, and cause of death if they are deceased. This applies to brothers and sisters also; and we must not neglect to get a picture of the types of ailments from which they have suffered. We often get a good picture of hereditary tendencies in this way. Find out, if possible, if there is or has been blood relationships between ancestors. Consanguinity plays an important part in hereditary tendencies as well as in making your prescription.

Now begin to record his past illnesses. What illnesses has he had? How about his recovery from each illness? Particularly note whether he reports himself as fully recovering from illnesses, or whether he says he 'has not been well since' any particular illness.

Now ask the patient to tell you in his own words how he became ill and exactly how he feels. Do not offer any interruption, lest you break his thread of thought. Leave space between symptoms so that you can fill in later answers to questions as it may be necessary.

Things we must not do:
a) Avoid all leading questions.
b) Never ask direct questions, that may be answered with a direct affirmative or negative.
c) Never ask alternating questions.
d) Avoid questioning along the line of a remedy.
e) While you are dealing with one symptom, confine yourself to that symptom. Never skip from one symptom to another at random, as it confuses the patient and scatters the physician's ideas.

If he comes to a point where he seems to hesitate, simply ask, 'What else?' Continue this system of interested listening until he (seemingly) has exhausted his story.

The mental symptoms rank very highly for the reason that they point to the man himself, and they may be classed under the generals to a marked degree.

The physician's degree of success in obtaining the proper symptom picture lies in his skill and patience. We cannot rush these patients through. We must be good listeners. Get the patient to talking, and tactfully keep him talking about the symptoms rather than wandering far afield. Then cultivate your powers of listening and give your powers of observation full sway like a criminal lawyer.

Then the strange, rare, and peculiar symptoms should be sought out.

Mental symptoms: To a great extent these are symptoms that must be observed from the attitude of the patient. Another reason for leaving these until the last is that during the examination you have probably been able to get the confidence of your patients to a greater degree and they will give you more fully their confidence.

The personality, the individuality of the patient, must stand out pre-eminently in the picture. This can be illustrated by likening the whole symptomatology to a complete picture of the whole individual, a whole personality. This embraces not only his physical characteristics, but the expression of his mental and emotional characteristics as well.

Let us remember the exposition that Conan Doyle so often puts into the mouth of his famous character, Sherlock Holmes. This worthy, in summing up some famous case in which he has acted the scientific detective, uses these words: 'That which is out of the common is usually a guide rather than a hindrance'. And again: 'That which seemingly confuses the case is the very thing that furnishes the clue to its solution' (Roberts 1936).

Close

Stuart Close in *The Genius of Homeopathy* (1924) in the chapter Examination of the Patient talks of the complexity of case taking.

> Nearly all of the objective phenomena possessing value from the standpoint of homoeopathic therapeutics are of such a character that they require the exercise of only the physical senses and ordinary powers of observation by the patient, his friends, or the physician himself. 'It takes nine specialists to make a physician'. The general practitioner must act in several capacities-as hygienist, sanitarian, pathologist, psychiatrist, diagnostician, therapeutist, and perhaps even surgeon and obstetrician
>
> It is well in some cases to briefly explain to a new patient the special purpose of a homoeopathic examination and to point out how it differs from the ordinary examination, especially by including mental and subjective symptoms and certain conditions that are usually ignored.

Close was born in 1860. In 1874 his family removed to California and settled in the Napa City, where he engaged in various occupations to earn his own expenses while further pursuing his studies. In 1879 he began to study law but continued this only about one year. The subsequent marriage of his mother with Dr. J. Pitman Dinsmore, for many years one of the leading homeopathic physicians of San Francisco encouraged him to study homeopathy. In 1882 he entered the Medical College of the Pacific in San Francisco and later he then went to New York and studied at New York Homeopathic Medical College. He was a therapeutic specialist along strictly Hahnemannian lines, and an expert in materia medica, devoting himself largely to chronic and complicated diseases. While a contemporary of Kent his writings emphasised and stressed Kent's work hence the discussion of his work in this chapter (Winston 1999, www.hpathy.com, www.wholehealthnow.com). In his case taking chapters the emphasis is upon rapport.

> We must first gain the patient's confidence and relieve him, as far as possible, from the sense of restraint and embarrassment. This is favored in a general way by a calm, dignified, but at the same time quiet and sympathetic manner on the part of the examiner; a demeanor confident, but not pompous; simple and direct, but not aggressive; cheerful, but not flippant; serious, but not grave or funereal.
>
> We should try to put the patient at his ease by adapting ourselves to his personality and mood. We should not confuse the patient by a too penetrating gaze at some objective feature which may attract our attention. We may learn to observe objective phenomena accurately without seeming to do so. The patient should be encouraged to tell his story freely and relieve his mind. We want the history and symptoms of the case from the patient's standpoint first. The best results are obtained by making him forget that he is under examination. One can be painstaking and systematic without being over-formal.
>
> We may start him in his narrative by asking when and how his trouble began, and we may instruct him to be as definite as possible in relating his history and in locating and describing his sensations as they seem to him. We should not laugh at him nor pedantically correct his errors. We should not ask 'leading questions,' nor 'put words in his mouth,' but let him express his feelings and observations in his own way.

There are plenty of practicalities.

As a matter of convenience in writing and keeping records it is well to divide the page into three vertical columns - the first for date and remedy, the second for the symptoms and the third for the modalities or conditions. This makes a page that the eye quickly takes in at a glance.

We should not hurry a patient in his narrative. We may quietly keep him to the point and prevent rambling and inconsequential statements (Close 1924).

All these authors emphasised the art and the science. The art was in the case taking. To quote from a contemporary source:

> Any repertory will be useless if the case is badly taken. Case taking is an art. It is the real art of medicine. The art comes first, before the science comes. This art can be learnt after a certain amount of practice only, but thoroughness, which is an integral part of it, can be practiced right from the beginning. When a case is well taken, our work is practically done. The master has made strict demands on the physician for the proper case-taking and they are as valid and necessary today, as they were in his own time. Nobody has improved on his ideas about it. If one is negligent in case taking or has taken incorrect symptoms, Repertorisation will give one the wrong answers. It will be like the birth of a monster instead of a normal body. It requires all the alertness, intelligence, ingenuity, care, and circumspection on the part of the physician. Rudolph Rale, writing in an editorial says, 'There is procedure in homoeopathic practice more important than a thorough knowledge of the right way to take a case. The ability to do this, ensures against humiliating mistakes and failure, prevents misconceptions of the sphere of Homoeopathic

therapeutics and paves the way to relief or cure where either is possible (Jugal Kishore 1998).

Researching the material for this chapter convinced me that these authors gave great advice on case taking. No doubt, in the years after Kent the focus of the case taking process and the evaluation of the symptoms, plus the emphasis on different aspects of those symptoms changed. Perhaps the type of patient coming to see them changed in those times. Constitution and mental aspects were stressed as being of higher importance. Because of some of these directives there was, and still is a tendency to ask questions such as,

What was the worst thing that ever happened to you?
Can you recall a time you were humiliated, please talk about it?
How did you feel? What did you do?
How do you react in similar situations now?
Who are you most like or dislike in your family?
What time in the 24hrs do you feel down or vulnerable?
On what occasions do you weep? What emotion do you find most difficult to express? Why?
What effects has consolation on you?
How are you with public speaking? or in crowds, etc?
In times of depression how do you look at death?
What complaints do you suffer after anger, grief, bad news, mortification, fright, etc?
What are your main issues in life? What about certain persons?
Tell me about over-conscientiousness, fastidiousness, meticulousness?
What is your character before, during, after menses?

To jump forward to the 21st century, there is no doubt that recent graduates from poorly training homeopathic colleges take bland cases because they ask these irrelevant questions at the wrong times and out of context. The patient came for help with travel sickness, or they came for their warts. Students get confused. Teachers tell them personality is important. They read this emphasis in Kent, Roberts and Close. They know they have to get the totality of the symptoms. So they use everything in their analysis. What is left then is a massive amount of uncharacteristic information and a lot of polycrests prescribed is the result. A bland result is death to the confidence of a new prescriber in homeopathy. This style of homeopathy done badly leaves everyone dissatisfied. Done well, at the right time and with an appropriate patient, the client feels heard, feels it has been thorough, and for them, such a constitutional prescription may balance out their ills and woes.

Getting Mental Symptoms

The importance of these symptoms established, the issue then becomes how and when to get them. Some homeopaths such as Borland have advocated and found it easier to bring out the patient's mental symptoms during or after the physical examination, since by this time rapport has been developed. Physical touch seems to bring the patient closer to the doctor mentally and emotionally (Gafoor 2010). By the time the case taking is half way through, the patient becomes more relaxed and cooperative and is ready to tell us all his or her inner feelings, doubts and fears. Schmidt however argued that mental symptoms should not be asked at the end of case taking because by that time the patient is exhausted and is not able to give out his innermost feelings clearly.

Either way the patient may inadvertently reveal an emotionally disturbed state by the way they answer our questions or even by an inflexion of the voice. Sometimes, a smiling patient may suddenly break down and weep bitterly when we have accidentally touched an emotionally sore spot. Sometimes the patient may avoid answering a question or hesitate, or they may give a vague answer or deflect around the question, or he may look down or look elsewhere while answering. All these generally indicate that they are trying to hide something.

The importance of mental and emotional symptoms cannot be stressed enough, though they may require great patience and tact to elicit. The experienced prescriber is able to find, in a vast majority of cases, an emotional or psychic element in the patient. But it has to be stated that homeopaths worldwide differ on their understanding of what is a mental symptom. The patient may try to hide or refuse to reveal some emotional factor. It may be some tragic episode or one which may have an element of personal shame. P. Sankaran argues that an important mental symptom is a change that has occurred in the personality and temperament of the patient. He argues these elements are very valuable because they often have a dominant say in the selection of the simillimum or they, at least, help us greatly to differentiate between competing drugs. Ironically, his son argues that it is the mental state not the symptoms that we should be searching for and this is further discussed in Chapter nine (P. Sankaran 1996).

P. Sankaran's instructions in tracing out mental symptoms:

1.	Mode of narration of complaint
2.	His attitude towards illness
3.	How the patient talks? The rate and quantity of speech. The maniac patient's speech is usually fast and in depressive patients it is slow, patient may pause a long time before

	replying to questions or may give short answers as also in the case of shyness and low intelligence
4.	Look for any neologisms - private words invented by the patient
5.	Any rapid shift from one topic to another - flight of ideas or general diffuseness and lack of logical thread may indicate the thought disorder characteristic of schizophrenia
6.	Accompaniments to the suffering, the state of mind that is produced during pain or suffering is often the state of mind of the patient in an uncompensated form
7.	Interests and hobbies- what would you enjoy doing the most? Why?
8.	Patients nature as a child, how he was as a child?
9.	Reactions in life situations. How he reacted in times of stress and strain in his life
10.	What are the qualities in others and in yourself that you cannot understand or tolerate. When are you angry with yourself?
11.	Person's occupation and area of work. Whether he has chosen himself or circumstances made him to choose it. How does he behave in his area of work? Any change of job and reason for that
12.	The situations that the patient has created in his life
13.	How do you stand waiting?
11.	How rapidly do you walk, eat, talk, write?
12.	In time of depression how do you look at death? Have you considered any way which you may end your life?
13.	Tell all about over conscientiousness and over scrupulousness about trifles
14.	What are the greatest griefs or joys you have had in life?
15.	What effect has consolation on you?
16.	On what occasions do you feel frightened or anxious? Have you noticed any change in your body and mind when you are feeling anxious? Like palpitation, pains, thoughts of fainting, losing control or going mad.
17.	Interview with friends and relatives
18.	The best technique is to watch what happens spontaneously. Then the other techniques are used only when you reach a dead end and do not know how to proceed further
19.	Any obsessional phenomena - any thoughts keep coming in your mind even though you try hard not to have them. Do you have to keep checking activities that you know you have really completed?
20.	Delusions, illusions, and hallucination - do not ask direct questions but observe from the talks and gestures
21.	Orientation of place, person and time

Best Practice Post-Kentians

Avoid

Direct questions
Suggestive questions
Questions where the patient must choose

Do

Begin with, 'What troubles you'?
Give placebo until you are sure of your prescription

Be

Receptive
Like a photographic plate
Restful and poised
A detective
Like a criminal lawyer

Have

A clear mind. Let them tell their own story
Develop rapport

Chapter 6

Best Practice Gathering Information

- Before Opening Your Mouth Remember
- The Purpose of Case Taking
- Attitude
- Method and Steps of Case Taking
- First Serve
- Observation
- Questioning and Silence
- Physical Examination
- Recording
- Own Words
- Importance and Underlining
- Legalities
- Time Management and Endings
- To Questionnaire or Not
- Difficulties and Specific Situations in Taking the Case
- The Last Word and Great Advice
- Being a Beginner

In this chapter you will be able to
1. Describe what information is required during process of case taking.
2. Know what is required of the case taker in order to get that information.
3. See the progression of homeopathic thought from its early underpinnings to contemporary practice.

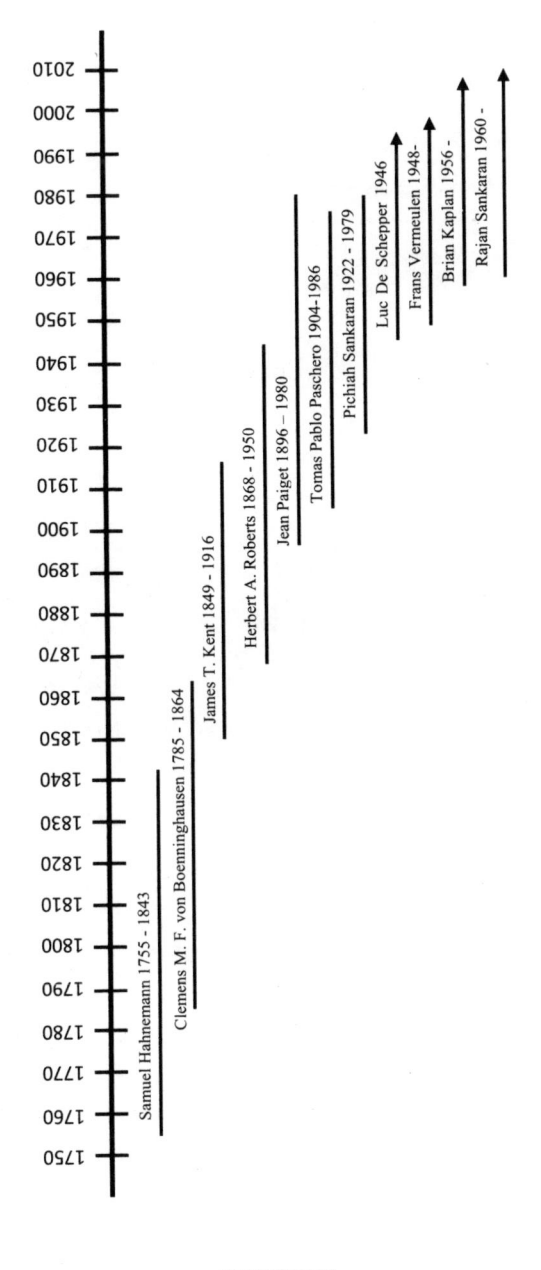

Timeline

- Samuel Hahnemann 1755 - 1843
- Clemens M. F. von Boenninghausen 1785 - 1864
- James T. Kent 1849 - 1916
- Herbert A. Roberts 1868 - 1950
- Jean Paiget 1896 – 1980
- Tomas Pablo Paschero 1904-1986
- Pichiah Sankaran 1922 - 1979
- Luc De Schepper 1946
- Frans Vermeulen 1948-
- Brian Kaplan 1956 -
- Rajan Sankaran 1960 -

Chapter 6

Best Practice
Gathering Information

A properly taken case is more than half cured (Garth Boericke)

To listen, to write, to question, to coordinate (Constantine Hering)

Just take the bloody case (Ken D'Aran)

This chapter represents a synthesis of all of those authors and writers discussed in the previous chapters. There is a collective accumulated wisdom from Hahnemann in the 18th century, through the 19th to the 20th century masters that create a historically derived best practice for contemporary homeopaths. It is so simple. Listen. Observe. Ask what the problem is. Relax. When it is over give the best remedy match possible, manage and monitor the case. In homeopathic colleges these days, students of year one and two are taught to take the case from this perspective. It is a blend that takes into account Hahnemann through Kent. For Hahnemann homeopathy was the simple process of matching the symptoms of a patient to the symptoms of the proving and as a consequence the case taking process is relatively simple (Kaplan 2001).

Recently I attended a folk festival in Queensland in Australia. It is not normally the sort of thing I do these days but I went because a number of homeopaths had volunteered to run a clinic. It was a marvelous opportunity to promote homeopathy and do good work and also for students to develop some clinical skills. It was also a lot of fun. The most memorable part of that occasion was a woman who came into the clinic complaining of some sinus congestion. I had two students sitting in with me. I said, 'Hi,' and welcomed her and got down to business. 'What is troubling you?' She said, 'I have been working in the bakery around the corner making doughnuts and the last few days I've been getting worse and worse sinus problems and now have a headache. There's a buildup of pressure and after that a discharge.' I asked her a little about that and a couple of other questions and then asked the student to go and make up some *Kali Bich 30*. There was this awkward moment where the student hesitated to go but eventually went and made up the remedy and we saw the patient on her way. When I came back into the room by students were incredulous, 'But you didn't ask about anything else,' they said. 'But you didn't ask about how they were feeling, about what was going on for her and her life. You didn't ask about her sleep or her state of mind, her constitution and what's happening.' It served to remind me that something which is so self-evident for myself now is never self-evident at the beginning, and I realize the distance that homeopaths come on their journey who have been practicing for more than five, 10 or 20 years. In this case the patient had an acute condition, even an indisposition that required five minutes of questioning to find a complete symptom, make sure that matched the characteristic keys of the simillimum and then prescribe. It was homeopathy at its efficient acute best. She reported the next day that all was well. Of course she'll be back another day with another acute or because she wants to delve into her chronic health, but in that situation it was inappropriate to go into any chronicity and in five minutes she was done. My students were a bit shocked.

Before Opening Your Mouth Remember

Reflection is a useful thing to do. Before beginning case taking take a moment to remember just what it is that you are doing. What are we doing? For what purpose are we doing it? The questioning must be aimed to discover the real disease disturbance as expressed by the patient through their symptomatology. It is a process of individualization, to look for the totality, to look for the big picture and the small picture, to look for both mental and physical symptoms. Remember the body doesn't lie and that the mind, while important is but a part of the human being.

From When the Patient was Last Healthy

These are most crucial words. It is this concept, hovering in the back of the case taker's mind that assists in the formation of great questions to elicit that relevant information. From when were you last healthy? When did this disease process begin?

> The unprejudiced observer...takes note of nothing in every individual disease, except the changes in the health of the body and of the mind...from the former healthy state of the now diseased individual...these perceptible signs represent the disease in its whole extent, that is, together they form the true and only conceivable portrait of the disease (Hahnemann 1922 § 6).

Search for that which is Peculiar

Hahnemann reminds us that the more striking, uncommon and peculiar (characteristic) signs and symptoms of the case of disease are the most important to be kept in view. Look for strange, queer, rare, bizarre and peculiar symptoms (§153).

> The homeopathician is always seeking that in the case which is peculiar, uncommon, characteristic, individual. That may be noticed in some casual expression of the patient as he talks, revealing his mood or state of mind, or the origin of his trouble; it may be found in the color, form, or expression of his countenance; or in his attitude, gait, or physical demeanor (Roberts 1936).

Practice looking for uncommon, characteristic, strange symptoms to make up the totality. Discount symptoms to be expected from the pathology present, such as anxiety in heart disease, paræsthesia in anæmia, œdema in nephritis, hunger in thyroid issues and gastric ulcers.

Search for Completeness

This can be thought of in a couple of ways. Traditionally it means:

Modalities
Causes
Onset
Pace
Sequence
Duration
Character
Location laterality, extension and radiation of pain or sensations
Concomitants and alternations

Or it can be remembered in another way:

Quis – who
Quid – cause
Ubi – location
Cur – what affects the complaint?
Quando – when
Quibus auxiliis – with what

The cause is so important to search for.

While taking the case I invariably try to find out from a patient the cause, source or origin of the illness or the circumstances in which it started. In the earlier years of my practice, when I used to enquire about this, my patients used to generally reply either that they did not know the reason or that the illness had started without any apparent exciting cause. And I used to generally accept and be satisfied by this answer. But nowadays I find that by persistent questioning about this point I am able to uncover and expose in about 75% of the cases a definite cause, source, origin and/or circumstance from which the disease has taken shape, (P. Sankaran 1996).

De Schepper describes case taking as detective work. You have to be Sherlock Holmes to understand who your patient really is (De Schepper 1996:113).

An accurate remedy should cover both the etiology and symptoms.

Sometimes, I have based my prescription mainly or solely on this etiology. I take the cause as the starting point as well as the most important symptom in the case. Generally we consider the cause as a very important symptom. If you know the cause give more value to it. Then secondly, mentals. If there are really good mental symptoms give importance to them, but peculiar mentals are the most important. In my own method I give grading as follows:

1. Peculiar mentals
2. Peculiar generals
3. Peculiar particular
4. Common mental
5. Common generals
6. Common particulars

> A good example of the inductive procedure outside homeopathy are the stories of Arthur Conan Doyle. They are an excellent teaching tool for case-taking. Sherlock Holmes was a master sleuth not only because he had a special genius, but because he tried to remain open to all the evidence, objective and subjective, reasoning from particulars to generals, and thus avoiding the hasty conclusions –'deductions' of his allopathic sidekick, Dr. Watson. (Stewart R, 1995 American Homoeopaths Homeopathy in America; Taking the case)

Among the parts of the symptoms - location, sensation and modality - I give importance to the modality. In summary disease is only an alteration in the state of health of the individual and this alteration is represented by symptoms. The homeopath must therefore ensure that all the symptoms recorded are actually part of the deviations from the originals or normal state of the individual and that therefore they form part of the disease-picture. It is useless to record details of the normal state of the individual because we are not going to treat the normal individual. We have also to ensure that the symptoms noted are fairly marked in intensity. In acute states the physician should consider only the symptoms of that state with the exclusion of the symptoms of the original chronic condition that the patient might have been suffering from (P. Sankaran 1996).

The Purpose of Case Taking

Ultimately the purpose is to record faithfully the picture of suffering of each individual patient in such a way that the indications for the simillimum emerge out of it. In taking the case, we seek to record details of the sufferings of the patient, including the chief complaint, present symptomatology, previous history, personal history and family history, along with the abnormal findings on physical examination, and a summary of the previous treatments taken and their results.

> While taking the case we have to remember that we may come across the most significant symptom or symptoms at any stage of the case taking while listening to the patient (or the relative) and so we have to be very alert and keenly attentive always. We have also to intelligently evaluate each answer so that we may frame the succeeding questions suitably. Generally speaking, nothing that the patient says or what we notice about the patient is completely useless or insignificant (P. Sankaran 1996). The purpose of the case taking is to develop the history of the main complaint, other complaints, and past medical history, including past surgical history, medications, vaccinations, and systemic history (Kaplan 2001).

Attitude

It helps to have an open-hearted viewpoint to help people but without over-sentimentality or a judgmental idealistic philosophy. Make the patient feel comfortable to answer questions without fear of judgment. Be neutral in appearance dress. Be able to adapt to the patients reality. Drop your own issues so as to be as present as possible to be able to question and listen to your client (D'Aran 2008).

Start with a blank paper and a blank mind with no preconceptions. It is possible that the first few symptoms of the patient may suggest to the homeopath a particular remedy but it is important to push these ideas aside until after the case taking has been completed. Objectivity can be lost (P. Sankaran 1996).

Furthermore, inform the patient just what we are doing. Let their and your expectations be congruent. Let the patient know you are concerned for their health and that homeopathy has the capacity to bring fundamental improvement to them. It is of utmost importance that the interviewer be interested and concerned with the welfare of the patient. There should be no implication of judgment. Avoid giving advice catch yourself before you begin moralising. Restrain your conversation also. Let them tell their case their way without interruption. The professional posture is one of a collaborative approach. Rather than the expert who understands and fixes the patient, better a mutual healing alliance. Try to create an equal relationship where they are given power over their healing. Hence the first question for many homeopaths is, 'What brings you here today?' rather than, 'How can I help you?' Be focused, inquisitive and caring.

P. Sankaran summarized it beautifully.

> Information provided by the patient voluntarily and spontaneously is of maximum value. Care should be taken never to interrupt since as a result of such interruption of his line of thought, what the patient was about to say might remain unsaid. All questions should be asked and doubts clarified only at the end without disturbing the patient's trend. Borland, that delightful teacher, has given some practical hints: For a successful

homoeopathic prescription the physician ought constantly to bear in mind the six following rules:

a)	To observe	b)	To question
b)	To listen	e)	To examine
c)	To write	f)	To coordinate

a) To observe without saying a single word, but with eyes wide open to notice the gait, behaviour, gestures, the smallest changes of expression, etc.

b) To listen to all noises, respiratory, digestive, articular, etc., and, of course listen without interrupting. If a patient talks, let him do so freely, otherwise he will reproach you for not having been able to utter a single word or, at the end of the consultation, he will come out with a long array of symptoms written in his notebook. Put him off until tomorrow if necessary but let him talk. First because to listen is a sign of politeness and, besides, you will let him do the extraversion so preached by the psycho-analysts. To be able to narrate one's ailments and feel that somebody is listening with interest and benevolence, constitutes a great relief. You know it.

c) To write and in the exact terms of the talker in order to be able later on to recollect his own personal expressions.

The attitude should be of 'Watchful expectancy and masterly inactivity' (P. Sankaran 1996).

Method and Steps of Case Taking

1. Observation
2. Listening
3. Interrogation and cross-examination
4. Clinical or Physical Examination
5. Laboratory Tests
6. Homeopathic Diagnosis

First Serve

When I see a patient, I always greet him warmly with a broad cheerful smile. The patient is in need of cheer and a cheerful smile will help him like a tonic. If we look serious, he may feel that we are angry, indifferent or hopeless. A smile costs nothing but can have a very beneficial effect (P. Sankaran 1996).

This is strong advice, but of course everyone has their own style and the advice from the literature is varied. After taking down the name, age, occupation and address of the patient, the physician can say, 'Please describe all your troubles from the beginning and give me all the details,' (P. Sankaran 1996) or 'What is troubling you?' or some such question and the client should be allowed to detail in his own words the description of his ailments.

Ask, 'What brings you to see me?' When they have finished, ask 'What else?' Keep the talkative patient on track with small comments and the quiet patient talking with questions like 'Anything else about…?' or 'Tell me more.' After the patient's story go back to each item and get the details they didn't tell you such as the modalities. Question them about any they have left out (Wright-Hubbard 1977). Let the patient talk until they run out of things to say.

Beginning the case is like breaking the ice. There are so many ways to do this. Kaplan's example starts with name and address and details or sometimes about the patient work. I find myself doing the same thing although sometimes the question that comes out of my mouth is, 'What do you understand about homeopathy' or, 'Have you seen a homeopath before'. The value of this question means that immediately I know where to pitch my questioning and any other information that the patient may have. Your work begins at the greeting. So much happens in that moment. Before the consultation start observing. All sorts of valuable material occurs before the patient is walked in the door. The way they talk on the phone, the structure of the e-mail, the voices in the background, the noise in the houses when they talk to you making the appointment can be as much a guide to the remedy is anything else is. In addition, remember to ask the receptionist there was anything that took place in the waiting room while they were waiting. Such information can be gold (Kaplan 2001). For best practice on how to guide a patient into the consulting room look no further than Kaplan (2001:53)

Explanations of the process are crucial. P. Sankaran says,

I have always found it very useful especially in dealing with intelligent patients to explain the disease to them. The patients are eager to know what they are suffering from and by explaining it to them we find that their cooperation is available to us in a greater measure. A patient who understands can cooperate better. And as you explain to the patient what his disease is, he feels greatly relieved because he understands what it is and has no doubts that the disease is something else, perhaps something very serious as he might have imagined or feared. After all, ignorance is a major cause of fear and it also magnifies the fear. And as this explanation removes the ignorance, it can even help the patient to recover. It also helps him to face his disease with more fortitude, courage and confidence. And explaining the disease process also instills in him more faith in our ability. In all my dealings with my patients, I always try to be hopeful and encouraging. Every matter has two aspects - a bright one and a dark one and so also every case. And I like in every case to throw maximum light on and emphasize the bright aspects and describe to the patients what the hopeful signs are in his case. As even the most hopeless case has some bright aspect, we can give the patient some encouragement. After all it must be accepted that medicine alone by itself may not be enough to cure. The patient's faith, spirit and desire to survive also help in the cure. I know even of cases which had been declared utterly hopeless and have eventually survived without taking any treatment. We should never destroy the hope of the patient even in serious cases such as advanced cancer. There is no use telling the patient that his case is hopeless. It is the hope in the heart of every patient which, to some extent, helps him to recover. One of the things the patient needs and expects from the physician is reassurance. It may be necessary to reassure the patient repeatedly or constantly. This can help sometimes more than the medicine and the physician should never feel tired of doing this. It is my policy never to criticise a patient. A patient may be full of faults and failings, he may not even cooperate or he may fail to carry out our instructions but even then I do not criticise him. The patient is like a child. In sickness he regresses to a childish state or behaviour and so we have to handle him like a child, firmly but tactfully. Even if a patient comes to me after a gap of many months or has taken medicine very irregularly and his condition is worse.

Sometimes the patient may leave our treatment and go to some other doctor. This, I do not at all mind. It is generally a good idea to make personal enquiries. For example, if the patient was directed to us by another friend we may enquire about the friend. Enquiry about the family set-up of the patient not only provides us with information which will be of use to us in our own work but also gives a sense of satisfaction to the patient. Anything that we want to ask or tell the patient should be told in an acceptable way. If, for example, I want to ask the patient whether he has suffered from syphilis, I always ask him whether there was any chance of his getting the infection. To summarize, I may say that all our expressions and actions should always be guided by the best of intentions. We must speak, act and do what is necessary and beneficial for the patient and make it psychologically acceptable to him. This way lies the road to success (P. Sankaran 1996).

In starting the process and getting the main complaint the question, 'What brings you here today,' or 'What troubles you,' is perhaps the best place to start. It is such an important moment in the consultation because, as Kaplan points out the patient has perhaps unconsciously decided that you are to be the person that he or she can trust enough to have an authentic conversation with. Your only role is to listen and perhaps bring them back and interrupt only as they wander into unnecessary jargon or meaningless details (Kaplan 2001).

Observation

Observation starts from the waiting room, or even before if the opportunity presents itself. Kaplan, De Schepper and many others give great examples of patients on the waiting room reading a book or fuming because of lateness. One is chatting to the receptionist and another is hiding behind the plant. One is pacing and one is chewing nails. The homeopath notices the greeting, the eye contact, the handshake, the complexion, the hair, the graying, the augmentation, in other words a multitude of factors even before the patient is sitting in a consultation (De

Schepper 1996:114). Moreover observe how closely they sit to you, the posture, the folding of the arms or other protective behaviour, leaning towards you, is there a list, how big is the handbag, is the mobile phone turned on or off. These days I always encourage clients to answer the phone if it rings during the consultation unless I'm really pressed for time. Once I was treating a man who came for some bleeding from his bowel which had been occurring for the last three months. In addition to that there was a clear discharge from his nose which had been there for much longer and seemed to be related to the amount of marijuana that he was smoking. He worked for an advertising agency and after a few minutes of the consultation the phone rang. Normally I just saw that behaviour as rude but before I had a chance to encourage him not to, he picked up the phone. The conversation went something like this. 'Hi there... yes I remember you, I know...I don't care, it's simple, do you dig me or not? I don't care if you're married...four o'clock then. Perfect.' I was stunned. In that brief interaction I understood so much about my client, his behaviour, ethics, values and morals. I learned even more when 20 minutes later the phone rang again and he set up a date with a different woman. 'I like chicks,' he said, 'And I like getting them drunk on red wine.' He did well on *Fluoric acid*.

How a patient sits, stiffly or withdrawn, still or restless provides great information (De Schepper 1996:114). I was treating a patient once with hepatitis C. She had a history of some drug dependence and I was weighing up whether to give *Sulphur, Avena sativa, Nux vomica* or whatever when suddenly she got up from her chair walked across the room and straddled the oil heater which was turned on. She remained straddling the heater for the remainder of the consultation without blinking an eye. I was amazed and I gave her *Hepar sulph*.

When the patient enters into the consulting room note the facial appearances and expressions of the patient plethoric, waxy, pale, puffy, edematous. Note whether they seem anxious or angry.

> Depressed patients may have vertical furrows on the brow, turning down of the corners of the mouth, sitting leaning forward, with shoulders hunched, the head inclined downwards and gaze directed to the floor. Anxious patients generally have horizontal creases on the forehead, raised eyebrows widened palpebral fissure, and dilated pupils. They usually sit upright with head erect often at the edge of the chair with hands gripping the sides and are restless (P. Sankaran 1996).

Moreover notice the gait, the clothes, the attitude, the smell and odour and where possible the mood and disposition. Furthermore observe closely any traits of character as shown in dress, cleanliness, neatness, pride.

> Writing on the value of observation, McKillop says, 'Observed symptoms are generally more reliable than those elicited by interrogation alone. I, for one, regard every patient as potentially incapable of telling the truth regarding his innermost nature and personal character. Even when they believe themselves to be truthful the judgement of most people regarding their own characters is apt to be widely off the mark. A symptom which does so correspond can be accepted with some confidence. I find that this tends to shorten one's case history'. Think of the great number of valuable prescribing symptoms that can be observed almost without uttering a word. On the physical side there are such signs, for example, as complexion, physical

conformation and deportment, speech, gait, proptosis, glandular enlargements, breathlessness, etc. On the mental side are such symptoms as loquacity, diffidence, easy embarrassment, timidity, tearfulness, anxiety, fearfulness, suspiciousness, impatience, haughtiness, egotism, excitability, depression, and many more. Again, observation can be used as a test of the reliability of a patient's responses to interrogation. If a reply is enthusiastic it can be trusted. This test applies especially to physical desires and aversions and to desires and aversions to certain articles of food. Particularly in children, the observation of the physician plays a vital role. As infants and children are not so articulate, we have to compensate by keener observation (P. Sankaran 1996).

The chief signs are those symptoms that are most constant, most striking, and most annoying to the patient. The homeopath marks them down as the strongest, the principal features of the picture. The most singular, most uncommon signs furnish the characteristic, the distinctive, the peculiar features. Fine observational skills are crucial in the case taking process of busy homeopaths. There is an equation between the difficulty of the verbal communication and the degree to which we need to rely on a few observational skills (Dimitriadis 1993). Observing the details not only the gestures, and the body language is also important. So much is known through observation. Is the patient trying test you with intellect, or impress you with the knowledge of the disease? Is this a way that they are attempting to test you or control you. Or is it a defense response because of being unable to access their emotional world. Is that pride or is there a rigidity. Do they launch into telling you about their sexual history and disclose intimate aspects of their life at the beginning of the consultation when one would have assumed that that would be not mentioned at all or come much later in the process. Do they answer your question slowly and stare off into space into the top left-hand corner of the room. Did they ask you direct questions about yourself, about your qualifications, about the homeopathic process, about if they will they be okay?

Observe their gestures, observe their accessories, jewellery, handbags, dress sense, colour combinations, the message on a T-shirt? Without being too superficial, this can easily augment the objective and subjective symptoms you elicit. The woman wears a T-shirt that says, *'Once I knew what I wanted to do with my life, but then I saw something sparkle!'* The teenager's says, *'Meat is Murder.'* Receptionists can provide so much valuable information to you also about the activities and behaviour of the client, hitting on them, ignoring them, commenting on the artwork, the fountain, the noise, the quality of the music or the age of magazines (De Schepper 1996:116).

Questioning and Silence

Allow the patient to follow their own path. If they sense that you are safe, they will gradually trust you with more sensitive and therefore more useful information. Be quiet. Stay silent. Shut up. Nevertheless ensure that the silent approach is OK with them. Do not interfere while they are speaking unless they wander off to some irrelevant matters. The process should involve active listening.

To direct a conversation and yet remain quiet at the same time is an art. As discussed previously leading questions are simply unnecessary. Leading questions may bring forth misleading answers. The patient sometimes gives the answer which they think the homeopath wants to hear. Ask only open questions, what do you drink? Do you drink? As opposed to do you prefer hot or cold drinks? Let patient answer in their own words. Some homeopaths add a disclaimer, 'No direct questions unless differentiating a sub-symptom later in the case taking'. Either way, it is better not to suggest answers or give alternatives. Similarly ask no questions that could imply judgment, and avoid labeling. Be interested, sympathetic but not prejudiced. Therefore, as a rule add no personal experiences of your own, no matter how similar your story is to theirs. It is their time and most resent having to share it. Stay on focus until they are finished. Keep remedies out of your head. Sometimes called the stage of interrogation or cross examination this involves filling the gaps left in the just previous stage in order to complete the symptoms with respect to their location, sensation, and modalities. This is the most difficult stage of case taking. It necessitates sufficient sympathy, patience, introspection and tactfulness. There is always a natural pause in the course of a consultation. The patient naturally runs out of things to say in relationship to their main complaint. This can be after 30 seconds in some cases or 30 minutes in others depending on the patient and the complaint. The question, 'Is there anything else?' or 'Tell me more,' is best practice. This neutral non-leading encouragement allows the patient to continue to talk about themselves knowing that the listener is actively there with them (Kaplan 2001).

Physical Examination

This is the stage of clinical examination, general examination and/or examination of various organs and systems. Many colleges around the world teach no physical examination to their students. Ultimately the role of physical examination depends on what kind of practice you have and in which country you practice (De Schepper 1996:124). In India, Germany and South Africa physical examination is taught as part of the fundamental skills of a homeopath. But in Australia and New Zealand it becomes more problematic because of the perceived scope of practice boundary that this crosses. Homeopaths in those countries have got in trouble for practicing 'medicine' and thereby breaking the law by conducting an examination.

In my own practice I rarely do any significant physical examination. Yet this is a constant criticism of homeopathic medicine that gets fed back from patients to professional associations. Because we are interested in the symptoms of the condition and not necessarily seeing the condition this confuses some of our clients. Often we will treat ear problems without looking in the ear. This makes no sense to a mother with a screaming child. It works both ways. A patient of mine years ago came because he had psoriasis on his penis. He was most insistent that I examine it. And he was disappointed when I refused and explained that because he had come with a diagnosis from the physician already there was no reason for me to examine it. Yet it is a fine balance between doing good homeopathic work but not crossing the line into the practice of medicine. When you have looked in 200 ears you tend to start to know what you're looking for. It's the same with tongues, pulses and blood pressure. Having confidence around using these tools often goes a long way to making patients feel comfortable in your presence. It helps them relax.

But some homeopaths prefer to ask questions, and find the peculiarities of the case from questioning rather than from observation. The information that comes from a physical examination is often crucial. The shape and colour of an ulcer, the specific colour of the eardrum, the furuncle or the boil, looking at the mucus, hearing the cough is important in identifying the closest match of remedy. De Schepper has some good advice in his chapter on case taking in *Hahnemann Revisited*. *'Look at the shape of the chest, the clearness of the skin, the state of their hair,'* (De Schepper 1996:124-126). It is also important not to necessarily trust what the patient says about their symptom given a lack of knowledge of anatomy and physiology. Getting the client to point to where the pain is important. 'My stomach hurts', could well be a pain in the abdomen. 'I am having tummy troubles', could well indicate diarrhoea or constipation. When the patient is telling the history always watch their gestural language to see if it matches the words. You should make them feel that they have your whole attention and that you will not be shocked or angered by anything he or she says. Gazing out of the window or continually writing notes will put off the patient. Never underestimate the power of communication inherent in touching your patient. It will give more comfort than your words of reassurance. Gentle and thorough physical examination is important in gaining a patient's confidence. The best totality of symptoms would include mainly those symptoms from which one can get no clue about or which do not depend upon the patients age, nationality, occupation, or pathology.

Recording

My memory is terrible. We cannot depend upon our memory in taking the case, and getting the case properly before us for analysis. The picture must be preserved in indelible form so it can be reviewed without leaving out any important symptom. Record all the important points in the words of the patient, both in what the patient says and in what is observed (De Schepper1996:117). When it comes to the layout of the notes, put the symptoms in a column at the left of his paper, leaving at least an inch blank between the items to be subsequently filled in as the patient reverts to that subject later when the physician questions about it. One may prefer to put facts pertaining to history on one sheet or in one column, those pertaining to actual physical symptoms in another, and mentals in a third, but this requires experience and adeptness. It is safer for the beginner to list them all as they come and sort them later in the working out of the case. Kent says, *Arrange your record of symptoms into three columns. The first one contains the dates and prescriptions. The second contains the distinct symptoms as headings and the third are the modalities. Otherwise, it's defective* (Kent 1900).

As you are writing, put a mark by or underline the symptom that you need to go back and ask about later to get more details or verify (De Schepper 1996:118). Leave gaps to go back and add or change sub-symptoms. Some have advocated using a bound book using the left hand page for recording symptoms and the right-hand page for the modalities.

For those that type and are comfortable with the electronic medium, all the homeopathic software designers (Archibel, Kent, HomeoQuest, Hompath, Miccant) have introduced various products to assist in case taking. One excellent innovation to assist in the process of writing the case is Jeremy Sherr's *Dynamic Case Taker*. If faciliates the typing of the case with shortcuts and autocomplete, and automatically sorts the symptoms out according to main headings, such as Mind, Generals, Dreams, Female etc, while still retaining the original free flowing format of the case. It also plots a graph of the timeline of the case, has useful follow up facilities for comparison with the first consultation, an index of each case for easy reference and a search for words feature.

Own Words

However the case is recorded, use their own words (De Schepper 1996). Enquire into each symptom leisurely, take your time and when they have exhausted whatever they had to say go over everything in detail. The main features can be noted down line by line with intervening spaces wherein further details of each symptom can be filled in later on by careful enquiry (P. Sankaran 1996). Ensure nothing is left out.

> Further, we have also to try to define and delineate each symptom. For instance, if a patient says he is worse at night, we want to know whether he is actually worse at night or worse lying down or merely worse by heat of bed, etc. If he is worse in the afternoon, we want to know whether he is worse in the afternoon as such or worse while sitting in the office or worse after lunch, etc. Thus, in dealing with his symptoms we try to elicit as many circumstances as possible which modify that symptom. This renders each symptom complete with its location, sensations, modalities, causation, duration, extension, etc., and the case becomes clearer and easier. In taking the symptoms, we attempt to record not merely a lifeless list of symptoms but to draw a picture of the suffering of a living individual and to try and understand the whole circumstance that has given rise to these symptoms. In other words we try to get at the background

of the patient's symptoms and in so doing we go through his fears and doubts, disappointments and emotional feelings and also his social, economic, domestic and other circumstances so that we get a better understanding of the patient's difficulties as a whole (P. Sankaran 1996).

Importance and Underlining

Some advocate the underline, when there is intensity, spontaneity, unsolicited information, when the symptoms are discrete, unexpected, out of context, or the patient is contradicting what they have been saying. The use of underlining to prioritize the symptom's clarity, intensity and spontaneity has been advocated since the beginnings of homeopathic case taking.

- One underline: Symptoms of greater clarity and greater intensity, yet still elicited only upon questioning.

- Two underlines: Symptoms of great clarity, moderate intensity, and volunteered spontaneously.

- Three underlines: symptoms with the highest clarity, great intensity, and given entirely spontaneously by the patient (P Sankaran 1996).

Legalities

I am astonished how in some parts of the world of homeopathy there is no discussion of the legal context of the patients notes. In Malaysia and India there are no privacy acts or simply unenforced ones or legislation to regulate this area. I strongly advise students to get a book by Michael Weir (2007) *Complementary Medicine Ethics and Law*. Read the *Medicines Act* in the country you practice. It is likely that the directives in that Act apply to the practice of homeopathy also. It is important even where there is no existing culture of litigation of doctors and therapists to remember that our notes are a legal document, so therefore keep them impeccably and up to date.

Time Management and Endings

Some people can talk forever. It is the ultimate problem with asking open ended questions. It is entirely legitimate to end the appointment after the patient's story and continue in another session if necessary unless they are in acute pain or distress. How many chronic cases is it possible to take in a day anyway?

Endings are complicated. Very little is talked about in relation to this important aspect of the relationship. Finishing with a loquacious patient is a delicate art. Depending on the clinic structure that you are practicing in you may need to exchange money or credit card details and make a new appointment. Take them to the door. Say goodbye. It is important to recognise but when you end the conversation and part company with a client after the first consultation it is only just the beginning of your relationship. It is important to do this as well as possible. It is vitally important to give your card with all of your details to the client and describe your availability to them for the management of their case in the interim.

To Questionnaire or Not

It is up to the individual. Some homeopaths do and some don't. Some started with one and now have thrown it away. *Extensive description of the precise kind of information needed in homeopathy and particularly the use of homeopathic questionnaires should be avoided. This makes the patient focus on insignificant details* (Gafoor 2010). I have provided Kent's in its entirety in this book, part of Schmidt's and Hahnemann's. Kaplan's is particularly good. With or without a questionnaire, from the perspective of best practice and keeping in mind the directives from the authorities from the earliest days of homeopathy, by the end of the case taking there should be:

a) The details of the patient

b) The presenting complaints

c) The history of the presenting complaint

d) Clarity of the cause

e) A history of previous illnesses

f) A family history

g) A personal history

h) A treatment history

i) Physical examination or lab work

j) A complete symptom to work with

Where relevant, an exploration of the rest of the health including:

k) The regional's

l) Any other pathology

m) General modalities

n) An understanding of the miasmatic expression

o) An evaluation of the overall energy available to the patient

p) An evaluation of the relevant mental symptoms and disposition

Of course it is then for the homeopath to begin the evaluation and analysis of the symptoms, the repertory work, the differential diagnosis, the selection of medicine, posology, decision on management strategies and prognosis.

Difficulties and Specific Situations in Taking the Case

One Sided Cases

There are certain cases where the symptoms are all one-sided and there seems to be no general disturbance expressed by the patient and few characteristics. Examples may be eczemas, warts, psoriasis or corns. There are also some cases where the patient seems to be apparently quite well but a blood test or examination and investigation reveal some serious internal disturbance such as hypertension. In a discipline that is essentially based on characteristic phenomena there are some problems in this regard. Happily, a thorough reading of the *Organon* of Hahnemann plus a growing familiarity with other methods assist greatly. If homeopathy is to embrace such conditions, it is necessary that we develop objective methods of remedy selection also where appropriate. We depend, sometimes too much on the symptoms of the patient and when they are cloudy or absent, unable to be detected with any characteristic colour we have to rely on Hahnemann's practical suggestions. There are times that giving importance to the patient's every word and therefore a lack of (or inaccurate) observation, deficiency of expression or absence of cooperation on the patient's part or a lack of understanding or interpretation on our part can lead us far away from an accurate prescription.

Aphorisms 162-184 in the *Organon* give clear instructions to homeopaths dealing with firstly, patients with clear symptoms but where we have an inadequate stock of remedies and then one-sided cases. At times we are presented with cases where there are no clear or usable mental symptoms. In addition at times there are cases with mental symptoms with no value. An example is a sense of depression that might be rather natural in a long-suffering patient who has taken much treatment with no relief. Furthermore there are cases we take of patients with incomplete symptoms and situations where we can elicit no cause or no concomitant. This can often be a case in the elderly or those patients that have had the complaint for a significant time.

Patients often come from other homeopaths having taken previous courses of medicines and the true symptom image of the patient may have altered or have been mixed up with the symptoms of drugs. In these cases those symptoms and ailments from before the use of the medicines or after they had been discontinued for several days might give the true idea of the original disease profile (Gafoor 2010).

Equally as difficult at times in the case taking is the situation where 'modesty conceals the facts'. Some clients experience the description of the symptoms accompanied with shame, humiliation and embarrassment. As Hahnemann encouraged us, this is the time for tact, delicate and skilful questioning. A legitimate strategy is to put patients at ease by alluding to the topic and adopting an oblique approach is entirely appropriate. But straightness is to be encouraged. If the client is truly secretive, hiding or lying to you this is usually very obvious (De Schepper 1996).

Some individuals are stoic and do not take much interest in describing their ailments. All homeopaths have stories of clients who refrained from mentioning important information, or the symptoms were described in vague terms due to laziness or modesty, or from a kind of mildness of disposition or weakness of mind. The patient may think that there is no need of telling everything about the health and disease.

Amongst the hardest patients to receive information from are intellectuals. People that intellectualise their feelings tend to relate to reality according to what is explainable to their minds. They evaluate or interpret their symptoms in terms of their knowledge and philosophy of life and explain away the very symptoms of most value to the homeopath. It is not only philosophers though but those who seek endless explanations. Some clients may adopt theories on diet keeping aside information about their desires and aversions and causing the homeopath to miss great data (Gafoor 2010). We experience these difficulties with patients who are depressed, who are academics, hippies, psychotherapists, psychiatrists, physicians, homeopaths, homeopathic students and lawyers (De Schepper 1996). Sometimes referred to as psycho-babble these clients are easy to spot yet hard to treat because they present their symptoms with such colour, too much colour and in the extreme, almost like hypochondriacs who give us explanations of their conditions and not pure symptoms.

Acute Case Taking

For the last word about best practice on taking the acute case read Kaplan's book *The Homeopathic Conversation* (2001), Chapter four. Many homeopaths find taking acute cases to be easier than chronic case taking. *In acute cases, the case taking is somewhat easier. The changes due to the disease being more recent and more marked, both the patient and those around him are able to observe and describe these symptoms clearly to us* (P. Sankaran 1996). For others it is exactly the opposite. Theoretically acute case taking provides clearer symptoms that are sharper and more focused and more characteristic and striking. Others find acute case taking most difficult because patients inevitably say that, 'I have the flu,' or 'My tummy hurts.' But mostly acute case taking is easier because the symptoms are fresh in the mind and the process of taking an acute case is exactly what clients are used to in the allopathic world. The first part of the process is to simply find out if the situation is part of an ongoing or recurring picture. This can never be assumed. Some develop clear approaches such as finding the three legged stool focusing on the never been well since symptoms and mental and emotional changes that supplement the location, sensation, modality and concomitants of the chief complaint (De Schepper 1996:128). What makes it all the more difficult is that sometimes these acute situations present to the homeopath over the other end of the telephone, or at the end of a long private consultation the client will suddenly say, 'Oh by the way my second daughter has developed a runny nose, can you give me something for it? My husband has a cold can you give me something for him?' It is usually the lack of time that the patient has for questioning which makes the situation extremely difficult. Of course, the homeopath who has been around for a year or two starts to rely on keynotes or specific prescribing, *Ferrum phos* for example for anything that resembles a fever, a flu or a cold. Another is *Sanicula*, nature's combination remedy, which has such a broad application in the treatment of children with acute conditions. It's the same with *Hypericum*, *Chamomilla*, *Rhus tox* and *Arnica*.

It is important to remember to differentiate between acute and chronic. Acute disease is defined by a definite beginning, period of progress, decline with a definite end, and self-limiting. This is opposed to chronic disease, characterized by an imperceptible beginning, period of progress, no period of decline, and ending only in death. Acute includes first aid situations, falls, cuts, burns, bee stings, influenza, chicken pox, food poisoning, grief from loss of a loved one, shock from an accident, one off situations of hayfever or headache. A real acute or first aid situation can become chronic if it is suppressed or not resolved. Chronic includes acute flare up of chronic conditions, asthma, panic attack, headache, or anything that reoccurs.

The simplicity of the genuine acute requires the homeopath to focus on finding that complete symptom. It can be almost mathematical, sensation, location, modalities, concomitants, anything peculiar? Prescribe. But it seems for most of the time most acute cases are not acute at all but exacerbations of a chronic state and this is where great care needs to be taken.

Similar and Dissimilar Disease

It is also important to remember that with acute exacerbation of a chronic state, or a true acute, the chronic symptoms will disappear into the background and be unable to be seen. This follows that principle articulated by Hahnemann that two similar diseases can never exist at the same time in a person and that the stronger will always annihilate the weaker. The chronic picture disappears into the background only to come back after the acute.

Infants

When it comes to the treatment of infants we have to rely on the comments of the parent or guardian and our observational skills, arching backwards in colic, any perspiration, the temperature. Most of the time I attempt to pick up the child, it's an opportunity to make any observations, detect any smell of perspiration and also the reaction of the mother. But clearly most case taking that takes place with an infant is through the parent. It is the general symptoms that are of most use and careful attention to questioning around this area is the most important thing. It is difficult to treat infants without any context of the family because first-time parents have increased anxieties about their children's health this can make the consultation unnecessarily complex.

Children

There are a number of specific considerations for case taking with children. Tumminello (2001) has written extensively on this area. Master, Santawami and Chauhan (2010) are also useful. It is Kaplan (2001) that points out the tremendous incongruity in homeopathy that we treat children as if they are small adults. Our provings are carried out on adults, and the assumption is possibly erroneous that remedies will act on children in the same way. The most important thing to remember is that the child's mind is not a miniature of an adult mind. The child's mind develops in a series of stages eventually to capacitive abstract reasoning. So for example an 8 yr old can comprehend analogies (getting an idea is like having a light go on in your head) that a three year old can't. The drive behind this intellectual progression is the unceasing struggle to make sense out of the world. While infants start with simple sense reflexes like sucking or grasping, in the adult world we have the capacity for a huge number of these activities from getting to know how to tie a shoe lace to much more complex concepts such as gender and race (Piaget 1997).

Again observational skills are very important and should start in the waiting room and continue until the child leaves. The choice of toys is important and the way they play or cleanup can be indicators towards the selection of the remedy (Kaplan 2001). Sometimes to the surprise of the parents I spend a lot of time on the floor with my children clients and play. After all, how often is it that you get paid to build a model plane or play cars or draw pictures? Very often I have had my better results with children when I've taken the case in their own environment. A boy diagnosed on the autistic spectrum was bought by very anxious Pakistani parents, one a doctor and the other a medical researcher. *Tarentula* created some very minor change but for some reason the third consultation had to be at their home. I arrived and sat down in the living room and was able to observe the boy through the glass into the lounge room while I was given tea. Eventually the boy came into the room did not acknowledge me but went straight to the fridge, opened it, took a can of Coca-Cola and drank it in one. I was astonished. 'He is drinking Coca-Cola', I said. 'Of course', they said, 'what else would you drink'. I was gob smacked. I went to the fridge and one whole shelf was devoted to cans of

Coca-Cola. I tried to negotiate on this point but it was pointed out that Coca-Cola is the one reward a devoted conservative Muslim family can have and I was told in no uncertain terms that removing the child from drinking Coca-Cola was not an option, non negotiable.

Kaplan (2001) encourages us to observe carefully and speak softly, make some physical contact, respect the child and ask simple questions. It is crucial to listen to the child's point of view.

Teens

I have recently been teaching in Malaysia and while most of my stories and jokes are usually met with bemused confusion, I had them in stitches with the description of the case of Max. Max was a 13-year-old boy who was diagnosed on the autistic spectrum. He was a very large boy and a little intimidating. Inevitably all of my questions were met with grunts and shrugs. He didn't like me and hated coming to see me in the clinic. His mother had struggled for his whole life on a grueling daily basis to get him into different schools, to integrate him as much as possible, to get him assessed by speech therapists, physicians, pediatricians, and she struggled dreadfully under the weight of this responsibility. One day she bought him to see me and as usual I chatted with her and asked him a few questions to which I received nothing but grunts and shrugs. At one point I asked Max, 'What is your favourite food at the moment', to which he just shrugged. His mother at this point intervened and said, 'Come on Max you told me the other day that you have a favourite food'. 'Piss off', he said. I was shocked, and all of a sudden I just had enough. And completely out of character I said, 'Max this is enough, from now on I want you to sit upright in your seat and answer my questions. Next, I do not want you to ever talk to your mother like that again'. I started to get on a roll. I could see that his mother was wanted to intervene. 'And another thing,' I said, 'You come here and you give me nothing I need you make more of an effort, can't you see your mother is really struggling, don't you think, you come here and give me nothing, she is stressed out and I am trying my best and you give us nothing'. His mother was trying to stop me at this stage and Max's eyes were getting wider and he was getting very uncomfortable but I think I had a few things to say which had been building up the number of months. 'And another thing', I said, and was ready to launch off into another rant when his mother started talking over the top of me. 'Alastair! Alastair!' She leaned forward and put her hand on my arm and said, 'Max said 'pizza'.' I died a thousand deaths and was abjectly apologetic. Every now and again they still come back to treatment.

Teenagers, like all reluctant patients are very difficult to deal with because in homeopathy we rely on symptoms so much. We need characteristic symptoms and vitality on which to prescribe. If the patient is reluctant or unwilling to give those to us then really we are hamstrung. So a teenager just being a teenager presents a very specific set of problems, but also a very special set of rewards when progress is made. It is important to have some sort of grasp on what is happening with music, sport, games, TV, movies to be able to engage in some meaningful way. That said, often when I ask a teen, 'What are you into?' and get a response I have absolutely no idea who the band is, or what the hairstyle is, or the movie is and the conversation awkwardly stops at that moment.

In addition, and where the legal and ethical considerations are taken into account, I tend to get that teenager by themself and let them know that whatever we talk about is confidential (De Schepper 1996). Over the years I have been a listening ear, a confessor, confidante, contraception adviser as well as homeopath to teens. Equally, although one can never be sure, a number of teenagers will walk away from my office shaking their heads and mumbling, 'Who was that idiot?' Kaplan (2001) suggests giving your card to the child or teenager so that they understand that they are having a personal relationship with you which is independent of the parent. It's great advice.

General Advice for Reluctant Patients
Be direct
Explain that you need specifics and sensations
Do not give yourself a hard time if they do not come back or don't take your medicine
Often the reluctance and reservations are a symptom worthy of exploration and repertorising
Do your best

Male, Anxious, Loquacious Patients and the Elderly

Whole books need to be devoted to the specific considerations needed to treat men well using complementary medicine. It is the same for anxious and loquacious patients and the treatment of the elderly. While everyone has an opinion, our profession urgently requires outcome studies conducted, evidence gathered and best practice guidelines formulated into these specific groups. When it comes to the homeopathic treatment of male patients in our clinics there is so much to say. In the West men are generally less interested in homeopathic medicine. The percentages of males and our practices are significantly less than women. In my own practice the percentage has been hovering at 38-42% consistently over the last two decades and I have written about this elsewhere (Gray 2010b). In my interviews and research with male patients and also with practitioners about the reasons why they treat so few male patients the message that emerges is consistent. Homeopathy and homeopaths fail to deal with the fundamental and underlying issues that male patients have whenever they see a healthcare specialist. They do not talk to them well nor describe homeopathy well. To a large extent, it is an admission of weakness or failure when a male patient stumps up at the doctor, naturopath or homeopath's office. This perception of failure cannot be underestimated. Male patients generally try to fix things themselves or hope that it will go away over the passage of time, 'If I don't think about it, it will go away'. Compounded with that is at times a sense of shame and a sense of suspicion. Too often the homeopath asks such a person to describe a sensation or a feeling for which there is no answer. This is a deeply uncomfortable situation to be placed in for a generally competent man. It is not that there is no feeling. Rather that there is no access to the language of feeling. For very competent males out there in the world who are managing this, doing that, building this, that sense of control and competency does not extend to the body especially as they head into middle age. I have found that by taking into account the underlying issues mentioned of failure, shame, and suspicion and making sure that my practice and my demeanor is as unintimidating to male patients as possible, I became very busy. Further, it is possible to manage this demographic of your practice by keeping the clinic space neutral. In other words, not too feminine with candles, flowers, Buddha heads. Miranda Castro many years ago in a series of seminars advocated that the space should be as neutral and as little about you as possible. For some men therefore, medicine charts and computers are better. And of course the case taking needs to be appropriate and pitched just right to the individual, not too chatty. The attire? Smart casual. Remember to focus strongly on the reason they are there, the presenting symptom.

Similarly talkative patients create for us numerous difficulties. It is an oversimplification to think that Lachesis or Phosphorus will be appropriate as medicines for these folks, because a quick glance at that rubric in the repertory highlights numerous other medicines. In actual fact the issue is, how to manage these people not medicate them (De Schepper 1996:118). Usually loquacious patients talk because they have to talk, they have to discharge because there is so much tension within. Either that or they cannot stand silence in which case that is worthy of exploration in itself. With elderly patients who are perhaps used to a much more doctor-patient style of consultation there are numerous considerations. Moreover for anxious patients, the most challenging of all, the capacity of the homeopath to manage them as they wrestle with our style of medication, and what is written on the labels (unfortunately *Arsenicum*, *Carcinosin* or *Syphilinum*) and guide them through the newness of what they are getting is a difficult and complex task. With all of these groups mentioned, until long-term confidence is established it is the chief complaint, or the reason that they came to see you that should be the focus during the case taking, even though you may know that the location that the symptom is manifesting is lower on the hierarchy of importance in the human body. There will be a natural progression from discussing the chief complaint to its cause and it's at that point that mental emotional symptoms may emerge (De Schepper 1996).

The Last Word and Great Advice

> There is a lesson to be learned in every case we see. Some cases present a challenge in terms of case taking, while others may be more difficult because of the absence of symptoms or a clear remedy picture. Most often, the difficulty is due to our own limitations: a lack of understanding of the person, a failure to follow up on important symptoms, or a tendency to lead the interview in the direction of what we think is the correct remedy. (Jacobs 1990)

> It's a dynamic situation, taking a case or interacting with another person. You have to be in a particular mode, when you are sitting next to that person. Trust is the most important thing. If you can remain in a state of not knowing, complete not knowing, and you just sit there, whatever happens will happen and you must trust that the exchange will give you the information needed. Whereas if you're in a state of panic, 'Oh, I must get it right,' 'Oh, I must find the remedy,' 'What's the remedy?' then this is the sycotic miasm, always having to be three steps ahead. After an hour, sometimes, I can be sitting there and not have the faintest idea what this person needs…When I take a case, I put myself into a more receptive mode for the first half hour. When the person comes to a stop, or dries up, then I'll just say, 'Anything else?' or repeat back their last sentence to them. Then perhaps, later on, I'll start using 'why?' questions, going back through the case, asking what exactly the person meant when they said a particular thing. But every case is different, sometimes you have to dig to get the information, other times it's coming so fast you have to steer them just to keep to the point. I'll do what feels right at that moment; that's where the intuition comes into it. (Mundy 1997)

> This is a matter of experience-an ability that comes with experience and with interest. If you are really interested in the case that you are seeing, I am sure you will observe a lot of things because you are immediately connected with the person who is walking into your room to ask for help. Everything that happens to that person is of great importance. And your observation must be correct, not a projection. I'm afraid many times homeopaths interchange observation for projection. That means they would like to see something they projected onto the patient, and they see it of course. The real secret is to observe without projecting anything on the patient and to get the real facts on the patient and work with those facts. This is very important for making a correct prescription. The moment that you start projecting, you can make any case. You can make a case for Causticum, you can make it look like Calcarea, or Sulphur, or whatever. (Vithoulkas 1999)

> I learned to go beyond the words into the way a person thinks and expresses himself. This is still primary. Now under the influence of other homeopathic teachers, in the interview I intervene less and less. I just listen with a faith that what needs to come out will come out. I have to be open enough to receive. Whether or not it fits into repertory or materia medica language is actually a limitation of freedom on my part. If I can understand the

patient and then make the homeopathic translation, then that is fine. If I keep a patient in a box, then I won't have a good response. I am learning all over again this process of case taking, especially learning the smaller remedies. My instincts tell me this whole range of things in homeopathy now is correct. (Gray 1999)

Hahnemann calls the totality, 'this image' (or picture). The word used is significant and suggestive. A picture is a work of art, which appeals to our aesthetic sense as well as to our intellect. Its elements are form, color, light, shade, tone, harmony, and perspective. As a composition it expresses an idea, it may be of sentiment or fact; but it does this by the harmonious combination of its elements into a whole a totality. In a well-balanced picture each element is given its full value and its right relation to all the other elements. The elements which go to make up the totality must be definitely and logically related. The Totality means the sum of the aggregate of the symptoms: Not merely the numerical aggregate the entire number of the symptoms but their sum total, their organic whole as an individuality. The totality must express an idea. It is the numerical aggregate plus the idea or plan which unites them in a special manner to give them its characteristic form'. Thus, we are searching for this 'idea' or 'plan,' this blueprint that underlies and unites the mass of symptoms presented before us. This concept is directly related to that of the 'Essence' of remedies, as formulated by George Vithoulkas. (Shore 1999)

Homeopathy is about process. If you can understand the process, and you have learned how to apply it, then you will be well on your way to becoming a good practitioner. The most important aspect that I have learned is to listen and to hear what the patient is telling you. Without good case taking you cannot get a good result. I develop an energetic connection with the patient during the interview and I become very sensitive to issues in the patient's life. I look for 'bumps in the road', and when I find them I look deeper into those issues which surround them. In this way I am able to perceive those factors which drive the case, and I am able to gain an understanding as to what the case is about and what is to be cured. (Ziv 2000)

The distinguishing characteristics, the key-notes, which form the individual and constitutional symptoms of the patient, are sensational symptoms, rather than functional derangements or structural disorganizations. And the method we pursue in relying upon these, in the absence of other indications, and of attaching very great importance to them, even where other symptoms are not wanting, is sustained by two substantial reasons. First, in many cases we can do no better, since few if any of our remedies either have or can ever be expected to have, direct pathogenetic symptoms to correspond to the innumerable ultimate forms of structural disease which we are often called upon to treat. Second, this method has been found reliable by much experience. The purely constitutional symptoms such as those of periodicity and the conditions of aggravation and amelioration, strictly

> sensational symptoms, being found to constitute infallible indications in the choice of the remedy, where all other guides are wanting. (Guernsey 1873)
>
> Another way not to do it is to be too ready with your prescription. If you take a lot of trouble with a case (when you know how!) it will given you very little trouble afterwards. (Conversely, if you take very little trouble to begin with, it will give you endless trouble, many times repeated). For you have fouled the clear waters by a wrong prescription, and how are you going to peer into the depths? You have no longer a true disease-picture to match. One bad prescription leads to several, perhaps to a hopeless mixing-up of the case. 'Curses and chickens' and bad prescriptions 'come home to roost'. If you are not sure, give a placebo, and wait. Hahnemann says a week's placebo to start with, anyway! (Tyler 1927)

Being a Beginner

To my mind the most important thing to remember about starting off in homeopathic practice is to allow yourself the space to be a beginner. Allow yourself the opportunity to be an amateur before mastery. Too many students and young graduates and homeopaths have massive expectations of themselves and their results. These have to be realistic. That is why it is crucial to get supervision as a mandatory part of being a beginner in the practice of homeopathy. All homeopaths, it doesn't matter how many years that they have been practicing, should be comfortable in asking for help. Recently I was in Malaysia lecturing and was talking about attending a Sankaran sensation method seminar. Some of the doctors there were astounded that I would go to a seminar when I am so 'experienced' myself. This is nonsense. We can all learn from each other and I cannot tell the amount of times that I have had a first-year homeopathic student set me straight on a number of issues related to a case that I was talking about or a problem that I had at my clinic. Being comfortable in asking for assistance is a professional posture that needs to be adopted wholesale. That assistance doesn't need to come in the form of formal supervision although that is entirely appropriate, but it can be a simple conversation with another homeopath on Skype or down the end of the telephone with a 'critical friend'. Pick up the phone. Experienced homeopaths are usually flattered to take that call.

Many homeopaths find themselves overwhelmed with the numbers of different styles of practice available or the overwhelming number of medicines. It doesn't need to be like this. It is important not to fly before you can walk and Hahnemannian and Böenninghausen homeopathy with its simplicity, elegance and replicability is a fantastic way to ground oneself case after case. This is such a legitimate framework upon which to ask questions about the condition, the disease, and to look for those strange, rare and peculiar, characteristic and complete symptoms. With this scaffolding and with the right books at your disposal an appropriate remedy will always be possible to find and apply. True, the depth of action of that remedy may well be an issue. Yet it is a great way to begin practice. With 10 cases, 100 then 1000 cases under one's belt, then more and more clients requiring a different method or more complicated presentations requiring more sophisticated styles of practice will emerge. Choose your style. Master it, and don't do anything else until it is integrated fully. Repetition is the mother of mastery. If you have a clinic where patients want to tell you 'the story,' and this is what is delivered then don't reach for any other textbooks. If it's Böenninghausen style then complement that with the appropriate books, use Hahnemann's *Materia Medica Pura*, the *Synoptic Key* of Boger or use *Systematic Materia Medica* from Mathur. If Kent style is being used then use the *Concordant* of Vermeulen or Tyler's *Drug*

Types. Get familiar with which textbooks complement what method and know that you don't need to reach for Sankaran's *Soul of Remedies* or Bailey's *Homeopathic Psychology* when case taking or prescribing in a certain way. These books will only be useful for other styles of case taking. Having eased into a style of prescribing, then with many cases under the belt, from that solid grounding, with those foundations creating a platform rooted in medical science and substantial homeopathic principles, then embrace enthusiastically and employ other advanced methods of homeopathy. From a purely educational perspective this makes pragmatic sense and creates confident graduates able to integrate new information.

Part Two

Getting to the Centre, Making Meaning and Learning from Other Disciplines to Find the Medicine

Chapter 7

Post Jungian Approaches to Case Taking: Homeopathy and Wounded Souls

- Introduction
- Historical Context
- Post Jungian Approaches to Case Taking in Homeopathy
- Dream Work
- Tattoos
- Psychology and Psychotherapy
- Art Therapy and Sandplay
- Archetypes, Myths, Fairy tales, Stream of Consciousness and Metaphor
- To Jung or Not to Jung
- Questioning
- Disclaimer
- Developing the Necessary Case Taking Skills
- Looking for Clues without Scaring your Client or Acting too Weird
- Conclusion
- Doing Nothing

In this chapter you will
1. Learn how ideas from other disciplines have made it into homeopathic practice.
2. Be able to discriminate when is the best opportunity to employ this approach and determine when to use it.
3. Understand what this approach demands of the practitioner.

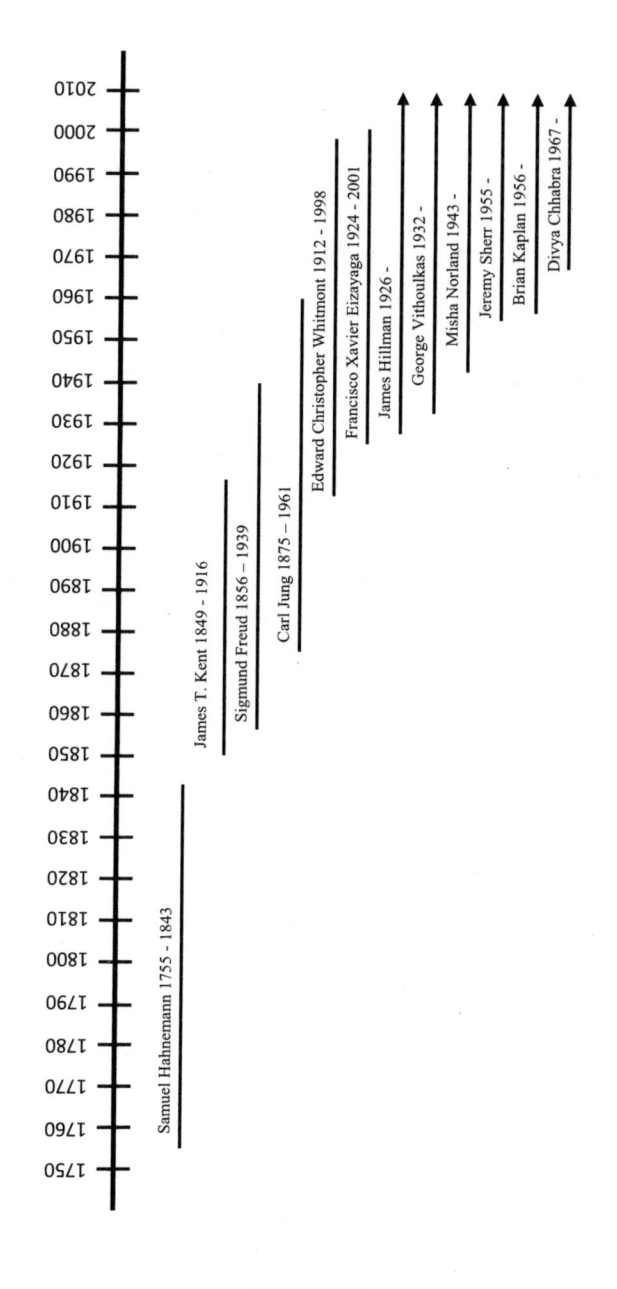

Timeline

- Samuel Hahnemann 1755 - 1843
- James T. Kent 1849 - 1916
- Sigmund Freud 1856 – 1939
- Carl Jung 1875 – 1961
- Edward Christopher Whitmont 1912 - 1998
- Francisco Xavier Eizayaga 1924 - 2001
- James Hillman 1926 -
- George Vithoulkas 1932 -
- Misha Norland 1943 -
- Jeremy Sherr 1955 -
- Brian Kaplan 1956 -
- Divya Chhabra 1967 -

Chapter 7

Post Jungian Approaches to Case Taking: Homeopathy and Wounded Souls

The body is the shadow of the soul - Marsilio Ficino

Introduction

Homeopaths that practice what is sometimes described as constitutional homeopathy, classical homeopathy, or traditional homeopathy, often forget that more homeopathic remedies are prescribed by chiropractors than by homeopaths, especially in the western world. This sobering statistic serves to remind us that the prescribing of those remedies is completely different and distinct to the traditional practice of homeopathy. Homeopathy is a philosophy and the application of that philosophy. But just as homeopathic remedies have been used by other professionals such as psychotherapists, counselors, and those professionals that work with the mind and body in their own disciplines and integrated to augment their own treatments, it is often forgotten that homeopaths have often borrowed from other disciplines to enhance their practice of homeopathy.

Whether they know it or not many homeopaths and users of homeopathy employ techniques that can loosely be described as Post Jungian. What is more, many homeopaths around the world have a fundamental set of unspoken assumptions that, when brought into the light of day, reveal the widespread belief that the Mind is the royal road to the simillimum. Other common assumptions include, that getting to the centre is better than working on the outside, and that by seeking the cause of the disease and its central, mental and emotional aspects, better and longer lasting cure takes place.

Homeopaths using Post Jungian theory in their approach to case taking are working on the hypothesis or belief that the presence of disease, whether physical, mental, or emotional, is indicative of a deeper problem in the psyche of the patient. This approach represents a move beyond the literal and into a realm of something else, different to vital force (Hahnemann), the simple substance (Kent), but to the realm of soul. For these practitioners, the patients eczema, depression, arthritis or insomnia are not perceived as belonging to the mechanistic scientific model that has held sway since the age of enlightenment but rather as signs and symptoms of a soul wounded. Moreover, this philosophical approach with origins deep in the past is found in most traditional medicine. It is predicated on the belief that treating only the clinical problems that the patient presents with may work in the short term but will not ultimately effect a cure, and that its results are merely palliative at best, and suppressive at worst, since it is not powerful enough to create the deepest level of change (Dethlefsen 1990, Ball 2004). Curative results are only considered possible when treatment is aimed at, and successfully touches, the psyche (or soul), the core of the patient's being. The language of the psyche and of the soul as identified by Jung, is to be found most purely in the symbolic world of dreams, fantasy, archetypes, personal mythology and in other forms of creative, symbolic and non-verbal self-expression. This represents a fundamental change and movement away from Hahnemann and Kent's understanding. Kent wrote and influenced generations of homeopaths before Freud and Jung.

To state it another way, the derangement of the patient's core self must be observed through its effect on the patient via the symptoms it produces rather than anything else. Hahnemann (1922) obviously also implied this at least 100 years before Jung in his Aphorism 15,

> The affection of the morbidly deranged, spirit-like dynamis (vital force) that animates our body in the invisible interior, and the totality of the outwardly cognizable symptoms produced by it in the organism and representing the existing malady, constitute a whole; they are one and the same. The organism is indeed the material instrument of the life, but it is not conceivable without the animation imparted to it by the instinctively perceiving and regulating dynamis, just as the vital force is not conceivable without the organism, consequently the two together constitute a unity, although in thought our mind separates this unity into two distinct conceptions for the sake of easy comprehension).

To paraphrase, in Aphorism 9 in the *Organon* Hahnemann says that health occurs when a free flow of energy moves through the body, keeping all parts of the organism in health so that the wearer of the skin bag, the owner of the body can employ the body for the highest purposes of our existence. Implicit in this idea is that symptoms are the expression of the vital force, the disordered vitality. Metaphorically, there is no point sweeping the snow away from the front door hoping to get rid of the winter. Winter is the issue. The snow is a reflection of that state. From this context Hahnemann's words can easily be re-orientated, re-engineered or reinterpreted in the light of the much more sophisticated symbolic language that Jung gave us and others have elaborated upon. Patients' symptoms collectively are understood as symbols of their deeper underlying state, which both the patient and the homeopath must then work together to carefully sift through and interpret. To access this largely hidden world we must look behind the curtain of the rational, compensated mind, and access the case both via the bright light given by the Sun as well as by the misty, mysterious light cast by the Moon. Understanding the patient's story, noting their pathology, seeking their symbolic patterns and treating them at the level of the soul wound is the quest of this approach to homeopathy.

Historical Context

In Hippocrates time medicine was still essentially holistic, and the unity of the physical, the psychological, and the spiritual were still presumed (Porter 2004). To our conscious minds the separation of the soul from the body began in the 17th century when mechanical models of nature were introduced and the human body was regarded in the guise of a machine. This movement gained momentum with the 'mechanical philosophers' such as Bacon, Descartes, Locke, and Newton (Porter 2004), mimicking the political separation of the spheres of influence of the Church and the State. It is Descartes who is attributed with having '…exalted rational thinking and banished the soul' leaving rational thought to reign supreme in Western culture (Elkins 1995). The development of homeopathy takes place at a crucial time in the evolution of medicine, where the rationalistic focus on the body separates from the mind. Hahnemann's homeopathy continues in the holistic vitalistic stream, that tradition. His allopathic colleagues launched themselves with their mechanistic world view into different waters seeking to understand the whole by reducing it to its parts. Reductionism had no place in Hahnemann's homeopathy.

It was not until the 20th century with the advent of psychoanalysis and the work primarily of Freud, Adler, and Jung that there was a significant shift back from the mechanical split and the beginning of the reintegration of the soul and the body in medicine. Even after this development, the practice of healing the mind (the province of priests and psychoanalysts) was clearly demarcated from the practice of healing the body (the province of physicians). Jung, a Swiss psychoanalyst who trained with Freud, is credited with pioneering the development of the use of symbols taken from the non-rational and intuitive realms of functioning as pathways to healing the psyche (Whitmont 1991). Jung's rationale for this approach to patients' cases lies in his belief that the unconscious mind contains a '...multitude of temporarily obscured thoughts, impressions, and images that, in spite of being lost, continue to influence our conscious minds' (Jung, 1990a) and that these images are the '...fundamental mode of operation of the soul' (Sardello 1996) and may be revealed in our daydreams and our nightdreams. The bridge from this psychotherapeutic view to homeopathic thought and practice was Whitmont. In his book *Psyche and Substance*, Whitmont (1991) explores homeopathic remedies through a Jungian lens, making one of the earliest forays into the symbolic perception of remedies which he refers to as 'remedy-personality pictures' and going beyond a remedy's pathological application. He further develops the concept of the remedy as archetype and works to close the division between medicine and psychology.

Post-Jungian Approaches to Case Taking in Homeopathy

Homeopathic case taking method is embedded within holistic medicine, a style of medicine which honours the unity of the body and mind, and Post Jungian approaches fit seamlessly within this paradigm. Homeopaths who practice on this level would concur with Hillman's (1997) statement that symptoms lead to soul and are '...the first herald of an awakening psyche which will not tolerate any more abuse'.

Taylor (2001) characterises homeopathic case taking as '... allowing your patient to take you where they need to go...'. The underlying assumption of this approach is that the authentic uncompensated part of the patient innately knows what they need to heal and will reveal their soul, wound, delusion, and/ or sensation if skillfully guided and largely unhindered by the homeopath. As Kaplan (2006) argues, homeopathic case taking is totally respectful to the patient as it is their subjective experiences, the stories of their illness and their life in general that homeopaths seek; patients are encouraged to tell their story in their own words and without interruption.

According to Sherr (2007) it is the disconnection between the patient's vital force and the soul that drives the patient into states of imbalance and disease, and once communication is lost between these two the vital force starts heading in the wrong direction and creating chronic pathology within the patient. Since it is the soul that is the intelligent driving force that maintains health for the human organism, the need for methods of accessing its messages and symbols is patent.

Misha Norland's (2008) description of his use of this approach is that he does all of the same things that other homeopaths do that are standard to taking a homeopathic case but that he differs in his perspective of the patient and his interpretation of the case. His work with a patient is based upon 'an awareness and respect for the patient's soul, out of which is born their individuality and their personal suffering' (Shah, 1993). Norland describes himself as being on a Holy Grail quest for the simillimum, seeing each patient as bringing their own unique expression into the therapeutic relationship (Jenkins 1999). Norland (2008) says that he is always looking for the repeating patterns behind the stories the patient is telling about their current life and about their past history, seeking the thread that links them all together for that is where the simillimum lies, in the remedy that links everything together. Or put another way, the tail of the simillimum must be in the past and the whiskers must be in the present. He regards the soul as being in the centre of the person's being and the aim of homeopathy to allow this to unfold naturally, so he focuses on treating the sickness of the vital force which has become an obstacle to the patient's self development. Since this process is largely a mysterious one, Norland argues that treatment methods cannot be predetermined but that as homeopaths we must '…be in a state of comfortable unknowing', and that we may only know the centre (or the soul) via the periphery and must access the centre by what we observe on the periphery.

Bridging the gap between the material (or conscious) and the immaterial (or unconscious) is undertaken by the use of archetypal imagery and moving deeper into myth and fairytale. He uses a 'poetic' approach to the study of materia medica, and he learns the remedies not only by their physical applications but also their history, and their myths. He uses gold as an example of this process, where gold enters into mythology and fairy tale and is depicted in the life of kings and the church as well as burial, commerce and ritual such as weddings. *Aurum*, the homeopathic remedy made from gold, is understood to suit patients who perceive themselves as the 'King' on some level, as leaders who have a duty and responsibility to their followers (Norland 2008).

How far is this from the origins of homeopathy? While many see this as a development and advancement of homeopathic practice, a natural progression, of deep and advanced work, many others within the profession have reacted against it. Very often it comes down to an understanding of what is perceived as disease. To see the aim of homeopathy to be to assist in someone's self-development is profoundly reasonable to some, and for others radical new age nonsense. To some, homeopathy is nothing other than Hahnemann's vision of the removal of disease, but for others these days, homeopathy is an opportunity for a journey, to explore oneself, one's issues of stuckness and old patterns. Homeopathy represents a brilliant way to cut loose the ties that bind to the past. Given the recent opportunity to deliver some lectures at an exclusive resort in Thailand and talk to the guests there, I was struck by the fact that the clients, overwhelmingly wealthy, at the top of their game, at the top of their tree, largest fishes in their ponds, the captains of industry and the makers and shakers of the world that we live in were also emotionally deeply afraid, wanted to talk and were desperate for contact. When I asked, 'What troubles you?' invariably their reply was that, 'I need you to help me on my journey'. I was expecting them to ask for help with their obesity or sinus problems. They didn't need Böenninghausen homeopathy, or specifics, or keynote prescribing, but rather a skilled listening ear.

Dream Work

In Kent's time the dream was nothing other that an aberration of mind, a discharge from the mind just like a discharge from the nose. A dream of a horse was a dream of a horse. A dream of a tidal wave was a dream of a tidal wave. In some cultures specific translations of these motifs abound, Greece being the most obvious. A dream of this or that was auspicious whereas another indicated misfortune. Freud and Jung's work changed all of that. A much more sophisticated understanding of symbols within the dream developed. The implications for homeopathy are actually quite important. In a proving situation, the prover may come up with a left-sided headache. But as well, that prover may dream of a waterfall, or dancing across boats, or a lizard being surgically removed from one's spine. What is missing in Hahnemann and Kent's provings and approach and is that they didn't explore these symbols. How could they? They didn't have a language to be able to do that. But we do now and these days when a prover has a dream of a coconut being chased by a dog a good supervisor knows that they need to explore that symptom and understand what it means to the prover. Of course this is exactly what we do in a clinical situation to assist in our understanding of the patient and make meaning from all of the symptoms. From this perspective that dream is gold. A good dream and especially a recurring dream in homeopathy is nothing other than a window to the cause, to the source. It is an unfiltered and uncompensated symptom and just what the homeopath needs in the clinical situation with an adult who can give us nothing else but filtered and compensated symptoms.

The use of dreams in case taking is one of the most well known and accepted methods of accessing the unconscious mind of patients for therapeutic purposes. For Jung, a patient's dreams had meaning just like everything else and he developed methods of using the information from dreams that did not involve asking the patient directly why they had a particular dream or what the secret thoughts expressed in it are, since, in his view, the patient does not consciously know the answer to these questions (Jung 1974). In seeking the unconscious mind of the patient, Jung considered dreams to be the '...most basic and accessible material for this purpose' (Jung 1964) or as Hillman (1975) puts it in exploring dreams we are trying to '... restore a view of the soul'.

Homeopaths using this style of case taking will ask the patient to recount their dreams, explore particular aspects of the dream, and use this process to gain an understanding of the patient, as a prescriptive tool, and also as an indicator of the move towards wellbeing as treatment progresses. Whitmont (1999) describes dreams as symbolic statements about the dreamer's psychological situation, and sees them as providing information for the homeopath on which issues need addressing and when they need to be addressed. This viewpoint is shared by Cicchetti (2003) who regards dreams as

'...an attempt on the part of the organism to heal itself...', and therefore an essential component of healing, as well as a vehicle for reaching into the inner realm and retrieving what has been lost. Dreams are the royal road to the unconscious (Kaplan 2001) and with the dream our defenses relax and the conscious mind throws up pure untarnished symptoms, suppressed memories and other aspects of our nature for homeopaths to observe. A woman recounted a dream to me. In the dream a spider is caught in a jar, it is huge and black and is crawling up the side of the jar to escape. She is freaking out and is trying to keep the spider in the jar, but it keeps coming. It is coming out. She sees some turpentine and quickly pours it into the jar. But the spider keeps coming. In the end she finds the lid and just as the spider is getting its huge hairy legs to the top of the jar she gets the lid on and slowly the spider sinks down the side of the jar into the liquid. Slowly brown fluid comes out of the spider like tea coming out of a tea bag. Then she wakes up with a start in a panic. On discussion, she had no insight into the spider itself, other than they were always female, and unpredictable and frightening. We moved on and talked about other things. In other areas of her case I learned that she had massive issues with control. She could not use public toilets (could not perform), lost the plot before exams (anxiety about performance) and had never had an orgasm (too much effort to perform, easier to fake it). She was afraid of letting go and all the scariness of not being in control. Then she put the pieces together herself. The spider, needed to be kept in the jar and not let out. She would not know who she would be if she let herself really go. That realization plus some *Lycopodium* led to some spectacular changes.

Actually, not all agree with the symbolic approach to dreams. A colleague of mine, Peter Tumminello has a number of cases in which he has successfully prescribed a medicine based on a dream and the motif in the dream. This idea never made sense to me. After all a tidal wave means one thing to one person and something else to another. In the same way a prover dreaming of a snail has a subconscious that grabbed that symbol for a reason whereas another prover who dreamed of a snail used that motif for another reason. The snail is surely irrelevant. However I remember one day he told me about a case of a person who in a recurring dream was clinging to the side of the boat in a wide expanse of ocean and responded well to the remedy *Silica*. *Silica* is one of the few remedies in the rubric, dreams drowning foundering in a boat. I was astonished one day in my own practice when a patient told me a similar dream except this time they were sitting on top of an upturned boat in the middle of Sydney harbour. All the other symptoms in the case, plus this one pointed to *Silica* and I gave it with success. How is it possible that a dream could possibly be linked or attached to a homeopathic remedy? Whatever the reason he and others are mapping thousands of dream motifs to specific remedies.

Tattoos

If dreams are useful then tattoos are gold. The tattoo is the tree lined avenue to the unconscious. 'What on earth made you stamp that mark on your body? Tell me about that scorpion? Is there a reason you have a wild boar with dripping tusks on your hip?' I remember a female client getting up to leave a consultation some years ago and as she did a snippet of a tattoo was revealed on her back. I asked about it and she revealed a black widow spider who's body took up the whole of the left buttock, the legs extending up and down her body from there. We returned to the chair and talked for another half an hour not only about spiders but what was going on for her in her life when she had it tattooed on her body, her father, her relationships with men.

Psychology and Psychotherapy

Thanks to the work of such pioneers as Jung and Hillman, who further developed Jung's work, many psychotherapists today work with the soul as the central organising construct that gives focus and boundaries to the profession (Elkins 1995). Hillman believes that without soul, psychology has lost its identity and becomes merely physical anthropology and statistics. Elkins (1995) states that medical and mechanistic models of psychotherapy leave little room for soul and as such produce soul-less results, meaning that very little healing takes place. He also describes psychotherapy as the process by which we assuage pain through '…nurturing and healing the client's soul'. Some homeopaths, and plenty of psychotherapists around the world employ an integration of both homeopathy and psychotherapeutic techniques. Many describe the exponential leaps the clients make within themselves, their personal development, and their symptoms with a combination of these two technologies (Elkins 1995).

Art Therapy and Sandplay

Art therapy is a modern method of psychotherapy that gets the patient to use art, drawing, and creativity to bypass their cognitive rational mind and to uncover their intuitive irrational mind or psyche. The rationale behind this method of practice is that it can be more effective than the talking therapies because patients are less able to hide behind language where they don't actually disclose anything useful, it gives the practitioner direct access to the patient's internal landscape, and, as with dreams, it can reveal parts of the patient that they were not consciously aware of (Kaplan 2005). Elkins (1995) believes that the soul and art are very closely connected and that 'art is the perfect container for the soul' because like art soul belongs to the world of imagination.

Brian Kaplan's *The Homeopathic Conversation* gives a few brief examples of finding meaningful and useful information in the drawings and art, and therefore the unconscious, of his clients. I can only concur. Many a time I have received useful clinical information from visiting the studios or looking at paintings and drawings of numerous clients. One in particular stood out. A woman, (she had been dropped on her head as a baby) who struggled intellectually grasping some ideas but was artistically quite superb came to see me. She was troubled by recurring headaches. I prescribed numerous remedies and we did make some progress, but we made far better progress the day that I went to the studio and realised that her art, which sold for hundreds of thousands of dollars in New York consisted of photographs of her own vagina being projected onto a wall. She would then paint these two metre high vaginas in various shades of black and vermillion. It signaled a reorientation in my questioning. Over the years I have had clients bring me images and art that have come from their unconscious and moreover poetry, songs and indeed any expression from the unconscious is a welcome augmentation in my practice from this perspective.

Sandplay is another useful technique which can give the patient and therapist a direct route into the symbolic realm. Figures in the sandbox are chosen and arranged by the patient who is encouraged to use them in role plays, interacting with each other and with the patient. Sandplay actively engages the psychotherapeutic tool of projection and releases the unconscious processes of the patient. It is equally effective with both adults and children and according to Kalff (1991) the series of images that take shape during sandplay aids in the process of individuation described by Jung which leads ultimately to wholeness. As with all Jungian and Post Jungian therapies, sandplay too sees disease in terms of an '...intellect which has lost all connection to feeling and the body (Kalff 1991) and places its healing emphasis on the reintegration of the mind, spirit and body.

Archetypes, Myths, Fairy Tales, Stream of Consciousness and Metaphor

Some homeopaths have advocated to a generation of students and practitioners that the role of the case taker is to encourage the patient just to deluge their symptoms thoughts and experiences, their sensations and feelings in an unending stream of consciousness (Chhabra 2002). It has to have value. It was good enough for Anais Nin and for a generation of writers doing their 'morning pages'. Other methods also employed, perhaps a little more controversially than dream work, are the use of metaphors, personal mythology or fairy tales, myths, fantasy and imagination. Tales and myths were considered by Jung to be means through which the psyche tells its story and as such were as useful as dreams (Jung 1990b). Jung also worked therapeutically with patient's fantasies because in his view life is '...spent in struggles for the realization of our wishes...' (Jung, 1974) and he believed that if we cannot fulfill a wish in reality then we will fulfill it in fantasy.

The use of myths and fairy tales in case taking may be an extension of dream work where the symbols revealed in the dream are related to themes, myths, or fairy tales that are already a part of the collective and can thereby be linked to issues the patient is struggling with. Cicchetti (2004) also advises observing the patient's language, bodily symptoms, fantasies, delusions, likes and dislikes as sources of their personal archetypal symbols. Such work is especially effective in taking the cases of children. I recall the case of a nine-year-old boy who had a sensation of a fish bone in the throat. His mother was a herbalist and tried all sorts of different preparations and as a last resort bought her son to see me. I prescribed *Lachesis* and then *Calc carb* with no effect. The mother brought the boy to see me one last time. It was his drawing of the house and then two figures within the house fighting that alerted me to pursue a different line of questioning. Finding that the mother and father were constantly fighting and that the son was prone to enormous fits of anger, involving locking himself in his father's office and smashing everything including the computer, highlighted *Hepar sulph* as a better simillimum. And it was. The fish bone sensation was gone within hours.

To Jung or Not to Jung

To pursue this issue further, the centre of the debate, the crux of the problem and the reason that homeopaths argue is because of a fundamental point. There is no agreement about what is health and what is disease in our industry. It must be addressed. There are plenty of opinions. Moreover one's prescription is predicated on what one sees to be diseased in the case, and what is perceived to be cured in the case both of which is determined by one's philosophy of what is health and what is disease.

English homeopathy in the 1990's, some American homeopathy, and the bulk of New Zealand homeopathy was dominated by these thoughts, assumptions and attitudes. And it's easy to understand why. The job of the homeopath became less about pleurisy, sneezing and discharges, asthma and warts but more about assisting people through their process, their individuation. Of course the colleges produced graduates who found patients to populate their practices with these sorts of issues and problems. From a historical perspective the history of homeopathy from the 1970's through to the 1990's is one where, to a certain degree patients stopped going to see the homeopath from a medical perspective to deal with their ingrown toenails, but rather patients went to see the homeopath because they were stuck, or because they couldn't let go. Homeopathy as a profession suddenly became much larger in scope with many patients demanding a system of medicine that was both transpersonal and transformative and one that embraced the growing trend towards reintegrating the spiritual in medicine (Johannes & Lindgren 2009). One of the issues that has emerged over those decades is that some homeopaths have applied this style of case taking to the wrong kind of patients. Homeopaths and their patients became confused with resulting jumbled cases, bizarre ideas about constitutional prescriptions and misapplied or distorted attempts at curing patient's souls. Many homeopaths found that the simplicity of Eizayaga's (1991) model of levels of disease has ironed out many of these issues and made homeopathy clearer for them. Other homeopaths have drifted away from homeopathy because they couldn't find enough patients who wanted to work on their personal issues homeopathically. One of the unfortunate results throughout this time has been that the public has an immense lack of clarity about exactly what homeopathy is.

From a personal perspective, one of the things I immediately loved about homeopathy, and what I was taught was that the case taking process involved me following my patient wherever they went. A lot of the literature tells the homeopath to ask a very general question such as, 'Tell me what brings you here today,' or, 'What's troubling you the most?' Such open-ended questions result in the patient beginning to tell the story. They say things like 'What I have is…', 'It first began…', and 'It makes me feel like…', and very often the experience is that after 10 or 15 maybe 30 minutes the patient has told all of their symptoms. But it is very interesting to notice where the patient goes within themselves in the telling of those symptoms. From this more sophisticated point of view, the case taker notices when the patient talks of home but only mentions his mother. That is something to be asked about or pursued at a later time in the consultation with something like, 'It's interesting that you mentioned your mother before, tell me about her', or better still, 'you haven't mentioned your father. Tell me about him?' This becomes a really legitimate question in pursuing the patient's disease. But to the unwary patient this is a very bizarre question, especially if it's a male patient, linear thinker, allopathic thinker or someone who puts one and one together to make two. 'Why on earth is this person asking me about my mother?' says the patient quietly to themselves, I came here to talk about my shameful warts.

A generation of homeopathy students in Sydney have watched a case of mine where a woman is talking about her eczema and history of acne. She describes her symptoms in detail, and she talks about when it first began, in her teenage years. As a throwaway line, she mentioned that her acne wasn't anything like as bad as her brother's and she used to tease him. 'You teased him?' I asked. 'Mercilessly', she said, 'after all I got teased really badly because I didn't have any teeth'. Suddenly the case has dropped a number of levels to a totally different place, and a whole bunch of information that I would never have found had I just focused on her presenting symptoms of eczema and acne. The story emerged that when she first got her teeth as an infant they came through as little black stumps, and with no enamel. They were all removed and she had no teeth until much later they came through. I use it as an example to teach students about the Hahnemannian directives of staying silent. But I also use that case as an example of following the patient wherever they go and encouraging them to talk. This is the point. From this Post Jungian perspective the homeopath is expected to follow the patient wherever they go and keep them talking. Not getting in the way themselves with their own self-talk, or prejudice or other ideas of what might be going on with the patient. The job of the homeopath is to shut up and allow the patient to go wherever they go. It is easy to see that this can then go into areas of the past, or the mind, or into dreams, or their fantasies in order to look for those deeper themes that might emerge in the case. Of course this is hard to teach. How do you teach this to students, and especially how do you teach this to school leaving students that don't really have much experience of the world, or any experience of working with people from a psychological point of view?

Questioning

It has been described by some as massaging information. How does one encourage a client to just speak? Clearly they need to be comfortable with you and in the space that you practice. Therefore those qualities of creating rapport and making people feel comfortable to talk are crucially important. Often it's information that comes without them knowing that they are giving it. Many homeopaths do this quite naturally and are maybe unconsciously competent in this area. But very few people are teachers who are consciously competent and can teach the skills. One of the ways that a case taker can prepare themselves before a homeopathic session is to reflect on just what do I want from the session. It is a great way to prepare for a homeopathic consultation. Many of the people that we are talking to are not observant, give us monosyllabic replies and are closed people.

Questions to Consider

How would your friends describe you?
What does ... mean for you?
If you had 3 wishes what would you wish for?
If this remedy could do anything what would you wish for?
Tell me about an event that changed who you are today.

> *When was the last time you felt very well?*
> *What dreams have affected you in your life?*
> *What's your first memory?*
> *What's the opposite of that?*
> *In pain what would you do to make me feel that pain – how would you recreate that pain?*
> *What do these symptoms stop you from doing?*
> *What do they mean?*
> *What are the people you dislike the most and what do they do?*
> *What are your energy levels?*
> *How happy are you – out of 10?*
> *What's the worst thing about this illness?*
> *What's the best thing about this illness?*
> *What would children find scary in dreams?*
> *What were you afraid of as a child?*

Some homeopaths advocate asking very large open-ended questions as the best way to deal with this sort of situation. Others have suggested painting the clinic in specific colours to allow people to feel comfortable to express themselves. Other techniques can also be employed such as talking about something entirely different, explaining what you do, even trying closed or pointed questions. However, usually the information that is gathered from such closed questions is unusable from this perspective. Quite naturally this style of case taking lends itself to supervision and daily self-reflection. From this point of view and approach to homeopathy it is such a natural and perfect question to say, 'Tell me about that necklace, it's beautiful', as a legitimate therapeutic gambit. From a medical, or medically orientated perspective this question is a nonsense. It's entirely appropriate to use our own experience from our lives in our questioning. Our questions come from somewhere. This is my experience, this is what I've learned along the way, you and I are in this together so let's explore it.

Again, from this perspective it seems incredibly sensible to ask the patient for examples of their art or poetry. And many insights can be gained into the patient's internal world, the wounds, their internal landscape and the damage to their soul, by seeing what comes out of their artistic and creative endeavours. It encourages patients to explore, and practitioners to pursue and foster an ability to look elsewhere for the information that might lead to the selection of a simillimum. Confidence needs to be developed by homeopaths and students in their ability to extract this kind of information. Furthermore, what is required is that the case taker cultivates their own innate skills and develops themselves as a person.

An example; a patient came to see me with a debilitating pain in her neck and at the front of the throat. The only thing that relieved it was incredibly hard pressure to the extent to which she would lie on the couch and jam a wooden spoon into the corner of the couch and push back against it with all of her force. The most aggressive massage was useless and gave her no relief. In the consultation she mentioned she was an artist and at the end of the consultation gave me an invitation to the opening of an exhibition. I went. What was striking about walking into the art gallery was that everything on the walls was black. Dark faces appeared coming out of layers and layers of black and every now and again at the bottom corner of one or two of the pieces of art was some colour and the colour was bright orange. The exhibition was called 'Dark Stone at the Centre of the Cosmos' and on reading the gallery's description of her work and what she said about it herself, it was really quite apparent that the remedy she needed was *Aurum*. All of the descriptions of the work were about reflection, blackness, falling, grace, redemption and God. She did really well on *Aurum*.

To me the lesson of this case is that it's important for the case taker to explore beyond the presenting symptoms. It's important to remember that the consultation room is an artificial place purely for the convenience of the homeopath. You come to see me, on my terms, at my time, when I want, and I expect you to deliver me the information that I want, as I want it, in the form that I want it. It's artificial. Better, is to get as much information around the case as you can because what is blocking the patient, what gets their juices going, what comes out of their creative space, what their predilections are, is what demonstrates to you most clearly the essential disturbance in the case and these aspects of the patient may not be visible or accessible in the consulting room.

Another example is that of an autistic boy in England whose case was essentially given to me by his father. We attempted to have a consultation in my office, at the time on the top floor of a natural therapy centre which had an 'A' framed ceiling. It was a disaster. The boy kept on smashing his head against the walls as he ran towards the corners of the room and we had to call off the consultation within a couple of minutes. What I did was to go to his school and we did the consultation there. I noticed a number of things, that he played by himself, that he was lonely, that he barely engaged with people, but what was striking was that at one point he ran up to me and put his fist into a boiling hot cup of tea that I had just been given and ran away acting as if he had no pain response. In addition to that whenever he walked upstairs on every fourth step he would lie down laugh and spin around. I eventually gave him *Belladonna*. His father reported that an hour after taking the *Belladonna* while he was in the garden weeding, he turned around as his son, who up till then had only ever used the word 'yellow', said 'There is oil in my face, I can't see, we're going down'. He also started to sleep better, and the disruptions to the family became greatly reduced. Art, graphology, writing, astrology, doodles, face reading all have the capacity to reveal the inside of the client. All of these things in the hands of a skilled practitioner can reveal aspects of their internal world, the wound.

Disclaimer

All of the above notwithstanding a word has to be said about homeopaths staying within their scope of practice. A sobering fact is that most homeopaths use counseling skills and yet few have any qualification in counseling. This can lead to trouble. Homeopaths climb into the lives of clients whether overtly or covertly, and have without doubt over the years made a hash of this kind of work and created some questionable reputations for the profession as a whole. Clearly to explore this kind of work in more detail further study is required. At the very least a weekend workshop, or preferably some sort of professional qualification in art therapy, music therapy or one of the branches of psychotherapy is an important augmentation to existing homeopathic skills. In addition, it has to be remembered that some textbooks support a specific style of prescribing. Best practice is to stick to Vithoulkas' *Essences*, Baileys *Homeopathic Psychology*, Cicchetti's *Dreams*

Symbols and Homeopathy and Whitmont's *Dreams a Portal to the Source*, and *Psyche and Substance*. Moreover it is not possible to use this approach with all patients. It is also too hard to use this approach wholesale in the city where for many clients there is no time, too many drugs and lifestyle hindrances for it to be effective.

Developing the Necessary Case Taking Skills

There is no agreement on how best to teach the skills in a homeopathic context. Students make various attempts at questioning that are often bewildering for supervisors and observers alike. With this approach it is still useful to begin with, 'What brings you here?' or 'How did you find me?' or 'How did you come to homeopathy?' or 'What interests you in complementary medicine?' and that immediately gives them room to go where they have to go. Again, the approach is to sit, just listen, because within that description will be plenty of symptoms with juice. One of the better examples I have is from a number of years ago. A man presented me with back pain. It was extremely unique back pain, was worse with stress but it was also worse from eating meat and milk but only sometimes. I explored the symptom in every direction I could but got nothing. He was a little edgy and I knew that he was holding something back. Things became a little awkward. On exploring further he told me that he sometimes had, 'a base chakra situation'. I didn't know what it meant. No one had ever said that to me before. Students watching this case invariably say that I should have asked him more about this because he was clearly withholding something. They usually think that he is gay and is not just admitting it. But to start asking a patient that has presented with a back pain and been in the room for 20 minutes talking exclusively about this back pain about his choice of sexual partners is a long bow for some. Hahnemann and Kent both remind us to employ tact and timing. Its an example where given an opportunity I chose not to go into that 'base chakra situation'. I could have said, 'Tell me about your reading on esoteric philosophy?' But for most people that is not a straight line. Even a question that we think is normal like such as, 'Tell me about your dreams?' is not a straight line for all clients by any means. A question such as, 'Are you in a relationship?' has got nothing to do with his back in the patient's view.

Looking for Clues without Scaring your Client or Acting too Weird

I am always at pains to encourage students to remember that,

> You're in second or third year of your study of homeopathy. That means your life has stopped, you barely see your family, you can't remember your children's names and the only thing that you live, eat and breathe is homeopathy. You cannot presume that your client is interested in anything that you're interested in. You have to remember that the person that walked in the door may know nothing. Perhaps the only thing they think they know about homeopathy is that it's herbs or it's natural or something. Therefore you cannot act weird. Do not act weird.
>
> Homeopathy has a poor reputation because of enthusiastic homeopaths asking totality of symptoms questions, constitutional questions to unsuspecting clients expecting to talk about their gingivitis not their grief. Some are ok with it

but many are not. The disconnect between a homeopath aiming for the centre, 'Tell me your issue, tell me your problem, when did this start, tell me about the base chakra', and the patient who is anticipating another style of questioning must be addressed by the profession as a whole. Of course education and explanation, clear communication and congruence of expectations are the key. This is not to say that the base chakra situation is unimportant. In this case I did ask him about it, but in the second consultation and after our rapport was thoroughly established.

Conclusion

Homeopathy, as a system of holistic medicine aiming always to treat the whole person and the totality of symptoms fits more neatly into a model that embraces similar therapeutic goals than it ever has with the orthodox medical model. Post Jungian approaches to homeopathy have a lot to offer the profession and are a refreshing shift away from a purely scientific model that seems somewhat rigid and narrow in its construct, and back to a holistic method that had a rebirth within the field of psychoanalysis in the 20th century but dates back many centuries earlier. These approaches are not without their pitfalls however, and practitioners must have a thorough understanding of how to implement this model, as well as be unprejudiced, spontaneous and open. Practitioners must stay out of the patient's way, and let the patient reveal their authentic self without judgment, interference, bias or excessive guidance. Also, not every patient will be ready or able to work in this way and the homeopath will need to adjust their approach according to what is appropriate for the patient in this moment. Nevertheless, at its best this methodology brings with it the possibility of healing for the patient on all levels of their being, thus granting them the opportunity to realise their fullest potential not only in the area of their health but in all aspects of their life.

Doing Nothing

What is clear is that the demands of a case taken that approaches a patient from this perspective are different to what is anticipated and expected of a case taken in a traditional Hahnemannian sense; fidelity in tracing the picture of the disease, an unprejudiced approach, sound senses, attention to detail. What is required of a case taker is to sit and listen and explore, as opposed to listen to the symptoms and then medicate. It is seductive, fun and is as Jeremy Sherr says, 'like a meditation'. The professional posture is, because I see your symptoms as a reflection of something else, let's explore this something else together, let's look at where you are stuck in your life, let's explore where the recurring patterns are, let's employ the use of a homeopathic remedy to push you through the pattern that you have been playing out over and over like a curriculum throughout your life. Both Misha Norland and Jeremy Sherr have spoken about how the process of case taking is essentially to do nothing. As Norland says in his lectures and classes, when you perceive symptoms to be symbolic, all you need to do as a case taker is just be there. As Jeremy Sherr says in his lectures, it requires nothing of you. Literally you do nothing, you sit, listen, do nothing, let it come to you. Ultimately it is a meditation. Case taking demands nothing of the person taking the case than to relax in the middle of not knowing. All a practitioner does is sit, observe, observe the phenomena. You don't know what will be relevant. Best practice determines that you do not evaluate the case as you're going. Rather relax, be with the person, take the case and evaluate later. Sherr has described it as letting go: to do homeopathic case taking is like my best form of meditation and that's why I don't bother meditating because to me every case taking is an exercise in meditation, like a Japanese tea ceremony. How to do it is to stay centered and loose and relaxed and be there at the same time. His professional posture, just do my best in every case and have faith that things will work out well (Kaplan 2001).

Best Practice Post-Jungian

Beliefs

Getting to the core creates better and longer lasting change

The body is a shadow of the mind

Psyche effects substance

Do

Be silent and be silent on the inside

Case taking is a meditation

Do Nothing

Follow the patient wherever they take you

Chapter 8

Learning and Borrowing from other Disciplines

- Introduction
- Police
- Human Resources
- Borrowing from Psychological Approaches
- A Relationship not an Event
- Rogers
- Empathy
- Unconditional Positive Regard
- Congruence
- Authenticity
- Other Strategies and Techniques
- Humour and Provocation
- Borrowing Further

In this chapter you will
1. Learn the areas that contemporary homeopaths have drawn from.
2. Understand the internal qualities of the modern homeopath.
3. Critically reflect on the value of self-audit.

Timeline

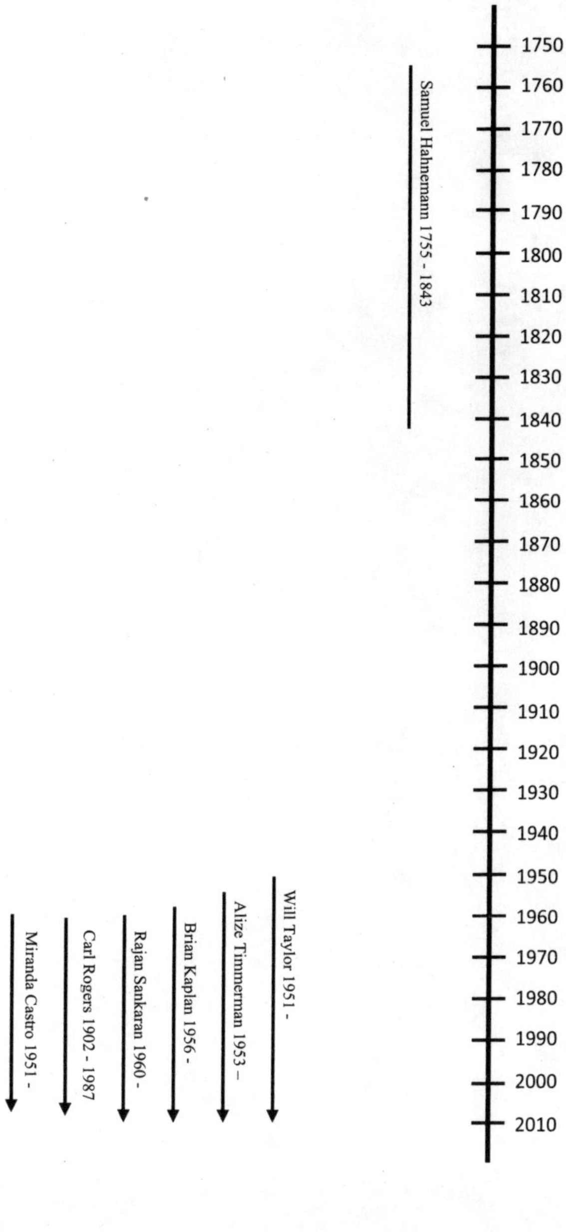

- 1750
- 1760
- 1770
- 1780
- 1790
- 1800
- 1810
- 1820
- 1830
- 1840
- 1850
- 1860
- 1870
- 1880
- 1890
- 1900
- 1910
- 1920
- 1930
- 1940
- 1950
- 1960
- 1970
- 1980
- 1990
- 2000
- 2010

Samuel Hahnemann 1755 - 1843

Will Taylor 1951 -
Alize Timmerman 1953 –
Brian Kaplan 1956 -
Rajan Sankaran 1960 -
Carl Rogers 1902 - 1987
Miranda Castro 1951 -

Chapter 8

Learning and Borrowing from other Disciplines

It has been the study for hundreds of years to find the best way to question witnesses in court, and as a result they have settled upon certain rules for obtaining evidence. Homeopathy also has rules for examining the case that must be followed with exactitude through private practice. JT Kent

Introduction

Just like the English language, homeopathic medicine, in order to survive has had to adapt and borrow from a multitude of different areas. It is speculated that Hahnemann borrowed from Arabic alchemy, from Greek medicine, and who knows from where he dreamed up his solution of potentising medicines by removing the matter and adding energy to them. In the same way Kent borrowed from Swedenborg to augment what he understood from Hahnemann. It has been no different in the 20th century and will no doubt be continued into the 21st. Homeopathy is as dynamic as everything else. Nothing stands still.

Kent talked of the homeopath as being a defense lawyer cross-examining the patient. Sankaran talks about the archaeologist. In my own lectures I describe it as the job of the historian. Homeopaths augment their practices by bringing the skills from their previous jobs or lives to the process. And why not? Those that are skilled in areas such as psychotherapy or marketing, those who were engineers or who have been grounded in some other orthodox medical or complementary medical discipline make better their homeopathic clinical skills when they apply their own synthesized and individual approach.

Borrowing from these techniques supplements and sometimes directs the quality of the information that emerges from an interview. When it comes to how to engage in the relationship homeopaths have gone searching in other realms. Borrowing heavily from the world of psychology, psychotherapy and specifically person centred therapy they have sought to deepen their relationship with those clients and to yield deeper and better information. Towards the end of the 1980's and the beginning of the 1990's, Pool, Townsend, Castro, Ryan and Carlyon in particular began to write about the therapeutic relationship, or the therapeutic alliance. Focusing less on the remedy and what could be extracted within the consultation, but more on the quality of the relationship with the client these writers talked to a generation of particularly English and American homeopaths. Culminating in the work of Kaplan in his seminal book *The Homeopathic Conversation* (2001) these professionals reoriented the thinking of many homeopaths. Kaplan's book is compulsory reading for homeopaths.

Police

One of the ways in which we can start to develop new skills when it comes to case taking to get good information is to look at other disciplines. Two of the closest areas to homeopathy are policing and job interviewing. The first is integrating some of the technical interrogation skills from the police. An interrogator like a homeopath is looking for useful information. While the investigator may be looking for a lie or a confession the process is actually not dissimilar. Online there is a wealth of information about police interrogation techniques. They teach us to look for when the body language doesn't match what they're saying or the voice is incongruent in some way. Further they encourage us to confirm what is being said by the position and movement of the eyes. Moreover they teach how to determine a lie. It is well known that people can only lie in a straight line. The way to check to see if someone is lying to you is to go to the middle of the story and ask them about it again, and again. It takes a very really skilled liar to be able to tell every aspect of the story from a different part of the story. For us it is not quite the focus in our consultation room. It's not about if they're telling the truth or not but it is a good way to get clear about the information. One of the things that Hahnemann suggests in case taking is keeping silent. Police training and the art of investigative interrogation adds to that, 'act dumb.' It is a great technique to employ, 'Look, I really don't understand, can we go back? Tell me again'. Choose a different part of the story for them to describe, and ask again and again.

Human Resources

Another augmentation has been to integrate the multitude of interviewing skills from the world of human resources. That is a discipline that necessitates placing the right person for a brief provided by an employer. Skillful and open questioning is required to determine if this person that has presented themselves in a specific way on paper is going to be right for this position. It is an art and science. Open questions lead to much more accuracy of information than closed in this world, just as it does in homeopathic medicine.

Borrowing from Psychological Approaches

It seems remarkable that given the degree and depth of the relationship that we have with our clients that such little work has been done on the true nature of the relationship. Kaplan argues (2001) and chapter 10 of this work will concur that the relationship is as vital in homeopathy than the close similar medicine. While a simillimum is of inestimable value in the treatment of chronic disease we know that the need to find it can lead to the homeopath shouldering massive levels of anxiety in the misguided apprehension that they have to get the remedy right and perfect in every case. Who needs to feel anxiety and guilt when one is at work? It is not a healthy professional posture, yet it is a strong sub-current within our profession and especially those practitioners who are new to the art. In his own work, Kaplan demonstrates Freud's understanding of the importance of the therapeutic relationship by presenting to us his own journey and vulnerabilities in a human and transparent way. His focus on what happens in the consulting room, rather than what happens when the remedy is given to the patient and they go away, appropriately places the relationship in its true context within the homeopathic process.

A Relationship Not an Event

In Aphorism 209 of the *Organon*, Hahnemann says something simply extraordinary.

> *After this is done the physician should endeavour in repeated conversations with the patient to trace the picture of his disease as completely as possible*

To my mind 'repeated conversations' (Kaplan 2001) do not imply one or even two consultations but more. Where does this belief that the homeopath has to find the remedy the first time come from? Where has this belief come from? What writer in homeopathic literature states this? Yet virtually all homeopathic students develop at some point this anxiety around needing to find the right remedy. I say in all of my seminars and lectures (until I'm blue in the face) 'relax'. 'Relax. No one is expecting you to get it right the first time. Hahnemann didn't and he is the boss'. This is not to say that patients should be encouraged to come back once a week and for there to be any unethical behaviour around the taking of money (Kaplan 2001). The point is that Hahnemann said over and over, when it comes to homeopathic practice Hahnemann said cure takes place with many anti-psoric remedies, and over repeated consultations. Moreover, if we look to the case books of the great homeopaths we know that they saw their client's repeatedly to assist in the treatment of their chronic diseases. Nowhere is it said that it has to be done in one go. It is not about a hole in one. Psychologists and psychotherapists don't do it, nor do counselors, physiotherapists or podiatrists (Kaplan 2001).

Rogers

Jan Scholten, Rajan Sankaran, Kent, Andre Seine and Brian Kaplan amongst many have all said the same thing. The thing that motivated their search and journey was to get better results in their own clinics. In Kaplan's case it was essentially to communicate better with his patients. He describes better than any other how the history, philosophy and practice of Carl Rogers influenced his work. Therefore it is not necessary for me to go into significant depth other than encourage you to read his book (Kaplan 2001).

The crucial point that needs to be made here is that the approach of Rogers differed significantly from analysts and therapists of his day because he had no interest in analysing or interpreting unconscious processes that his clients were experiencing. In other words the therapist does not need to make the client aware of his or her inconsistencies, their role is to listen to the unique experience of life and mirror that back to the client. There are significant synergies with homeopathy in this approach as this mirroring provides an environment where the client is able to grow and understand themselves and not do it within the timeframe of a conventional psychoanalyst with his or her own agenda. As Kaplan (2001) describes, this is non-directive, client and person centred.

There are some significant assumptions in this approach and one of the most important is that there is a belief that it is the purpose of a human life and role of the being to individuate (Townsend 2002). In other words there is a belief underpinning these ideas and method that self-knowledge, personal development and knowing oneself is the reason for being here and this journey can be facilitated with the listening of a skilled ear and a good practitioner.

Rogers argued the techniques to be employed were empathy, unconditional positive regard, and congruence. Kaplan, and others immediately realised the complementary and overlapping skills of this therapy work and homeopathy. Another way to put it is, the role of the person centred therapist is to be homeopathic with their client (mirroring), and the role of the homeopath to be homeopathic and prescribe homeopathically.

We all have been battered in the homeopathic world with accusations of peddling nothing other than placebo. It is implausible scientifically therefore it doesn't work (Shang 2005). Curative results could only be an unheard of and misunderstood aspect of the placebo response at best, or peddling snake oil at worst. All homeopaths at some time have had to question whether they are in the business of giving nothing and charging money for it. Of course they all dismiss their hesitancy when they get a great response to the homeopathic medicine given on the fifth or eighth prescription when if it was a placebo response it would surely have improved on the first, second, third or fourth. Then are the spectacular results with the chickens, the cows and the treatment of infants that could in no way be ascribed to some sort of elaborate placebo response (Kaplan 2001:100). My own healing response and the reason for me studying homeopathy was a result that could in no way be considered or written off as a placebo response. So it is important to realise that when we talk about counseling skills and the therapeutic relationship and homeopathy that it is not to diminish the remedy as important. As Dr Peter Fisher said in a Sydney lecture, *Our job as homeopaths is to maximize our relationship with the client and leverage it to get clear symptoms in the case resulting in a more accurate medicine*

Homeopaths at the beginning, and at some point in their practices reconcile themselves to knowing the clinical efficacy of their prescriptions. The purpose of the case taking in the context of Rogers client centred therapy is to fully understand the patient as much as is possible. But the difference is important. It is not about understanding with the intellect. It is not about analysing the case from this perspective or that perspective. Rogers and his followers know that by being present for the patient in the consultation and maximizing that experience, the homeopathic prescription will be as easy as falling off a log. I have seen students wrestle with the amount of materia medica that they are supposed to know. I have seen students, and practitioners of homeopathy anxious and worrying day and night about their prescriptions. One I spoke to recently is fortunate to have found herself at a clinic that provides her with a great number of patients. While seeing a lot of people, every one of those prescriptions is providing huge anxiety for her as she tries to get it right. In the few days that I spent with her in her practice I forgot the number of times I encouraged her to drop the emphasis on the technical parts of what she was doing and emphasized *her* as being most important. Just be there. In my conversation with her, as in all my conversations with students I encourage an honest self-audit of the qualities required of the case taker to ensure that this fundamentally crucial part of the process is going well.

Empathy

This is the capacity to identify yourself with a client when you're sitting in front of them, essentially to put yourself in the shoes of a patient in both an intellectual and emotional capacity. Will Taylor (2001) and Kaplan (2001) have written on this quality.

- That must have been a difficult time for you
- You must have been pretty upset by that
- That must have been painful for you

These are perfect examples that enable the patient to know without question that you are there with them and for them. This is different from sympathy. A fundamental difference is about maintaining a boundary that is clear between yourself and the client. Knowing when you have lost yourself in a consultation is a very important skill to develop, because it means that at that moment you slipped from non-prejudice to prejudice. Once I rang a friend to meet for a drink after work and was startled to hear her clearly upset as she picked up the phone. I asked what the problem was and she said, 'Oh it's okay I always cry after seeing clients'. And she did, every day. She took on so much, identified herself so clearly with her clients that she required this emotional release to establish some equilibrium again. The sensitivity, which at one moment was a perfect quality to be a good homeopath, was a double-edged sword for her and it was the quality that within two years was the reason for her burnout, and leaving the profession. From this perspective it has to be said that homeopathic consultations can be brutally hard. As we know from our nursing, massage therapist, counseling and psychotherapy colleagues, they all run the gauntlet of burnout. It is a very hard professional posture to keep one's heart open in the face of pain. Quite understandably some health professionals develop a hardness over the years, in the emergency room where they are working or the women's shelter dealing with trauma, or abuse, or the other shadows of human existence. Somehow the posture that we have to adopt to be in the helping professions, to do good work, and have longevity is to have an open heart but not to open (Ram Dass 1985).

Unconditional Positive Regard

Another quality of client centred therapy that has a homeopathic counterpart is unconditional positive regard. This is non-prejudice in 21st century speak. A therapist should strive to have positive regard to the goodness in all clients and is therefore not to judge them in any way (Kaplan 2001). As mentioned in chapter 1, how is one to teach this or develop the skill if it's not there already or there naturally. Patients tell me every day about their recreational drug use, needles, cocaine, bowel habits, excessive relationships with other people, addictive behaviour to alcohol or food, salt, Coca-Cola, pornography and their sex lives. For some reason, it is easy for me not to judge any of that behaviour. On the contrary, my prejudices often go in the other direction. I notice that I judge people that drive SUV's. I judge people that leave the air conditioner on when they leave the house, I judge political systems that allow for 100 story buildings to be built in a desert environment, I judge people that make decisions to build desalination water plants run on brown coal. I judge people who leave their children in cars in order to go into the casino. I judge people a lot. But for the most part I am aware of judging them and if I find myself on the rare occasion in judgment in the clinic I refer the client the next day. I often wonder what is the best way to teach this and I think the answer is to travel. By taking oneself out of one's familiar environment and into an uncomfortable one you learn about yourself. We fall back on our default settings, the learned behaviours and we challenge those. Another way to develop non-prejudice and unconditional positive regard is to participate in provings. This heightened situation allows one to observe very clearly oneself or the person doing the proving if you are a supervisor. This cannot be underestimated. As well as traveling, provings, meditation or some spiritual practice is a useful strategy to work on the skills of professional neutrality with warmth.

Congruence

The other quality articulated by Rogers necessary for practice is congruence. It has to be said at this point that 'congruence' is often used in different contexts. Elsewhere in this book I have used it to indicate when things feel dissonant and not resonating, when you know something is not right, when it is incongruent. However Rogers uses it differently, describing congruence as genuineness, realness and authenticity. Kaplan says,

> In my opinion it is an absolute requirement to be as genuine as possible at all times of the consultation. The alternative is to hide behind a mask of a professional facade. There is nothing more

disconcerting to a patient in the feeling that a doctor or homeopath lacks authenticity at any time during the consultation. If he senses that you're not being genuine at any moment a consultation will be ruined (Kaplan 2001:105).

Of these qualities, empathy and warmth are important to have but authenticity is essential.

To paraphrase Kaplan and Rogers, what is being expected of you is to be there with your client fully in a consultation, to be aware of your feelings, and if those feelings necessitate it, then express them. This at times requires some courage, some self-disclosure, different skills that we are taught by other homeopaths not to employ in the consultation. It is correct not to use these strategies when using a different style of homeopathy. But in a client centred or humanistic approach this openness is crucial. Moreover, it yields fantastic results especially when you notice yourself feeling agitated, board, annoyed or frustrated. These authentic interventions, to my mind are as profound as the techniques we will talk about in the next chapter on Sankaran's work focusing on hand gestures as a way to the energetic sensation. In fact, the use of the Freudian slip, empathy, unconditional positive regard, warmth, congruence and authenticity with a healthy dose of courage allow the chronic disease of the patient to manifest itself for you in the room perfectly.

Authenticity

I remember the case of a woman who rang up twice before the consultation to ensure there was air conditioning in the room and to fine tune the directions to find the clinic. When she turned up, she walked in, an older, 70-year-old woman with a green Woolworth's supermarket bag. This was striking and I said to her, 'Hello, welcome, what do you have in the bag?' 'Oh', she said, 'I have a heater, just in case'. I said, 'Really?' and peered into the bag. In the bag was a power adapter and a four plug power lead. I asked about that. 'Oh, I take these everywhere, just in case, you never know when it can be too hot or too cold'. Gold.

Ultimately this technique is founded on the belief that a patient's symptoms are a piece of the story, a slice of the curriculum that they are here on the planet to examine, study and complete. The idea clearly is that health is a journey and that with homeopathy we have a way to facilitate that journey. We hold the hand of the client as they take a few steps through their journey.

To me it is so interesting that when talking about this approach, the language required to describe it is so different from the language and skills articulated in Chapters 2-6 in this book. What are mental symptoms? What are the keynotes? What is a specific remedy for hypertension? What we are saying here is that those are events. Those are nouns. From a client centred perspective, symptoms are nothing other than an expression of the flow of energy, they are symbolic and health is a journey. It is a verb not a noun. Ultimately this patient centred approach attracts some different kinds of homeopaths to those who see the homeopathic system as essentially a technique to get rid of symptoms. As Kaplan says, and as Gray's (2009) research confirms, busy and thriving homeopaths have a number of things in common. While we might think that great homeopathic results are what leads to thriving practice, this is not the case. The quality common to all, is that busy thriving and successful homeopaths are tenacious, have persistence, and for personal and financial reasons *had* to make their practices work. A close second quality is that their success rests on the capacity to communicate and relate to their clients. Third was that they spoke of some sort of inner work, growth work, spiritual practice, internal work, be it meditation or some such practice. As I asked a colleague once, *'Does psychotherapeutic training make you a better homeopath?'* 'No, but it makes me a better person'.

Other Strategies and Techniques

The skills learned in neuro linguistic programming can be useful especially in the hands of a skilled therapist (Kaplan 2001). My own personal experience is that the skills I learned in my training in gestalt therapy have been invaluable and I employ them in many situations. These days some homeopaths are using voice dialogue and family constellation work to facilitate their consultations. Moreover, we know that many homeopaths take themselves off to kinesiology classes in order to find some external authority to validate their own knowing about whether a remedy is valid or not.

Humour and Provocation

In addition to these skills and techniques that can be learned in workshops or informal training there are some other qualities that are useful to bring into the consultation room. Kaplan talks of the value of humour and provocation. Of course humour works both ways because it can go horribly wrong when used inappropriately. I remember the time when a very proper and upright English lady came to me for her osteoarthritis. She was reserved to say the least, and I was struggling to get much meaningful information. I asked her about the cause and the origins of her symptoms. She vaguely implied that they had started from some possible back injury. I persisted on my line of questioning and finally found out that she had had a bad fall once in the garden and landed on her coccyx. I asked how she did it, and she related to me how she had been pulling a weed out of the garden, a very reluctant weed and she eventually cartwheeled backwards into the compost heap. The image of this very proper woman with her affected accent legs in the air in the compost heap in a leafy northern Sydney suburb was too much and I split myself laughing. She was mortified and quite rightly admonished me. Interestingly from that piece of authenticity our relationship deepened and I assisted her with her arthritis in the following years. Like Kaplan, I often laugh in the consultation and don't feel guilty about it and I know from feedback that most patients love it. We have fun and in fact both laughing and crying is a common occurrence in the clinic room.

Kaplan also talks about the use of provocation and directness as a legitimate therapeutic intervention in the consultation. If used authentically this is infinitely useful. It took me a decade at least to find my own voice and authority in the clinic. Like so many things I've no idea how to teach this. Actually a client said something to me once that made me realise that I had been too compliant and soft at times with my clients. A Spanish man consulted me. He had been pushed along by his wife and ultimately his problem was that he smoked too much marijuana. He worked trading on the Japanese stock exchange and so he worked strange hours and of course spent a lot of those hours by himself on the computer relying on his friend marijuana. His wife wanted me to cure his messiness and he actually genuinely wanted to come off the marijuana. I tried this and that and over a period of months gave different remedies. He was doing okay but not really making spectacular strides in those months, spent some time smoking less and sometimes working more than usual, in other words nothing spectacular but adequate homeopathic improvement. My approach was to say to him, 'Look at the side-effects that too much smoking of cannabis can create, bladder problems, memory lapses, motivation issues etc.' He went along with it and my medicine. One day he turned up for his consultation in an Armani suit and looking a million dollars. His hair was full of lustre, his skin was fantastic and this posture was different. 'Isn't homeopathy just amazing', I said to him as he came downstairs, 'You look fantastic'. 'This?' he said pointing to himself, 'Oh this wasn't homeopathy, I went to see a tarot card reader'. 'You're kidding', I said, 'tell me about that?' 'Well while I was at the markets on a Saturday a few weeks ago my wife suggested I get a reading. I sat down with the tarot card reader and she was doing my cards and then suddenly she stopped and looked me in the eye and she looked down at the table and she looked back at me in the eye and she pointed and touched this card and pointed at me with a finger, and said, 'Do you smoke dope?' 'Yes', I said. 'Stop smoking dope', she said and she thrust a finger into my chest. 'So I did'. I love that story because it reminds us that the practitioner at times is the voice of authority and when it comes to lifestyle issues it is entirely appropriate to draw a line in the sand and say, 'Stop doing this behaviour'. For more on these and other techniques go no further than *The Homeopathic Conversation* (Kaplan 2001).

Borrowing Further

I have argued in Chapter seven that borrowing from Freud, Jung and Adler's use of dreams and the symbolic world that we are able get different and useful information, to understand the patient better. Free association or stream of consciousness (Chhabra 2002) has been advocated by some homeopaths as a great way to understand the patient. Kaplan (2001) argues that for the most part we don't have enough time for it in a homeopathic conversation. Nevertheless some use it as a tool of getting to the unconscious or the energetic imprint of the disease. In addition, there is the Freudian slip, the slip of the tongue. These are not accidents but are often the truth bursting through the cracks when for whatever reason the defenses of the patient are down. Some, such as Alize Timmerman have become interested in other techniques such as family constellation. Some have found voice dialogue and have integrated their use in the homeopathic process. To my mind the idea of integrating the work of Reich and his understanding of the mind/body connection and integration of bioenergetics articulated and made more elegant by Alexander Lowen simply augments homeopathic practice. As Kaplan (2001) says, what these two authors teach us is that the muscular tension of the body is a valuable pointer to the psychological state of our patients. The scaffolding we have is there for a reason. Also the sexuality and sex life of the patient must be addressed and talked about in the homeopathic conversation.

As mentioned earlier the homeopathic clinic is no place to be modest. To be appropriate and to time one's questions is crucial but they still must be asked at some point. Buber is another whose work in a different discipline is easily integrated to the homeopathic context. His emphasis on the I-Thou relationship and its healing effects make perfect sense. The willingness to understand more about the realities of a relationship between two people and specifically a healing therapeutic relationship cannot be underestimated.

What is of crucial importance is whether these techniques should be taught to undergraduates who have yet failed to grasp the basics. Allowing easily influenced homeopaths into substantially advanced homeopathic work has little value for our profession, and results, and only succeeds in strengthening the bank balance of the dynamic homeopathic teacher looking for the next new thing to deliver. Only the very skilled practitioner should undertake voice dialogue work (Kaplan 2001). Without a doubt this is valuable work and not only deepens the relationship but also elicits greater information. But the patient must be safe and protected and the homeopath skilled and qualified when doing this kind of work. Where this goes wrong is where the enthusiastic homeopath inappropriately applies a technique on a very mentally ill or unstable person. Patients with well-hidden dissociative disorders or multiple personality disorders in the hands of a passionate, enthusiastic but untrained homeopathic practitioners is an accident waiting to happen. Numerous stories abound of poor patient outcomes and negative press about homeopathy as the result, as well as complaints to professional associations. This is not to say that these techniques are not useful but care must be taken. Homeopaths must stay within their scope of professional and personal practice.

Questions for Self Audit

What did you do before coming to homeopathy?
What job did you have?
What skills have you bought with you?
What are they?
Identify them clearly

Best Practice

Qualities required
Empathy
Unconditional positive regard
Warmth
Congruence
Authenticity
Courage
Love

Chapter 9

Sankaran and Sensation

- Introduction
- Debate
- Case Taking from the Beginning; Spirit of Homeopathy
- The Purpose, the Method and the Techniques
- Sensation and Going Beyond Delusion
- The Levels
- Sensation is Non-human Specific
- Case Taking in a New Light
- Conclusion
- The Requirements of the Case Taker using Sensation Method

At the end of this chapter you will be able to
1. Identify the historical development of Sankaran's ideas.
2. Critically reflect on the major issues.
3. Know where to go for further reading and reflection.

Timeline

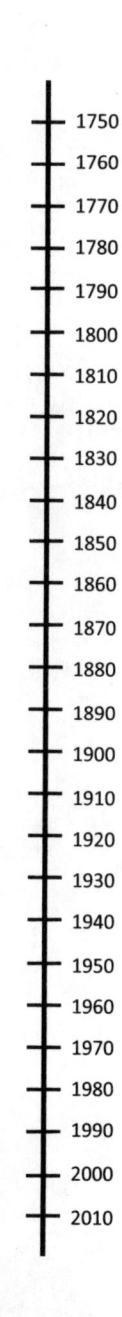

—	1750
—	1760
—	1770
—	1780
—	1790
—	1800
—	1810
—	1820
—	1830
—	1840
—	1850
—	1860
—	1870
—	1880
—	1890
—	1900
—	1910
—	1920
—	1930
—	1940
—	1950
—	1960
—	1970
—	1980
—	1990
—	2000
—	2010

Rajan Sankaran 1960 -

Chapter 9

Sankaran and Sensation

Introduction

This chapter explores Rajan Sankaran's insights into case taking over the course of all his books and looks at his ideas and suggestions. Having examined Hahnemann, Kent, Schmidt and the Post Jungian perspective, as well as looking at the lessons of other professions, it is possible to examine these new techniques and deeper understanding in an appropriate context.

Sankaran's focus and the intention behind his work has always been to find a method, or a system that produces consistent results that can be reproduced in case after case.

> Symptoms would indicate this remedy, these symptoms would indicate another remedy. There was confusion because if you chose one set of symptoms you came to one remedy. In the same patient if a homeopath chose another set of symptoms they would come to a totally different remedy. So there had to be something deeper to this. And then we tried to understand that all symptoms and especially the mind symptoms, they are the expression of a particular way of looking at and of reacting to reality that each individual has (Sankaran 2010).

Sankaran advocates looking at patients more deeply than previously and as a consequence the consistency and predictability of his results increased significantly. At the heart of the issue is the perception of the client.

> For example, you look at a mountain, you can see it as the name of the mountain or as the facts of the height or the dimension, or the approaches of the mountain or you can have an emotional experience of the mountain or the mountain can trigger off some imagination in you, like you're flying or you're climbing or you're on top of the world of whatever. But behind this perception also is an experience and if you allow yourself to go into that experience then you come into a different level of experience. (Sankaran 2010).

He extrapolated this metaphor and image to the homeopathic case and has as a consequence created two radical propositions.

> You can see a case as diagnosis or you can see the symptoms as different parts or you can see the patient as an emotional being and who he is and how he, whether he's an angry man or a sad man or so forth. Or you can try to understand, how does he look at reality, how does he see things? But deeper to that, how is his inner most experience which kind of brings together the body and the mind where there is no separation and not only is no separation between body and the mind but then at that level he speaks of a language which directly connects with some mineral, plant or animal in nature which seems to be expressing or speaking from within him. So at that level one could make a direct connection between the patients language and the language of the source and at that level the remedy selection became very predictable. But in order to come to that, one had to develop

two different approaches. One was the technique of taking the patient, guiding the patient, staying with the patient as he or she goes into a journey of discovery of witnessing what the inner most experience is. And at the same time we had to find ways and methods and techniques of doing this on the one hand and on the other hand we had to develop the materia medica from an entirely new paradigm. Not of individual remedies but of groups of remedies as in nature with the kingdoms of the minerals, plants and animals.

The process has involved a great deal of mapping, of the periodic table, and the zoological and botanical maps of nature.

Each kingdom, each sub kingdom and see this whole map. So we had to develop the map on the one hand and the techniques of case taking and by doing this, now we have come to a certain level where this whole system, this whole method has a foundation has a whole framework of techniques and of materia medica understanding that it can be used practically in a very effective manner and now we have colleagues all over the world practising it, using it, giving feed back of the results and developing it (Sankaran 2010).

Debate

Listening to Sankaran speak and reading his work reveals that he sees the job of the homeopath as different to simply removing symptoms via similars. But as a consequence of the publication and dissemination of these ideas around the world there is a substantial divergence of opinion. At the Links Heidelberg Conference in 2007 he was introduced as the 'Sensation in Homeopathy'. He has a massive following around the world and a generation of homeopaths are versed in his method and are getting and publishing good results.

Yet on the other hand we cannot get away from other feedback about the use of the method. Not *his* use of the method, but the consequences of other practitioners who have often been prescribing on half information, guesswork, speculation or at worst, a lazy doctrine of signatures. Irrespective of the value of the method we have clear feedback about what people feel about it and their reactions.

As a practitioner, Ken D'Aran with 29 years practice experience, who also teaches at various colleges and is a student clinic supervisor reported,

> I have experienced a number of situations that now concern me regarding the teaching and practice of Sankaran's 'Sensation' method especially when introduced to undergraduates of homeopathic medicine. The first concern is the bias towards the 'mentals', encouraging the student/practitioner to interrogate the patient, to bring out an assumed basic 'feeling' behind their condition. Though noble in theory and in some cases absolutely essential to probe deeply into the mental state of a client so as to address and if necessary prescribe on or just identify the issue so as to refer to an appropriately trained and qualified professional in regression or other psychological therapy, the majority of presenting cases are not 'ripe' for such interviews and are often left shattered, intruded upon and dismayed by what they now think is 'homeopathy', never to come back, never to refer to, tainted by a bad experience.
>
> What also concerns me are the 'medicines' prescribed in this method are often not traditionally proven or clinically verified by the profession. They are not known to be based on 'likes will

cure likes' but often based on symbolisms, and thus are simply 'generalisations', vague themes that the practitioner/student may recognise, like in 'flower' essences, astrology, etc., basically speculation, interpretations of mythology, totemism from ancient tribal people, or just new age theories and metaphysical assumptions. Thus they are often not prescribed on what they can cause (like cures like). The assumption apparently being that if they are 'potentised' they must be homeopathic!

In Australia homeopathic students are not generally trained sufficiently to undertake such deep psychological assessment, regressing the patient to basic primal feelings. The danger is a naive trust that the medicine is a 'magic remedy' that will make the client all perfectly healed. Contrary to this, I see clients unravelled and left with erroneous ideas about what homeopathy is (D'Aran 2010).

Furthermore, as a patient reported,

The concepts and philosophy associated with homeopathy really resonated with me. I was keen to experience it first hand from both a personal healing level and with a view to perhaps study it as well. Unfortunately, the experience was disheartening and disappointing to say the very least. From my limited knowledge I understood homeopathy to be a gentle, holistic and supportive modality. Instead, I found the actual consultations to be aggressive, invasive and confronting. I felt exploited and violated. I left feeling disillusioned and with any previously positive impressions of homeopathy absolutely shattered.

It has to be agreed that this is a tragic, unfortunate consequence for homeopathy. Anecdotal stories suggest it is not an uncommon experience. We have in the lecture room an elegant, brilliantly articulated new system, but at the coal face some mixed messages. Implicit in Sankaran's work is that the homeopath should attempt to get to the centre of a case, not the facts, but the inner most experience. Moreover, the subsequent implication is that to be able to perceive a patient's *experience* requires examining our medicine profiles in a way like never before.

Case Taking from the Beginning; Spirit of Homeopathy

However it did not start out that way. When Sankaran's first book hit the shelves of homeopaths in the early 1990's there was a considerable stir. For the first time, a homeopath was describing something so eloquently and elegantly and that was also so self evident, that was intuitively known to virtually all homeopaths, a description of homeopathy that met a 1980-90s mind/body medicine understanding. Homeopaths were excited. In that early work he described the job of the case taker to find the remedy as getting to the very heart of the case. It still involved an application of the principles of homeopathy. 'Our firm grasp of the principles alone can guide us in proper case taking' (Sankaran 1991).

The Purpose, the Method and the Techniques

> The purpose of case taking is 'tracing the picture of the disease'. The idea is not to try and fit the patient into some remedy or idea, but to trace out the true picture of the disease. The way to do this is to bring out the individuality of the patient. In this aphorism, (83), Hahnemann is stating the cardinal principles of homeopathy which is that disease is an individual affection, and that each patient is an individual, suffering from his own unique

disease. When we want to draw someone's picture, we first note his individualizing features. Similarly, 'tracing the picture of the disease' requires us to clearly bring out the individualizing features of the case. Only when you bring out the individuality of the patient, can you really claim to have taken the case. Now, we have both the aim of case taking, which is to trace the picture of disease, and the method of case taking, which is to individualize the patient.

There was nothing new or startling here, just described exceptionally well.

What are the requirements for case taking? The only requirements are an unprejudiced mind, an observing mind and a mind that draws a very accurate picture. We must not fit people into slots; instead we have to just let the picture come out, without imposing our own ideas on what we see. We must try to bring out and understand the true feelings of the patient not in terms of remedies, but in terms of human understanding. Case taking is the process of perceiving and recording the inner experience of the patient. It is not merely writing down whatever the patient says. This does not mean that we have to theorize or symbolize what we see, but just trace the picture as we see it.

This case taking strategy was based on his understanding of disease. Each disease had a core, a centre. Moreover every remedy produced a specific central disturbance,

Though different provers will have different organs involvement depending upon their susceptibility. The central disturbance supports or causes these peripheral organ effects. The central disturbance is like a stick which is constant but on which different creepers grow, depending on where it is situated. The stick is responsible for the growth of the creeper, but the same creeper can grow on different sticks. Our job is not to cut the creepers but to remove the stick that support them. If you cut only the creepers and leave the stick intact, some other creeper can grow on that stick (Sankaran 1991).

He articulated and introduced the idea of the central disturbance, clearly stated that local peculiarities also indicated the central disturbance and encouraged homeopaths to discover the central disturbance of a case which was often hidden by features of peripheral pathology.

We can easily understand that, as time passes, more creepers get added, the stick gets further hidden from view, and recognizing it becomes more and more difficult (Sankaran 1991).

In an acute case or one of recent origin, or in the case of a child, the central disturbance is less obscured from view and symptoms are spontaneously forthcoming without much effort on the part of the physician. In a chronic case, where much time has elapsed, the central disturbance is more obscured. He wrote that two factors contributed to obscure the central disturbance, the symptoms of the situation of the patient and the symptoms of the pathology. He relied heavily on an interpretation of Aphorism 211 of the *Organon*.

... The state of disposition of the patient often chiefly determines the selection of the homoeopathic remedy, as being a decidedly characteristic symptom which can least of all remain concealed from the accurately observing physician.

For Sankaran in the 1990's, the mental state had to be judged against the situation, the person's characteristics versus characteristics of situation and homeopaths had to eliminate situational features in the case taking and analysis. He rightly pointed out that remedies had fixed totalities; they are the same in any country, culture, or situation. If this were not so, we would have to have a different materia medica for different subgroups. *We would need one for Swiss females and one for Tibetan males.* A remedy is the same anywhere although the expressions may be different. In addition, homeopaths were encouraged to eliminate features of pathology. *The pathology on a central disturbance is like clothes on a person. There can be no pathology without central disturbance, just as a shirt cannot stand up without a person being there.*

He taught a generation of homeopaths to search for the centre and eliminate anything unnecessary. He argued the best totality of symptoms included mainly those symptoms that did not depend upon the patient's age, nationality, occupation or pathology. As the totality gets more and more focused and the marks of situation and pathology are removed, the clearer will be the indications for the remedy. Therefore, for the purpose of finding the remedy,

> Choose mainly those symptoms from which you can get no idea whether they belong to a Russian grandfather who has cancer or an Australian child who has as cold (Sankaran 1991).

He eloquently argued the homeopath was an archaeologist finding the original structure covered by the layers of earth. Just like the archaeologist, the job of the homeopath was to separate what has accumulated, from what is original. Just as we have heard, Norland, Sherr, Kaplan and others argued that when the homeopath begins this search, he does not know what is going to emerge. He just has to keep separating the false from the true. This has to be done very carefully. Homeopaths learned from Sankaran,

> One must not remove parts of the original monument itself in the process, nor should one be too cautious and not remove all the earth that has accumulated. In case taking, this would mean that we are not to try and explain away something on the basis of situation and pathology, which may be a part of the original disease. An expert archaeologist may be able to make a good guess about the identity of the structure even after uncovering a small part of it. But a scientific and thorough archaeologist will uncover the whole structure before he gives his final verdict. Similarly, initial observations or symptoms may give a clue to the remedy, but a good homoeopath will examine all aspects and elicit the whole picture clearly before he decides on his prescription (Sankaran 1991).

Crucially he pointed out a source of strong confusion with homeopaths and students alike. All features of a remedy need not be found in every case and that all the characteristics of the patient must fit into the remedy selected. In addition, he articulated the superficiality of relying on essences or constitutional types for all cases.

> This point is worth stressing again and again because unconsciously we expect some definite symptoms of a remedy to be found in every case of that remedy. For example, if the patient is to be Pulsatilla, we expect her to be mild, weeping and thirstless...we say Lycopodium is a coward or Natrum muriaticum dwells on past disagreeable occurrences. When we make this kind of statement, it is like saying that we would rule out this remedy if that feature were not present. We must not fall into this trap. Remedies are combinations of several traits; it is not mandatory that all traits be present prominently in all cases. It is not for us to see whether our picture of a remedy will fit or match all the patient's characteristics. If they fit well into

one remedy, we have to give that remedy even if our favourite symptoms of that remedy are missing in the patient (Sankaran 1991).

Case taking involved tracing the background, searching for peculiarity, sifting the common or uncommon and focusing on intense and striking symptoms. Moreover, he gave other useful hints that have been adopted and are now commonplace.

1.	Ask questions in the opposite direction. If you want to confirm that the patient is really mild, you ask him: 'Do you get angry?' Often, even a mild patient will say: 'Yes.' Ask him next: 'When did you last get angry?'
2.	Always confirm symptoms from relatives and friends.
3.	Never accept what the patient says at face value.
4.	Look at the hidden expression behind the symptoms.
5.	The symptom expressed with spontaneity, clarity and intensity is of highest value.
6.	If the patient is markedly irresolute, this symptom will be best elicited when you ask him about cravings and aversions.
7.	Try to confirm the essential parameters of the person.
8.	Try as much as possible to avoid asking the patient directly about his nature.
9.	If you cannot elicit characteristic symptoms in the patient's present state, you have to go back to the time when the last characteristics existed.
10.	I give a standard questionnaire form which asks questions about the patient's past history, present complaints with modalities, etc., personal and psychosocial history.
11.	The expression of characteristics can often be easily provoked. For example by making the patient wait beyond his time of appointment: Is he patient or impatient, mild or rigid, or is he restless or calm?
12.	Beginners in Homoeopathy often feel the need to put question after question; especially if the patient stops talking, they immediately ask the next question. This should be avoided.
13.	The patient should feel that the doctor is someone who cares, whom he can trust and to whom he can reveal everything: only then will he really open up.
14.	What the patient asks you is more important than what you ask him.
15.	If you come to a dead end in case taking and just do not know how to make the patient talk, just ask him to describe one typical day in his life, his routine from morning to night, you will find many leads from this narration.

He articulated the science and the art. In case taking, the internal state of the person in front of you is gradually revealed. It is simply an effort to understand the person in front of you and one can use any technique to suit one's temperament. While he elaborated on observation and repeated much that the older masters said, he is the first homeopath to encourage the patient to manifest the disease in real time; in the room right now.

> Observe how he conducts himself, how he has filled in the questionnaire, how punctual he is, how he is dressed, how he enters, how he sits – at the edge of the chair or behind, what his hands are doing, what his feet are doing, his facial expressions, his manner of communication and how he reacts to the person he has come with. If he has brought some medical files, how well he has arranged them, how he has brought them, has he brought them at all. Every single thing has to be observed: his movements, his postures, his speech, the way he explains himself and what atmosphere he creates in the room. None of them really indicate the remedy, but the state and frame of the patient's mind. This will be confirmed by other information later, but during this initial observation, looking and feeling are important. One good way to begin an interview is to put your observation back to the patient and ask him if he is experiencing this. From here you can get straight into the heart of the case. For example, you might say: 'You seem to be tense, what is bothering you?' or 'You seem to be in a hurry'. He is caught unaware and the answer spontaneously jumps out; now, if you attempt to go behind the answers, you will straightaway find something very deep in his personality.

This is a technique that the patient cannot escape from and immediately deepens the relationship and the level of communication. Also, more valuable and unadulterated information emerges. Another strategy was to seek the patient's nature as a child. He argued,

> We could understand the mind of the patient in an uncompensated form if we knew how they were as a child, because in childhood they compensated much less. You may be able to find in him the same nature now as in childhood but in a more compensated way. The remedy is often the same. You can use his nature as a child as a clue to understanding his nature now (Sankaran 1991).

He encouraged homeopaths to look for clear reactions in life situations, how the person has reacted in times of stress and strain in his life.

> The true nature comes out in times of stress; whether he is bold or timid, whether he wants to escape or stand up and fight, or is suicidal and depressed, or elated and joyous. I believe that the nature of reaction during and after a stressful situation reveals the uncompensated state of the person more than at other times.

Crucially he encouraged us to seek the central feelings of the patient. While some examples made clear sense:

> ...a girl said: 'Doctor, why are you not giving special attention to my case? What have I done?' Here you can see quarrelsomeness and lamenting, but what is the feeling? Her feeling is that she is not being appreciated, in comparison with others, a feeling of being neglected and jealousy. I gave her Calcarea sulphurica.

Others required artistic leaps that some were able to seamlessly integrate into their practice.

A lady developed a problem of pain in the shoulder and inability to move her joints after the death of a neighbour. I could have taken it as 'Ailments from grief' but I found that this lady was quite a reserved and shy type, and the neighbour was the only person in the building with whom she was able to communicate because the neighbour spoke the same language as the patient. From this, I got the impression that the death of the neighbour had created an anxiety in this lady as if she had lost a crutch, a support; so, I took the rubrics: Delusion, he walks on knees; Delusion, legs are cut off; Fear of strangers (because she was unable to face new people; she wanted to be in the company of familiar people only) I also took the rubric: 'Delusion, beloved, dying'...Baryta carbonica (Sankaran 1991).

Throughout the 1990's and into the 21st century, Sankaran taught and demonstrated this new style of homeopathy worldwide.

Before I went on a trip to Europe, a patient came and said to me: 'Doctor, please come back soon and for heaven's sake don't settle in Europe, since we will be lost without you.' Again, in this case one might be tempted to use the rubrics, but it is better and it is more important to be able to see what is the patient's view of the present situation that is making him say that. It is obvious that he feels frightened of being left alone just like a child lost in the wilderness and that the person who is to protect him or to support him goes away and betrays him. He will not come back and when he does not come back, he is finished and is left to the wild animals to be eaten. It is that idea of being frightened and alone in the dark in the night, in the forest with animals, in the terrorizing world with the only source of support going away, nobody to hold on to, nobody to protect him, that makes him shriek out and ask that I should come back as soon as possible. This might sound theoretical. But one has to observe the expression of the patient's face, the tone of his voice to be able to notice the urgency of his plea and the fear that makes it come out. The rubrics one could use are:

— Clinging;

— Praying;

— Delirium, crying, help, for;

— Fear of being alone at night;

— Delusion, that she is alone in the wilderness;

— Begging;

— Religious;

— Delusion, wife is faithless (wife, a trusted companion, will leave him and go away to somebody else).

In this way, from one expression, one can see the entire gamut of the symptoms that characterize a Stramonium state. The idea is not to point to the list of symptoms that one could derive from one expression, but it is to show that all these symptoms come from one single perception of reality and that one should be able to see the same perception behind all the symptoms and expressions and especially be able to see that even from one single expression one can get straightaway to the person's central delusion, to his central perception of reality, which is the heart of case taking. To explain a bit further, one could say that now we can see that all symptoms of Stramonium are in fact one symptom. That there is no difference between the clinging of Stramonium and the religiousness of Stramonium and no difference between religiousness and praying, praying and begging, between begging and entreating, between entreating and fear of darkness, fear of darkness and desire for light and company. The whole Stramonium expression is actually one thing and it is one thing that we are trying to understand both in the patient and in the remedy, and not the conglomeration of symptoms that make the totality (Sankaran 1991).

Sankaran also heavily emphasized the dream for the same reasons that Norland, Mundy, Sherr and others did in the 1990's. These represented important uncompensated feelings because in the dream one's capacity to suppress is at its weakest, and those feelings came out through symbols. When dreams were placed alongside other observations about the patient, they showed up in sharp contrast and these were integrated into the 'picture of the person'. The state of mind of the mother during pregnancy was sought, as was the exploration of the intense, real and extreme situations faced in the life of the patient. The questions and posture he wrote about indicated a sophisticated understanding of the Mind. In addition, he acknowledged the recurring patterns and stuck postures that patients developed in their lives and sought to understand the situations that patients had created in their lives. The scripts, life curriculum, the actors and the dramas of life were asked about. 'Indeed, the best case taking is done through silence, not questions'.

For Sankaran, what was required was to be free from prejudice.

> Prejudice means judging the present on the basis of past experiences, which leads to a fixity and rigidity of thinking. Prejudice is like darkness, it cannot be pushed away. It can only be removed by bringing in light. Light is the awareness. The same applies when we look at ourselves. Again we experience

preconceived notions about ourselves and these prevent us from knowing who we really are and what is going on within us. In the same way these notions prevent us from really seeing what is going on outside and in other people. To be unprejudiced demands letting things be as they are, and observing without fitting them into any category. Life demands this of us and so does Homeopathy. In fact we are required to be fools, to know nothing.

Furthermore, he argued, case taking demanded stillness of mind, openness and space.

If you are able to create this, then the case will come to you. The person sitting in front of you is unique, there was never anyone like him before nor will there be anyone like him in the future. How exactly does he think, what are his exact feelings? We have to understand how he views his life and the space around him. This will come to you, not from intellectualization or analysis, nor from rationalization, but from unprejudiced observation; you can then perceive his exact and true feelings (Sankaran 1991).

In *The Spirit of Homeopathy* he described the process,

'The first thing I do when I see a patient is to observe everything about him. It is not only observation of details such as how he dresses, talks and walks but it is also the impression that he makes. As I go on with the case taking, I note his every gesture or act and every peculiarity of his nature as narrated in his history. Slowly, I build the picture of a person in mind and, in the formation of this image, I try to depend upon his uncompensated features. Initially, his general appearance, such as whether he is excited or calm, dependent or independent, hurried or slow, strikes me. Later, I start noticing specific things.

There is humility there also.

I am very skeptical about my own judgments. That is a key to success. The scientist or physician who is willing to prove himself wrong will be successful. The more certain you are, the harder you need to try to prove yourself wrong. I am not talking about remedies at all. The more I keep remedies out of my mind, the more successful I will be.

The job was to understand the situation of the patient, the background, the occupation, the family life, social relations, cultural and economic status as well as childhood environment. At the same time observe how the patient has reacted to the situations around them. These observations about the patient, the way the feelings are expressed, whether they be excited or dull, weeping or cheerful, slow to answer or hurried, mild or vehement, should be carefully noted (Sankaran 1991).

With all this information, we have to use our human understanding and ask the following questions to ourselves:

— What are the patient's conditions for feeling OK (at peace with himself and others)?

— What are the basic feelings about himself or his situation that necessitate such conditions?

— What are the other expressions of such a vision of himself in terms of his feelings and actions?

Sensation and Going Beyond Delusion

On hearing the lectures and reading the books homeopaths quickly integrated these concepts of delusion, roots, perception and compensation. Good results were often the consequence and curricula began to change as students were made to learn the central delusions of remedies, sometimes at the expense of the less interesting lists of symptoms or even keynotes. What is more, homeopaths were delighted to almost be given permission to shift from mechanically repertorising cases after selecting a few characteristic symptoms, to using mental and general symptoms, from there to understanding the central disturbance, perceiving the mental state and unearthing the concept of disease as a delusion. The *Substance of Homeopathy, The System of Homeopathy* and the *Soul of Remedies* soon followed. Moreover the ideas began to change and to those staying abreast of Sankaran's own development, it involved a deepening understanding of miasms, kingdom classification and finally the development of a system of prescribing where all these concepts fitted into place, to discovering the common sensation in each of the remedy groups and families and more recently to an understanding of various levels of experience, to vital sensation. The scaffolding of the system was to understand his concept of levels.

The Levels

In his later works Sankaran provides various examples of the levels in practice. A simple example would be, when I stand and look at a landscape from a window I notice things. There are the names and facts, trees, houses, rivers. But I also feel it, experience an emotion or mood, and I sense it also, my imagination may become engaged and I am able to abstract about it.

1.	Name	The most superficial level at which homeopathy is practiced is pathological prescribing, or giving a remedy based on the diagnosis of the disease condition. Question: So what exactly is happening?
2.	Fact	Question: What brings you here, tell me about it? 'This is what I have'.
3.	Emotion	Feeling: What it is? (Common feelings, anger, fear, sadness.) Peculiar and characteristic feelings. Question: How does it feel like? What comes to your mind? A situation that had a big effect on you? How did that feel like? Prescribing on the emotional state of the patient. 'It makes me feel'
4.	Delusion	Delusion: The situation. How is it experienced? Dreams. Here the patient is able to express his false view of reality, which he takes to be real. This false view of reality can be a core belief or attitude caused by past traumas, inherited tendencies, or even past lives, which affects the way the individual responds to his current experience.
5.	Sensation	Sensation:Kingdom. (Sensitivity/structure/victim-aggressor.) Subkingdom/family. (Precise nature of the issue.) Source. (Precise degree, depth and quality.) Question: What sensation do you experience in that situation? What are you showing by that gesture of your hand?
6.	Energy or Universal level	Energy: Observation of energy patterns.
7.	The Seventh Level	

For another example, we can apply this idea to homeopathy itself. I can, 1) name what I am doing, 2) provide the facts (I am examining the homeopathic landscape), 3) have feelings about it (frustration, disappointment, excitement), 4) experience delusion (it will always be like this, I am constantly having to justify myself, I am surrounded by enemies), 5) experience the sensation (my spontaneous survival strategies to this situation), and 6) the energy of it (my energetic experience of it).

> In the third step we put in the adjectives or feelings or emotions. In the fourth step we create situations out of our imagination -situations that may or may not exist - or situations we may have or have not experienced. This has to do with delusion. When we reach the stage where we can abstract, we are able to convey our delusions, sensations (mental and physical) as well as describe some kind of energy in the form of patterns and shapes. In this way, in learning art, we have progressed from what can be only named to something that has no name but only an energy pattern. The levels also apply to the experience of any event or phenomenon.

Having articulated this undoubted truth and understood that each patient's experience of disease manifested at any one of these levels Sankaran's next question was,

> Of what use is this concept in practice? What will be most obvious to those who used the Delusion theory and realised that it yielded better results than prescription based on mere collections of symptoms, is that the levels of sensation and energy are deeper and closer to the Vital Force. Prescriptions based on sensations, and those that take into account the energy pattern experienced by the patient can yield far better results than did those based on Delusions. So how does one get to these deeper levels, how does one recognise sensation and energy, what sense do we make of these when attempting to understand the patient, and finally how does one use these to find the remedy?

To understand the application of the idea it is important to note that in each case, the deepest level the patient takes us to spontaneously is the level at which he experiences all phenomena. This is the level of his or her consciousness. In any case therefore, all relevant experiences, the chief complaint, exciting cause, stress situations, dreams, interests and hobbies, will be experienced by the patient at one and the same level. This is significant as far as the process of case taking is concerned, as well as in selecting the potency.

Sensation is Non-human Specific

Sankaran writes,

> Energy is universal and immaterial. All things, living and non-living, possess energy. Energy can be manifest in the form of different patterns, all part of a common, universal pool, yet each one with its own peculiar shape, direction, speed, form, etc. Energy patterns are common to kingdoms, so that certain plants, animals and minerals can have the same energy patterns specific to them, yet all belonging to the common pool. The energy of any substance is that which is common to that substance and to the entire universe. At the energy level therefore, it is difficult to differentiate the kingdoms. A specific energy pattern could manifest itself in a member of any of the three kingdoms. Sensation is more specific to kingdoms. Each kingdom has its unique basic sensation. With the mineral kingdom the basic sensation is structure, and in the consciousness of each mineral substance this basic sensation of structure is expressed in a way quite unique to that substance. With the animal kingdom the basic sensation is survival, and again in the consciousness of each animal, this is experienced differently and in a way unique to itself. With the plant kingdom the basic sensation is sensitivity,

and each plant family has it's own peculiar kind of sensitivity.

In cases of diseased human beings the Vital Force is deranged so that man's consciousness is altered. This altered consciousness is similar to a specific mineral/animal/plant consciousness from the Universe. Homeopathic remedies are prepared from plant/animal/mineral sources among others, and when these substances are potentised to a degree far beyond the material, there remains in them nothing but the spirit or energy of the substance. These remedies, when administered in accordance with the Law of Similars, are capable of bringing back the altered state of man's consciousness to a level where he is able to achieve the 'higher purposes of his existence' - in this way health is restored. In a diseased individual, the altered state of consciousness is similar to the consciousness of a specific plant/animal/mineral substance (remedy source) from the universe. The diseased individual and the remedy source have in common the energy pattern and basic sensation. These, the energy pattern and basic sensation, are therefore non-human specific. This means, that they are shared by human beings and other substance(s) in the Universe. On the other hand, emotions and delusions could be human specific; they may be experienced only by human beings and may not be present in the consciousness of any other substance in the Universe (Sankaran 2010).

This idea, this step has immense implications for homeopathy. Sankaran argues that he is still using homeopathic remedies based on the idea of similarity, but others argue that he is doing this based on the similar energy pattern, not on similars from a proving. It is an important difference.

Case Taking in a New Light

Whatever one's point of view, a real consequence is that case taking from this perspective has the aim to reach to what is non-human specific in each patient. The patient begins with the name of their main physical complaint. From there one has to cut through the various levels and reach to the levels of sensation and energy. While traversing the various levels, one picks up (i) peculiar symptoms (sensations, modalities, concomitants, mental symptoms, delusions, dreams, cravings, aversions, etc.) and (ii) sensations/words/expressions that have the potential to lead to the next level. At each level there are various sub-levels and to get from one level to the next one has to ask an appropriate question. Another technique is to observe the energetic expressions.

> I noticed that patients often used hand gestures to describe sensations. And as I started paying attention to these gestures I realised that only sometimes were these indicative of sensation; at other times they could indicate the delusion and at still other times they were only patterns that could not be reduced to either a nervous or emotional experience. Like sensations, these patterns too could not be localised in either the mind or the body; they were too general. Further, what the patient was conveying through these was mostly movement, sometimes together with form, shape, color and speed. These patterns seemed to me to be representative of energy (Sankaran 2010).

Conclusion

The consequences of the method and the changes to what is necessary for case taking are huge.

The concept of the levels and this new approach to case taking have so far yielded for me and some of my colleagues, very encouraging results. We are able now to prescribe remedies we might never have otherwise used. But I would like to add that these ideas continue to evolve and techniques continue to get more and more refined. It is a work in progress. As with 'An Insight Into Plants', I feel there are sufficient results to convince me that there is at least some truth in the idea and it has much potential. As long as we have failures, we need to look deeper, to look wider and to continue to evolve in our concepts and techniques. In this way we can hope for better and more definite results in our cherished and chosen task of restoring the sick to health (Sankaran 2010).

So we are left with a dilemma. Sankaran's work contains so much of practical value that it cannot be dismissed, but there is much misinformation most notably by those who have not read his books nor attended seminars about the work. This is an equally legitimate point. Students turn up in student clinic armed without any books except for Sankaran's *Schema*. Homeopaths call the professional homeopathic association when they move to a new country to become accredited and registered, but can't or don't know how to use a repertory, and then argue they are being discriminated against when they are politely told they are unable to join, and argue they do 'advanced homeopathy'. When a patient comes to see the homeopath and says, 'Yes I saw such and such a homeopath for my arthritis and all they did was interrogate me and I left feeling brutalized', then it is fair to question just what was that homeopath doing, just what were they taught, and what were non professional homeopaths doing in a seminar teaching such advanced work? These issues were recently put to Sankaran on a visit to Australia.

AG

Well, essentially there's two things which I suppose are a concern to me, and they come from a change that has taken place in my understanding of homeopathy of late. Recently in Australia the education system for natural medicine has changed and one college in particular has bought up all of the private colleges of homeopathy. It's quite possibly fantastic because they're committed to natural medicine but it's interesting because of course now the homeopathic department that's responsible for the development of the next generation of homeopaths here in Australia has to make its own way, find its own budget and all the rest of it and we have to develop the best curriculum. So that said, one of the things that has just come up over and over in all of the colleges that I've taught at around the world is what on earth we do when Rajan comes to town and talks. Its fine while he is here but what do we do once he leaves? It's folks like myself or, who else, Carmen Nicotra in Sydney or Ken D'Aran, Pauline Wilson in New Zealand who are left to pick up the pieces. And there are a lot of pieces. We've got these classes of students that have a lot of questions about the method. So essentially the questions is...have you considered what is the best way to teach sensation homeopathy? I really understand and hear you when you say that traditional homeopathy and Sankaran method are the same and you see them as not being separated, but how to teach it? How about that for a question?

Silence for at least a minute.

❑_❑

Umm. I can answer that question. I think that there are many view points about homeopathy and I think that they're all right and I think it's something that different people can look at in completely different ways and there is truth in all of it. I can only speak from the way I look at it and I, I do believe that the approach with the kingdoms and the miasms and the levels, just make it easier to practice to understand what we already know. It puts things in a more systematic, in a more accessible manner and it also gives possibilities beyond what is very very well known. This is my personal view and I'm obviously quite in favour of it but that doesn't necessarily mean what I say is right. It's what I experience is what I've found, it's helped me a lot and the most important thing that this development has come on the ground of traditional knowledge; it is based on it. So when I talk about a plant family of Anacardiacea it's not really different from what we know about Rhus tox, Anacardium, it's only a generalisation of that. Or when I talk about the terror of the Solanaceae, we all know this about *Belladona* and *Stramonium* and so many others, *Capsicum* or whatever it is. Similarly this knowledge of family and kingdoms is derived from what we know already, it is a generalisation, it is derived from that. I've done repertory work and it came out what is common and then generalised it and used that generalisation in other remedies of that family. It's actually quite simple.

AG

That's how you've got to those family qualities through extensive repertory extractions, right?

RS

Yes. And they're necessary. I did the same with the mineral kingdom. I did the same with the animal kingdom and if necessary I did provings where it was necessary to fill up the blanks and to know more, so to be really honest my entire background is coming from repertory and materia medica.

AG

That's very clear because we know that's how essentially you've done your extractions and come to the family qualities.

RS

That is part of the story but also it is this repertory and materia medica that I use every day in my practice. Rubrics are flowing into my head when the patient talks. They come automatically. That's what I did for 25 years so naturally when the patient talks I know the rubrics come.

AG

That's right.

RS

That helps me. So I definitely don't want a divorce between this and that and I want to see. When I see a patient and I see what the symptoms are I must have the rubrics supporting me from one side and I must have the kingdom supporting me from the other side. It must come together. Even if it is close for example with the patient we just saw and we just talked about stiffness and tightness. I know that this is very close to *Rhus tox* from my traditional knowledge; the same knowledge that helped me understand Anacardiaceae and then I just have to expand a little and I know there is a remedy Mangifer which is good for cervical spondylosis and it falls in the sycotic miasm of the Anacardiacea which the patient is expressing is beautiful. It's all together in my head, it's unified. But it is possible that people without the strong foundation of materia medica and repertory can be lead astray.

AG

Indeed because remember 30 years ago what it was like to study homeopathy for the first time. I mean this is the question that I'm faced with is how best to train a homeopath in the 21st century.

RS

So my question to that, in my view, this is completely subjective. It is that I believe that's because the systems, the kingdoms, miasms and levels help us to understand the homeopathy better, patients better, materia medica better, we should have to teach both of them parallel where one completely feeds the other. For example when you teach *Tarantula* how can we not mention that most of these symptoms of *Tarantula* are spider symptoms. So we say *Tarantula* is this this this, this quality, these ten symptoms of *Tarantula* for example the rhythm the music, the dancing, the difficultness, the cunningness, the foxiness, whatever it is, the impulsiveness, the violence, but these are also qualities of the spider. And then we need to generalise the spider qualities, describe what a spider is, and then come back to Tarantula and say what is it that differentiates *Tarantula* as an individual spider as opposed to general spider qualities, this will make issues very very clear. And then you will need to describe other spiders as well and then you'll need to study what is the classification of spiders which is basically into two, Aranomorphae and Mygalomorphae and there is an essential difference. The same story with *Lachesis*. When we study *Lachesis* we know that many qualities of Lachesis are qualities of serpent then we study snakes and we can then classify snakes into three or four main categories the Elapody and the Chrotolidy for example and then we understand so beautifully that the Chrotolidy is one that strikes and disappears. The Elapody is one that strikes and holds on and then we can understand the Elapody like *Naja, Black Mamba, Elaps corallinus* etc in one way and then you can understand the Chrotolidy like *Lachesis, Crotalus horridus, Crotalus cascavella* another way. And then the whole thing becomes clear. So many remedies come, so this way of studying materia medica within kingdoms and both of them feeding each other is in my understanding the ideal way to teach homeopathy.

AG

But hang on that's only one part of homeopathy. That's our tools, the technical parts and understanding our medicines. For example, Misha teaches sensation method from day one in his programme. So how would you ideally go about teaching case taking given what you know about gathering information from Hahnemann through to Vithoulkas and then to now what you're suggesting with sensation method?

RS

I think also in the case taking we need to also find a way. Again, this is what I do in case taking, I do exactly what we do traditionally is I take the case, I understand the physical symptoms, I understand modalities, I understand cravings, aversions, dreams, desires, sweat, sleep, position in sleep, so many factors that nothing is left out. But in addition to this we also think that one should go a little deeper into the experience of the patient and to see where this experience finds common ground in the mind and the body in the symptoms, physical symptoms and you will see that there is one experience that kind of brings all of this together and when you reach that depth, then the certainty becomes much much more.

AG

What are the qualities therefore that are crucial to teach a student when it comes to search for that level of depth.

RS

I think that at the first he must be conversant with what is basic. That means he must be conversant with what we know as traditional homeopathy and then he can be taught to go deeper into the experience of the patient.

AG

But we have an issue here. Because the students you have at this seminar are not conversant with the basics. Many are naturopaths with little homeopathy. Some have no medical sciences at all. You see those skills that you talk about, today for example, those skills of silence, of reflection, of listening, of observation and essentially of meditation; those are skills that are not traditionally taught in a homeopathy school or a medical degree. These skills you're asking students to employ, some have them but they haven't learnt them in homeopathy school.

RS

Again?

AG

What are the requisite skills of a good case taker and how can they be taught? Let me explain more. You see one of the things that happens with teachers is they forget what it's like to be an amateur, especially when they're a master and one of the jobs of teacher is to remember what is was like to know nothing One of the things that we face with modern students that sit in your lectures is that they get a handle on these advanced concepts sometimes before they've developed the skills of even knowing how to trace the image of the disease, you know those aphorisms of Hahnemann. So what is it, what makes, what are the skills that we need to teach confident and competent case takers?

RS

It is so much easier for me to describe cases rather than, I think I will describe you a case, that will be better. Can I?

So this was a patient I saw just a couple of days ago so it's fresh in my mind, I can remember it and his problem is he's a 35 year old male and his problem is insomnia for many years and he says its killing him, it is ruining his life and he's been like that for last ten years and he can hardly sleep at night. He's been to sleep therapists, he's been to five different homeopaths, he's been to alternative and so many... And because of the sleep disturbance he gets dizzy, blurred vision, he feels weak, he gets depressed, he cannot work and life is like almost coming to a standstill. So I ask him, describe what happens and I think the first quality that we need to teach the students is just to listen, just to listen, what is he saying, without any idea. And he says, I am nervous, I anticipate, I get embarrassed and even if there is anything exciting the next day like a competition or an examination or an excitement or even if there is something pleasurable, I am going to go out with a woman, I can't sleep. And even after the event I can't sleep because I'm still excited and so forth. Then he tells about his story, there's a big spiral in my mind, I can't push it away, I have guilt, I have this, I have dreams of spiders and delusion of spiders and I have fear of doctors because I had some problems in childhood and he says since I am from an ethnic background in a white community I felt very very not accepted and there was racist people there and so forth. I was victimised, I was isolated I was alone, I was ostracised and even the staff of my school treated me so badly because of my colour and I was hiding in a corner and there was no friends, it was like walking into a pack of lions. What we need to teach the students is to hear behind the story, the story may be anything, that he was ostracised, that he was victimised, he was racially discriminated, he was persecuted, treated unfairly, this is his story, this is what happened. But the question is, how did he experience it. To try and hear this, the experience behind the story, this is what we need to train, for herein lies the state of the person not in the story, not in the expression, not in the emotions. So how do we know then that, what is the expression, is because we need to teach the students to see what is common between the various things of the person. So if you feel that here is the story of victimisation and her e is the story of comparison and competition and this is animal but then this same experience must be found in a completely different area. Are you open? So we must teach the student not to get fixed with an idea and to be open to that which doesn't fit. So it looks like an animal so then I ask him, what do you like to do? He said the thing that I like to do most is swimming. And describe swimming: he says, swimming is like freedom, I feel freedom, rhythm, it is beautiful, it makes me feel alive, it is just me. The trees, the wind, my body, I feel so good. It is like ecstasy, it is like paradise, it is like bliss, it is like running by myself in a beautiful sunrise. So here, on the one hand he was describing being victimised and racially discriminated which looks like animal but when he talks about swimming, there is no discrimination, there is no racial, there is no competition, no comparison, no survival, no victim...it is just a sensory experience, almost a drug like state. So therefore that victimisation and racial discrimination is a fact that happened to him and not really his experience, his experience must be something else. Then he says, I was profoundly affected by the poverty and the homelessness in India, it was so...and so overbearing and then he talked about so many things but the main words that he used was it was overwhelming, everything was overwhelming, I was hyper-vigilant. So what we see common in his...is everything is overwhelming him, whether it be pleasure, pain, anxiety, whether it be anticipation, whether it be victim aggression thing, whether it be poverty or whatever, everything so much over whelms him and excites him that he finds no rest and the opposite is swimming and running where he is alone and he can shut out everything and he is in bliss because nothing excites him, nothing overwhelms him.

Now to hear this, to hear the commonality of what's happened, what is really his essential problem, what is it that he could remove, then he will be healthy? What is his chief complaint telling us? What is his insomnia talking to us of? To bring everything together and to see the commonality. This is the tool that we need to develop. And I ultimately in this case, it's quite interesting that the remedy we can think of from traditional homeopathy is *Coffea* because *Coffea* is the main remedy for insomnia, from too many thoughts and excitements and the whole idea of drinking coffee is overstimulation. So it's a really simple case but I didn't give him *Coffea*, I gave him something slightly different. What did I do? I said this is the *Coffea* family no doubt, Rubiaceae, but his miasm is not tubercular like *Coffea* but it is more like cancer, everything is going out of hand. He's so desperate, he can't control it, he wants to kill himself. It's a cancer miasm and in cancer miasm and the Rubiaceae family is *Galium aparine* and then I read a proving done by Misha Norland of *Galium* and the first word in the mind is overwhelmed. Overwhelmed by everything. This is the first symptom of the proving and then I read the proving together with the patient and he said ' I could have written every word of this'. That was the whole story so, these are the things we need the students to teach, to teach, listen, to listen behind. What is, who is the patient, who is it who is having this? Not what he is having not what situations he underwent, not what emotions happened to him but who is he who's talking? To observe the tread that runs through the entire story and the case and to listen behind and to identify and recognise that which is the patient. I think it's not difficult.

AG

I understand, this is the depth of the new method. So what are the differences between old fashioned sensation, location, modality, listen, keeping silent, writing everything down. With what you have just said in this case there's no difference so far. Just keeping silent and attention to detail, all of those things. But there's something else and that is its quite a courageous leap, courage is required to make a leap from Hahnemannian homeopathy to sensation method because immediately more, much more is required of the practitioner. They've got to be prepared to sit and be in a relationship and actually quite possibly be confronted with the unknown. Who knows what is going to come out when you ask a patient to describe which is quite possibly something which is unconscious to them. It seems to me that courage is a quality which is also needed.

RS

I would imagine also but I think it's very easy actually.

AG

Right right. Let me ask something else then. See one of the things that you know naturally, as does Misha as does Jeremy, is that it doesn't matter who they're talking to, they just relate to them and that's a skill that not everyone has. Just the ability to comfortably sit and be with somebody as they tell their story and not get involved in the story. One of the things which in an education institution teaching formal degrees in homeopathy is how do you teach that?

RS

I think you can actually. It is a skill no? What the psychotherapists do. They do the same thing. It can be taught. But to be honest, I teach students and they learn it quite easily. I don't see the difficulty. So many people. They pick it up, in fact they pick it up really easily. And maybe there are some people who have the ability to pick it up even more easily than others. There are maybe people who work at the fact level, maybe they don't want to pick it up but there are a huge number, especially those that come to learn homeopathy, are already having the background to do something deeper. I find most students and most homeopaths are quite perceptive in a way.

AG

Let me ask you another long question! So have you found, what are the things that are required also to make a leap or to make a change from Hahnemannian homeopathy through to the sensation method. Is it that there is a fundamental difference? I know you said there's not, but I think there is, and it's that from a traditional perspective homeopathy is the application of the law of similars from a proving. Now what you're saying and the implication from your work is that homeopathy is the application of something similar in its nature from nature. *Drosera* is given because it's the same energetically, as opposed to *Drosera* given because it does similar symptoms from a proving. I think that's a massive leap and one that lots of folks aren't prepared to take. You know, you got an email from Ken in Sydney, he's a fact man but you see he teaches, he's taught a generation of homeopaths in Australia and teaches really good homeopathy. Do I get him to teach first years and just Böenninghausen method or what do I do? Do you see some of the issues that I'm wrestling with, It is my responsibility now to really just, really get clear about how do we do this right? And so that jump. That is a jump. Similars from a proving is different to similars from nature.

RS

There are two answers to that question. The first is: at some point I believe we have to accept that there is no difference in the way because the proving is not coming from air it has to come from the nature of the substance. There cannot be any other. Otherwise, I mean what's the difference between say *Drosera* and *Lachesis* and a remedy. *Drosera* must represent *Drosera* the plant and *Lachesis* must represent *Lachesis* the snake somehow. Otherwise there's no sense at all.

AG

That's true but traditionally we give *Drosera* because in the proving it creates a certain sort of a cough.

RS

What I am saying is that the symptoms of the proving of *Drosera* must essentially represent the survival strategy of *Drosera* itself. The energy of *Drosera* is the only thing that can come in the proving. Number one. Number two, and this of course I have confirmed and verified in several provings; that the person exactly describes the quality of the source when asked deep enough. I mean is it a coincidence that *Thuja* has got the symptom that he's made of wood and that he's fragile and that he'll break into pieces and that's exactly the bark of *Thuja* tree. Is it funny that *Baptisia* that comes from the legume family has the symptom of parts getting split up and thrown all over is just peas and pods. I mean these are not coincidences any more

AG

But now this is very similar to signatures. I mean remember in Ireland you and Misha talking about that sensation method is not signatures.

RS

No, not at all.

AG

It's hard to describe it in any other way sometimes, when you talk to students or members of the public.

RS

It is not signature.

AG

Or critics of homeopathy

RS

It is that the survival strategy, the existence of that particular source of nature will be reflected in the proving. There is a symptom in *Lachesis*, tongue darting in and out like a snake, it's a proving symptom. Can we say that this is completely divorced from the snake? Then how do we not say that that proving symptom is a signature?

AG

Because not all snakes have it?

RS

Every snake, every snake has to put the tongue out?

AG

Clearly you're comfortable with that idea

RS

But there's a huge difference with being. What is a doctrine of signatures is saying that the proving represents the source completely. And there is no other way than that the remedy is the source incarnated. The spirit of the source. In a way we cannot see even. For example this patient described the movement up the stairs like this: 'I arch back and pull myself, I arch back and pull myself, I arch back'. This is how she's describing. I did not know that this was. It was on the internet. So when you say signature, it means, like what you see. People are so gross about it. They say when I teach *Chelidonium* and I...something yellow comes out, it's good for jaundice...doctrine of signatures.

AG

But this is what's happening and one of the things is, you know, and it is a consequence with some of this work with families over the last ten years is we've got people saying, Lac delphinum has these qualities as a remedy because of all of this projected anthropomorphised nonsense about what people fantasise about what dolphins are like and what they do and ultimately what we think dolphins do.

RS

This is grossly wrong.

AG

It is.

RS

But if you study carefully that particular source and take out specific qualities of it then you will see that those qualities are found in the patients. And it would be really fantastic to see that. Not gross. Not, when the patient said, when I walk, I just go like this and like this and like this so I gave him *Kangaroo*. This is nonsense. In order that the patient gets *Kangaroo*, not only we have to walk like this but he must he have the entire constellation, the entire group of symptoms of animal, of mammal, of particular the species of kangaroo and the kangaroo itself in ways that we don't even know.

AG

See you remember, I mean you couldn't forget, back in 1999 that Vithoulkas interview came out, remember? Where he went for you and Jeremy and Jan and quite superficial criticisms of the method and you know new provings and the rest of it. Do you agree with one of the things he said, that one of the problems, one of the reasons that homeopathy is struggling now after the big boom in the eighties is because of some poor practices with what we do within the profession. You know things like we were just saying about dolphins because of whatever or jumping like kangaroos. I mean we do in Australia, we've got people in that room today who will be prescribing like that. I know it's not what you advocate. It's a real problem, really superficial stuff.

RS

Superficial. Superficial homeopathy is also a problem. Something has to be understood in depth and I can say one thing for sure that there is absolutely no doubt in my mind that the remedy represents the source completely and therefore qualities of the source are as useful information about the remedy as the provings are and they should complement each other and in fact one is the mirror of the other. It's just the mirror of the other. And I also agree with you that sometimes this can be done superficially and sometimes taken too far and especially with people without grounding in the foundations it can be taken very very far, more than necessary and that can be very harmful. And I'm trying to antidote that in a way. I'm doing something very interesting in the last month and I think that that will help someone.

AG

You see for me that last comment at the end of the day that you made was a really important one, you know just to ground everything.

RS

What did I say?

AG

You just said it is really important to work from the foundations, medical science, Hahnemannian homeopathy, sensation, location, modality, and then you can fly. Really really important.

RS

So what, I'll tell you what I'm doing at the moment. I'm starting an online course from March. It's called Wednesdays with Rajan and I'll be teaching every Wednesday for one and a half years. It will be on the computer so people can watch from everywhere in the world, unfortunately probably not in Australia.

AG

Why? It's only four hours difference.

RS

I will be starting at 8.30 or something. At night. That's late.

AG

That's starting 12.30. On breeze or Skype or what platform?

RS

It will be on something called live web or something. It's like a television. So you can log into it and you can see me speak and there is a dialog box in which you can type your questions and I can read and everybody can read it and then I can answer the questions and then you can ask me questions afterwards which I will answer by email. This is the program. And over one and a half years the main idea of this doing course is very simple. It is to integrate traditional and sensational homeopathy. That is what I will do. Because for me this is completely integrated into my practice and I want to teach that through, I'm going to teach through 100 cases. And all I'm going to teach is integration. I'm going to use in that course repertory, materia medica and the new matter all together and to show that's how I work.

AG

I think that that's a fantastic idea.

RS

I felt the need to do it, so you can imagine that I must have the same apprehension that you're expressing.

AG

I think you know, you've obviously had some feedback around. Well you know, what it's like in the west for example when you're not a doctor, to try questioning. You would have heard stories about people brutalising their patients with really inappropriate questions. And so, it's really important to clarify aspects of the method and it's a great thing. Because what happened in the mid nineties, in Spirit, Substance, the idea was essentially to find the delusion, get into the mind and forget about the presenting symptom. And then happily you really quite clearly changed, well started to say no, no, no, remember the presenting symptom. Remember that's the portal into the case. That's what you were saying, that's what you are saying. I think that's really important. It's good.

RS

But it's changing again. I'm taking another step and that step is integration. Bringing it together with the tradition. I fear the same thing and I want to show it. Even with this seminar I began with the concepts but now tomorrow and the day after I will bring it back to show that it's the same thing but its expanded. The course I am doing. I'm doing this more as a service rather than something that I don't know if I will have the energy because it's a lot of commitment one and a half years every Wednesday to sit there and answer all those emails afterwards, it's not easy. But it's something that's satisfying me a lot because I want to bring my practice into the teaching. Because what happens that when you go into a seminar, you don't want to teach *Calcarea carbonate, Natrum mur.* Because you feel that it's not worthwhile for them you know that they paid money and they don't want *Natrum muriatricum* and you want to teach them very exotic things. It's a natural tendency. Because it's also something you're excited about you know. You give *Calcarea carb* to the patient, they got better, it didn't excite you. It doesn't matter it was cancer, it was just *Calcarea carb*. So I want to bring the reality of practice into the teaching and that's why this is not going to be a seminar of three days, it's going to be an extended one and a half year thing. Therefore, the real facts, the ground reality has to come out here.

AG

Well tell me about something else then because in my work one of the significant things that I've been doing and emphasising is this: it looks from your practice and the way you teach that the emphasis is definitely on finding the medicine, the central piece, finding the remedy. That is number one. The second thing is we know some things about homeopathic students, especially in Australia, New Zealand, England, America and the west. They're not very confident and they're anxious. Compared to an osteopathic student or a physiotherapist you know and one of the reasons is because it's so daunting, there's so much pressure because when the patient comes in they've got to find the remedy. So in reality in my practice, all I do is have relationships with my clients and I do my best and if I get it right I have a little dance and it's good but if I don't then they come back next time and we work further and further towards the central issue. So it's more of a relationship than a medicine, than a holy grail. You are certainly still emphasising the remedy in your work.

RS

I think the remedy is very important because I know that I do the same as you. I don't find it right the first time each time. We have to work, sometimes it takes a couple of years also. So we have to work each time but ultimately one day we have to find the remedy for the patient. Until we do that, things don't really move. But I don't encourage the student to be anxious or worried about it, I say just be easy, be calm, be relaxed and see what happens and it will come. And usually this strategy works. And I, to be honest, I think that one of the reasons that the whole development of these systems came about was because there was a lot of confusion and one didn't know because you take a particular set of symptoms, you come to a remedy, you take another set, you come to another remedy and there was not the certainty in the practice. That was the reason the systems had to be developed otherwise homeopathy was perfect and you could take the symptom, put it into some repertory programme and out came the remedy, I wouldn't need to do anything. And I think the systems and understanding of the kingdoms and stuff, does increase certainty in practice, if it is done the right way. And at least when the patient talks and you come to something, at least you have a map to know where to go and what to do. And if that's backed up by traditional homeopathic knowledge and rubrics and materia medica, you are fairly certain.

AG

You see in Australia most homeopaths need the bread and butter, to earn a living out of their practice. I think its hard with three hour consultations. Most homeopaths aren't medically trained. We do good medical science, but we are professional homeopaths, not medical. And to run a practice often it's quick prescribing, knowledge of keynotes and things like that helps with earning a living. So sometimes it's hard to know what to say to students.

RS

But I don't think this method takes three hour consultations all the time. I can do it in half an hour, sometimes 20 minutes, 1 hour, 1.5 hours. Some cases are very easy, it comes very easily and some cases take longer where it's rare and I think at a student level and a beginner level you will get rather easy cases. When you get more experienced, more difficult cases will come which may take a little longer. But it doesn't necessarily mean that cases take longer. If you develop a new practice you can see it very quickly. So I don't think time is an important thing. The second thing of course is that I often found that if you don't give the time that is needed in the first consultation you are going to suffer for a long time afterwards but if you put in enough time and effort and take what it needs, it may need half an hour it may need two hours it may need six hours, I don't know. Mostly doesn't need that long, but if you have the space to give the time that's needed and say 'I'm going to really get to the depth of the case, doesn't matter what time it takes' then first of all its quicker and secondly you don't have to waste time in the follow ups, it goes so smoothly. Because after I do the new case I reached such a comprehensive understanding of that case that I don't need to think about it for six months. That it. So I the time spent in the first case is really an investment and I don't see a substitute for it.

AG

So essentially the whole strategy is 'understand the patient, understand the patient, understand the patient'.

RS

Yes that's it.

AG

Leave the remedy stuff until the end, it will come.

RS

It will come automatically to you, you just have to focus on, what it is that the patient is going through, what is really going through him? What is really behind all the...expressions, what is he essentially, what was he essentially from his childhood until now? What is he presenting now in every aspect of his life. You have to keep the focus single mindedly on that and with every expression you have to go deeper and deeper and deeper till you touch the level which is common to the whole, it's just simple like that and sometimes it comes so easily, in five sentences. I've practiced in hospital OPD, every Monday from 9 until 11. In two hours I have to see sometimes 60 to 80 patients, out of them 15 or 20 are new. I get less than 2 or 3 minutes to see a new case. The success rate is very high over there. First of all, patients are simpler and secondly you have to just put your focus completely on what's there in the moment. I enjoy that practice like that.

AG

It's good.

RS

You have 3 minutes sometimes, 2 minutes. You have to get to the, get very, and with practice you can do it, you can get to it very quickly. It's the same thing like anything else, in any state or art. I saw once, once I saw, I was in the medical college and I went to the surgery department and I saw the house physician...the surgery department was under training, he did a hydrocele operation and it took him like 40 minutes to do it and there was so much blood and ten stitches and then, then the next case was also a hydrocele and this was done by a very skilled surgeon. It took him less than four or five minutes, there was one stitch and not a drop of blood, it was so fantastic. So as you practice, you just, it comes naturally but you have to do it right. For any reason we can't do it not right, in a sense we can't do something we don't believe in. I don't like that idea. I am short of time so I'll do it. I know it's not right but I'll do it anyway because I don't have time. This doesn't, it's not right.

AG

Good, that's very useful. What I have to do is write curriculum and at some point introduce, family, sensation, case taking. You know? And it's important that we get it right. One of the things that we're trying to do in Australia or in this college is create a more formal structure for teaching rather than what a lot of homeopaths around the world get, especially in America. You know, seminar, this, that, you know cobble a homeopathic understanding together.

RS

That is what I'm also attempting to do through that Wednesday thing. For the first time I am trying to teach a course, in which everything will be systematically organised you know, first this, then this, then that, first the conception, the case taking then the repertory, materia medica, then the kingdoms, the whole course is laid out. I think I even have it, integrating the knowledge or remedy and kingdom knowledge and systems complement each other. Concepts, case taking, kingdoms, families, animals, minerals, repertory, cases, remedies, materia medica, potencies.

AG

Fantastic. You've put a lot of work into that, fantastic.

RS

It is the integration between sensation and repertory and materia medica. And I am writing a book on it, it's called *The Simplicity of Homeopathy*.

AG

Nice. What about The Soul of Remedies, do you still use it in – with its focus on 'feeling'?

RS

No. The *Soul* somehow remains useful even to me because everything there is true but now we understand it even deeper but it doesn't negate what is written there. It is highly useful that book. Because I wrote it from what I saw you know, it cannot be wrong. But now we understand it deeper, in terms of the family, the kingdoms.

AG

Do you feel, do you think that those maps of nature that we are using, the family kingdoms, the periodic table, do you think that we are getting close? Do you think that the work has charted enough of the plant families and the animals remedies? Or is there still lots of work?

RS

No, no, a lot of it but we have at least a skeleton. At least. And that's very useful in practice but we have a long way to go. It's not going to get completed in two, three lifetimes also but at least it's a beginning. I have a lot of failures in my practice and so I know there is a long way to go, in understanding concepts, understanding families. Every failure teaches us that we are deficient, that we are incomplete. Every success gives us hope and encouragement.

AG

In my development, what I remember was essentially, aim for the centre, at all times, shut up and aim for the centre. But what it lead to in my early years of practice was lots and lots of polycrest prescribing. And all I gave was Natrum mur and Lycopodium and you know, 1980's essence prescribing, and so this, the sophistication that you have developed with all of the maps that we have now means that it's possible. You know to go for the centre and not prescribe bland polycrests. I think it's very important.

RS

And we must also keep open to the peculiar symptoms at the same time. I had two weeks ago, I had a patient who had severe headaches, they were proceeded by blurredness and like a dimness of vision and then she'd get severe migraine attacks. And I looked up these peculiar some symptoms that she had, led to *Iris* remedy, beautiful. It was so strange, the exact symptoms that she described of *Iris*, it was there. That's it. So why should you neglect it. IF the patient is giving it to you on a platter and describing very very peculiar symptoms, do look in the repertory and go for it.

AG

Rajan, thanks so much.

The multiple consequences of Sankaran's quickly evolving work will reverberate round our profession for years. Of it's value there can be no doubt. But it also seems that it is not finished nor a complete system yet. The details, intricacies and internal logic all need some substantial ironing out. It's integration into, or separation from, traditional Hahnemannian homeopathy is still to be determined, and the timing and level to which it is taught and pitched is undecided. In addition, it needs time to settle, and most of all needs verification in the clinic. A profession is based upon best practice, evidence, research, critical thinking and evaluation. There is not enough water under the bridge or honest rigorous debate yet to accept wholesale the sensation method.

The Requirements of the Case Taker using Sensation Method

Time

Allow space and time to wander

Follow

Be a fool. Know nothing

Look for the expression of energy

Look for that which is non-human specific in this case

Part Three

Patient-Centered Medicine and the Relationship

I invited a friend and colleague, Ben Gadd to write a chapter for the third part of this book as I felt it important to confirm for the contemporary homeopath that case taking is not simply about getting information from a patient in order to do something to them. Homeopathy is afterall more than the dispensing of medicines. It is intended that this third part bookends the directives of the old masters and reminds homeopaths of the sophisticated nature of the therapeutic relationship that they engage in. This is all the more necessary as the climate of evidence based medicine impacts on all areas of based medicine.

Part Three

Patient-Centered Medicine and the Relationship

Chapter 10

The Therapeutic Relationship in Homeopathy – Ben Gadd

- Why a Therapeutic Relationship?
- What Patients Want from a Consultation
- Common Elements in the Therapeutic Relationship
- Homeopathy and Psychotherapy
- Homeopathic and Allopathic Consultations
- Placebo
- Empathy
- Patient-centeredness
- Therapeutic Alliance and Compassion
- Impact of Homeopathic Process and Philosophy of Disease

In this chapter you will
1. Learn what is meant by a therapeutic alliance.
2. Understand a patient-centred approach.
3. Familiarize yourself with the literature and understand the qualities of the case taker from this perspective.

Chapter 10

The Therapeutic Relationship in Homeopathy – Ben Gadd

In his guidelines for case-taking, Hahnemann demands freedom from prejudice, application of sound senses, attention in observing, refraining from interrupting, and the use of open-ended questions (Hahnemann 1922). While homeopaths adhere to these techniques as the foundation of taking a history, case-taking has expanded beyond this skill set, with an understanding of a range of therapeutic techniques that are useful in interactions with patients.

Since Hahnemann, with an increasing knowledge of the benefits of the therapeutic relationship, there has been growing interest in the idea of the homeopathic consultation as beneficial in itself; for example, patients may state that they feel better after the consultation, even before any medicine has been given. Indeed, many patients regard their involvement in the process of telling their story as empowering, enlightening, and therapeutic.

The therapeutic relationship is difficult to define: it is a complex phenomenon, incorporating various dimensions ranging from behaviours and skills to social, institutional, and cultural contexts. Emerging from psychoanalysis, the key idea is that it is the relationship that is central in helping the client change. In complementary and alternative medicine (CAM), this change is most likely to be in the area of wellbeing. In its basic form, the therapeutic relationship can be defined as 'the mutually beneficial, professional bond that exists between a health care professional and their patient' (Wagner 2006:13).

Empirical research into the role of the therapeutic relationship in homeopathic consultations is minimal despite studies that clearly show that the role of the relationship is an important one that has a positive impact on clinical outcomes. Research into therapeutic relationships comes mainly from psychotherapeutic disciplines, and while clearly applicable to homeopathy, an increasing emphasis (or overemphasis) on the importance of psychological understanding of cases may mean that we have uncritically embraced some of these ideas, without determining if they truly apply to the homeopathic understanding of disease and healing, or developing our own robust knowledge base in this area.

This chapter will explore some of these ideas, looking at why the therapeutic relationship is important, and at the research in this area. Some of the similarities and differences between therapeutic understanding in homeopathy and psychotherapy will be looked at, as well as research looking at the differences between allopathic and homeopathic consultations.

Some of the underpinning concepts that are important to understanding the therapeutic relationship in homeopathy will be touched upon, including placebo (or self-healing responses), empathy, patient centredness, and therapeutic warmth. Not all of these attributes are essential to homeopathic consultations, but undoubtedly they can contribute to some of the positive outcomes in homeopathic practice. Moreover, homeopathic understanding of patients means that some of these therapeutic features are a natural consequence of homeopathic case-taking, while the trend towards evidence based and technology-based medicine may, for some patients, unfortunately minimise the therapeutic effect.

Why a Therapeutic Relationship?

I was already feeling a lot better yesterday... you see I get better just from seeing you, even before you give me the remedy. (Patient quote)

There are many benefits to a therapeutic relationship in any health care encounter. At a basic level, gathering a patient's history and health information occurs with greater ease within a therapeutic relationship. Patients are more willing to disclose, particularly sensitive information, and a number of studies show that patient satisfaction is higher. Research shows a positive correlation between effective patient-practitioner communication and improved health outcomes (Cape 2000, Kaplan et al. 1989, Martin et al. 2000, Stewart 1995).

The therapeutic relationship can help to develop trust in the patient, create a safe space for the disclosure of information, a sense of being listened to and understood, and enhance treatment effects. Therapists more able to form a strong alliance with their patients show statistically significant better outcomes; the relationship can be seen as a medicine of sorts, with important therapeutic effects for patients. Consultations can be seen as treatments in themselves (Baldwin et al. 2007, Marnocha 2009, Mercer 2001).

At best, the homeopath can become a therapeutic resource for his or her patients through the process of case-taking and homeopathic enquiry. By developing the skills of the therapeutic relationship, the practitioner becomes an active ingredient in healing (Balint 1957, Budd 1994, Hyland 2005).

What Patients Want from a Consultation

So they [homeopaths] kind of get context before rushing to tell you what's wrong. (Patient quote, cited in McIntosh & Ogunbanjo 2008:69a)

When I first went to a homeopath, it seemed remarkable that the practitioner was interested in who I was, my background, influences on my health, my disposition and temperament, responses to environment, the weather, and so on. After all, I had a skin condition, so how could all that information possibly be related? My dermatologist had never been interested in such details.

Patients often turn to complementary medicine after having tried everything that conventional medicine has to offer (Zollman & Vickers 1999). While most people are looking for a solution to a health problem, some come frustrated with past health consultations or poor relationships with practitioners. Complaints include rushed consultations, being asked too few questions, a lack of enquiry or emphasis on context, and poor bedside manner (McIntosh & Ogunbanjo 2008).

Evidence shows that communication is highly valued in primary care consultations (Cheraghi-Sohi et al. 2008, Scott

& Vick 1999, Vick & Scott 1998). Patients want relationships where they experience trust and the right amount of autonomy, caring, and expertise (Epstein 2006). Caring, from the patient's perspective, is seen as involving effective communication, getting needs met, and the practitioner being respectful and empathic (Quirk et al. 2008).

There are several studies that consistently demonstrate that patients who choose homeopathy value the length of consultations, a whole-person approach, being treated like an individual, and telling and having their 'story' listened to in depth. Also, patients value equity of the relationship, mutual respect, shared decision making, and taking more of an active part in their health care (Eyles et al. 2009, Luff & Thomas 2000, Marian et al. 2008, McIntosh & Ogunbanjo 2008, Mercer & Reilly 2004, Ratcliffe et al. 2002, Rise & Steinsbekk 2009, Steinsbekk 2005, Vincent & Furnham 1996, Wensing et al. 1998).

The resulting homeopathic medicine from my first consultation produced an immediate improvement in my skin condition, but more than that, I left the consultation with a new understanding of how all my complaints were connected, a sense of wellbeing, and a feeling that I had been listened to by a health care practitioner like never before.

Common Elements in the Therapeutic Relationship

When I started studying psychiatric nursing, I was amazed at the variety of therapeutic techniques available: person-centred approaches, supportive psychotherapy, interpersonal psychotherapy, exposure therapy, cognitive restructuring techniques; a whole range of techniques that place different emphasis on context, learning, and the relationship between practitioner and patient. As my training went on, it dawned on me that some people were good at forming relationships with their patients, while others just didn't seem to be able to do it, no matter what therapy they used. Better practitioners seemed to get results no matter what techniques they used.

Research into the therapeutic relationship is complicated; therapist effects are difficult to study and data difficult to interpret (Frank 2002). Most research in the area has been done in the field of psychology and psychotherapy. For example, the following factors of the therapeutic encounter may affect treatment outcomes in some way: client characteristics; therapist characteristics; therapist reactions, perceptions, and feelings about the client; therapist direct influence skills/behaviour; counselor and interpersonal skills/behaviour; therapist self-disclosure; client autonomy; client perception of the therapist's credibility and persuasiveness; client willingness to participate/hopefulness for change; affect towards the therapist; and client participation (Karver et al. 2005).

Literature on the therapeutic relationship tends to examine one or more characteristics of clinicians, such as empathy, listening behaviours, communication styles, etc., then correlates these with outcome measures, typically patient satisfaction. The difficulty of this is that in all likelihood a healing relationship, for example as developed by homeopaths, is more than a sum of its parts, and so needs to be studied as a whole system (Quinn et al. 2003).

Di Blasi et al. (2001) showed in a systematic review that enhancing patients' expectations through positive information about the treatment or illness, while providing support or reassurance, significantly influenced health outcomes.

Research in medicine shows that verbal behaviours positively associated with health outcomes include empathy, reassurance and support, various patient-centred questioning techniques, encounter length, history taking, explanations, positive reinforcement, humour, psychosocial talk, friendliness, courtesy, and summarisation and clarification (Beck et al 2002). Therapist attributes of being flexible, honest, respectful, trustworthy, confident, warm, interested, and open have been found to contribute to the development of a therapeutic alliance (Ackerman & Hilsenroth 2003).

Research into different therapies shows that there is little difference between different schools of therapy, leading to the conclusion that there are common factors at work which explain these results (Asay & Lambert 1999, Blow & Sprenkle 2001, Blow et al. 2007, Catty 2004, Eisler 2006, Horvath & Symonds 1991, Lambert 1992, Messer & Wampold 2002). Success in therapy results from a number of factors, the most important of which may not actually be due to the therapy itself, but to client variables and extra-therapeutic influences (e.g., patient motivation, maturity, ability to become productively involved in therapy, social supports) (Bohart 2000).

Relationship factors however are important for improvement, and common factors (or core conditions) in different therapeutic disciplines are described in the person centred approach of Carl Rogers: accurate empathy, unconditional positive regard, non-possessive warmth, and congruence or genuineness (Rogers 1951, Rogers 1957). Expectancy and placebo also appear to have an influence (Asay & Lambert 1999).

Mercer and colleagues have undertaken studies into the therapeutic relationship in homeopathy at the Glasgow Homeopathic Hospital; empowerment (defined as coping and understanding one's illness better as a result of seeing the doctor) is also correlated with positive health outcomes (Mercer 2005).

Homeopathy and Psychotherapy

Homeopathy can learn from psychotherapy. Many good homeopathic case-taking skills mirror good counseling skills, such as active listening, providing empathy, positive regard for clients, and a curiosity in the patient's way of viewing the world. Psychotherapy can help us to understand elements that are important in the therapeutic relationship. Transferable skills can benefit homeopathic practice - and arguably better practitioners utilise good listening skills, as well as the use of clinical supervision to explore therapeutic use of self, impasses, stuck cases, and so on.

There is a potential problem though, when we move towards wholeheartedly integrating psychotherapeutic or psychodynamic concepts into our homeopathic framework. At its fullest extent, this integration somewhat mirrors psychoanalysis' use of the therapeutic relationship as a diagnostic tool. Yet we have a fundamentally different model of understanding disease and treatment than psychotherapists (Adams 2009), meaning the skill sets may be complementary, but are not interchangeable.

I may appreciate when the patient requiring *Aurum* tells me that he has a fear of high places since he is certain that he will fall, because it seems to symbolically represent his unconscious dread of falling from his high position of responsibility. However, there is no need to speculate about unconscious phantasies and symbolic meaning. Much more reliable is turning to the proving to find the symptom, 'dreams he was about to fall from a great height' (Hahnemann 2007 symptom *CD413*).

The danger of an overemphasis on the therapeutic relationship is that it may result in a delving into the mind that becomes one-sided. An overemphasis on psychological symptoms is not holistic; it results in a Swedenborgian notion of the hierarchy of man that is not individualised to the patient.

Modern psychological understanding of cases can become speculative and judgmental (Bridger 1998). It follows a modern trend of believing that the cause of disease arises from disturbances in the mind, or dysfunctional ways of viewing the world. Of course, conjecture as to the cause of illness is not new; it was this that drove Hahnemann to discover homeopathy in the first place. The resulting system of homeopathy had no requirement for speculation about the causes of disease, which Hahnemann cautions us against (Hahnemann 1922 §6).

Homeopaths have different requirements for understanding the mind than other therapists. Homeopathy pays little attention to common symptoms, so that, for example, delusions in a patient with a psychotic disorder are not unusual, and so are unlikely to be a characteristic symptom from a homeopathic perspective. Different symptoms, taking grief as an example, will be considered differently within different frameworks. In psychiatry, pathological grief may be identified from understanding normal bereavement and its relationship with related disorders, such as major depressive disorder

(Stroebe et al. 2000). For the homeopath, understanding grief may depend more on the extent to which it is an aetiological component of the patient's complaint, and what characterises that particular grief state in that individual. Grief, after all, is no more diagnostic than a fever, and requires characterising before it becomes useful in finding the simillimum.

Moreover, there is a danger of using psychological techniques in case-taking that are in fact not therapeutic. As a student of homeopathy, I remember observing a practitioner who used silence as a main therapeutic technique, on the grounds that she was a 'blank page' who could absorb the patients' projections that would lead her to identify the homeopathic medicine. The result was a string of long and increasingly uncomfortable silences, whereby patients became obviously frustrated with not understanding what the practitioner wanted, and why no one in the room was saying anything.

Psychotherapeutic techniques, then, can add to the skills of the homeopathic practitioner both from the perspective of improving the therapeutic relationship, and of improving the quality of case-taking. However, practitioners should be competent to practise these skills, and use them in a way that is consistent with homeopathic philosophy.

Homeopathic and Allopathic Consultations

It is much more important to know what sort of patient has the disease than to know what sort of disease the patient has.
(William Osler cited in Porter 1997:682)

In a comparison of primary care physicians or general practice and homeopathic consultations, the context in which the interaction takes place is relevant (Peräkylä et al. 2005). For example, discussion of eating and drinking patterns is different according to the context in which the information is sought (Lindfors & Raevaara 2005). In an allopathic framework, such information is sought to understand potential contributions to poor health; in homeopathy, it is sought also as an indication of patterns of individual susceptibility and of homeopathic pathogenesis.

Studies comparing homeopathy and general practice consultations have shown that homeopathy patients in general are more oriented towards ideas of holism and the importance of their own individual perspective, and that this affects their narrative (Ruusuvuori 2005a). Homeopaths when compared with general practice physicians demonstrate more empathy and more neutrality with regard to patients' opinions and a greater range for showing compassion (Ruusuvuori 2005b). Studies of routine medical consultations often show avoidance of 'empathic opportunities', either by ignoring them, or by returning to a diagnostic exploration of symptoms (Platt & Platt 1998, Suchman et al. 1997).

Mishler discusses the idea that there are two separate voices in consultations (Barry et al. 2001, Mishler 1984, Mishler et al. 1989), the voice of medicine, in which a technological model of medicine, and physician control or dominance, is compared with the voice of the Lifeworld, in which patients can verbalise meaningful and coherent accounts of their problems. In the former, the practitioner asks response-constraining questions that follow a logic of enquiry based on a biomedical model (by stripping the context). In the latter, there is a connection between the questions, and the content and internal cohesiveness of the patient account. Listening to the voice of Lifeworld involves asking open-ended questions, and minimal interruption. Focusing on the voice of Lifeworld brings greater reciprocity to the relationship. Homeopathy, by necessity, seeks internal consistency, and hence an understanding of the Lifeworld, as part of identifying the totality of symptoms, just as it searches for coherence in homeopathic provings.

Interruption of patient narratives is obviously a factor resulting from time constraints. In one study physicians redirected the patient's opening statement after a mean of 23.1 seconds (Epstein et al. 2008; Marvel et al. 1999). After redirection, descriptions are rarely completed. Haidet and Paterniti (2003) note that once interruptions occur, the patient soon learns that short biomedically oriented answers are preferred and starts to leave out other details that they think the practitioner is not interested in. This means that patients' agendas may go unvoiced (Barry et al. 2000; Heritage et al 2007). Emotional wellbeing is sometimes not asked about in conventional care, even in situations where treatment is known to provoke psychological problems (Ford et al. 1996).

While much research has been done into allopathic consultations, there is much less empirical research into homeopathic consultations. Di Blasi and Kleijnen (2000) observed a number of homeopathic consultations and identified that there was evidence of sharing and partnership building, with the homeopath creating a safe space to express feelings and the therapist's ability to understand the patient, and the maximising of placebo effects.

Placebo

The doctor knows that it is the prescription slip itself, even more than what is written on it, that is often the vital ingredient for enabling a patient to get rid of whatever is ailing him. (Cousins 1980:58)

For a thousand years the action of the placebo has made vast numbers of patients feel better; have we today produced a consultation in which the placebo does not act? (Thomas 1987:1202)

The logical conclusion from the variance between a meta-analysis showing homeopathic remedies are no better than placebo (Shang et al. 2005) and outcome studies showing significant clinical improvements in large numbers of patients (Spence et al. 2005, Witt et al. 2008), indicates that the analysis of Shang and colleagues is unsound, or that homeopaths are particularly good at utilising placebo effects to produce outcomes that others seem unable to produce.

In homeopathic trials, placebo responders have shown clinically significant improvements in their conditions (Whetherly Jones et al. 2004a), moreover, two interventions may have different effects on outcome even though they are both equivalent to placebo in clinical trials (Vickers & de Craen 2000).

The latest scientific evidence indicates that placebo responses arise from active processes in the brain that are mediated by psychological mechanisms, such as expectation and conditioning, where the environmental and psychosocial context of treatment is important (Benedetti 2008, Busse & Lemanske 2009, Price et al. 2008). Placebo is an essential part of the double-blind, placebo-controlled, randomised clinical trial as a comparative measure. It is usually tolerated as nuisance noise and generally considered as inconsequential or with contempt (van Weel 2001). Some authors suggest that placebo responses can hinder the development of new treatments, as high placebo response rates can invalidate the effects of a therapy. A consequence of this is a call for further understanding of placebo so that its effects can be minimised (Enck et al. 2008).

An alternative way of seeing the placebo effect is as the self-healing capacities of the patient, as a therapeutic effect in itself (Di Blasi & Kleijnen 2000, Kaptchuk 2002). Walach and Jonas define placebo response as the effect that is the result of the meaning of a therapeutic intervention for a particular patient and context. If patients receive clear and positive communications conveyed with trust, credibility, and confidence, then healing is more likely (Walach & Jonas 2004).

Research shows that placebo effects are due to a variety of factors, such as:

- Patient characteristics (e.g. treatment and illness beliefs, desires and expectations, preference for intervention type, memory of previous experiences, somatic focus)
- Treatment characteristics (e.g. colour, size, shape of drug, frequency of dosing)
- Practitioner characteristics (e.g. beliefs and expectations, optimism, enthusiasm in suggesting treatments)
- Patient-practitioner characteristics (e.g. therapeutic alliance, length of consultation, assurances of recovery, communication of concern, compassionate care, opportunity for dialogue, agreement about the nature of the problem)
- Nature of illness (e.g. subjective symptoms, chronic conditions with a fluctuating course often influenced by selective attention)

(Di Blasi & Kleijnen 2000, Kaptchuk 2002, Price et al. 2008, Turner et al. 1994)

If placebo response accounts for self-healing capability, then it is perhaps surprising that more attention has not been given to how placebo effect can be enhanced in consultations. Understanding placebo is a way of understanding the normal healing response (Reilly 2001) and so is aligned with many CAM therapies that attempt the same.

Empathy

Well, he just didn't seem interested in what I had to tell him. He might know about kidneys but he didn't want to know what I was worried about. (Patient cited in Platt et al 2001:1079)

Empathy comes from the German word *Einfühlung*, meaning 'feeling into' the experience of another person (Feller & Cottone 2003). Empathy is defined as the ability to imagine oneself in another's place and understand the other's feelings, desires, and reactions. In psychiatry, it has been defined as the capacity to put oneself into the psychological frame of reference of another and thereby understand that person's thinking, feeling, and behaviour (Wynn & Wynn 2006). From a homeopathic perspective, empathy is aligned with the principle of similars, and in searching for the simillimum in case-taking, homeopaths may engage in unintentional empathy.

Empathy is a core determinant of quality in medical care (Neumann et al. 2009), and yet there are many studies showing poor consultational empathy in conventional settings (for example, see Evans et al 2007, Ring et al. 2005).

Carl Rogers defines empathy as 'to sense the client's private world as if it were your own, but without losing the 'as if' quality' (Rogers 1961:284), emphasising the importance of not merging the experience of the client with one's own experiences.

Empathy is an attribute related to the understanding and communication of emotions in a way that patients value (Hemmerdinger et al. 2007), an appreciation of the other's troublesome feelings (Ruusuvuori 2005b). It is regarded as essential for the development of the therapeutic relationship and is responsible for improved satisfaction, increased diagnostic accuracy, and improved outcomes (Horvath & Symonds 1991, Krupnick et al. 1996/2006, Mercer & Reynolds 2002).

Basic empathic skills include recognising when emotions may be present but not directly expressed, inviting exploration of these unexpressed feelings, and effectively acknowledging these feelings so that the patient feels understood (Suchman et al.1997). In studying how practitioners demonstrate empathy, it is '... not only by making accurate comments about a patient's feelings, but by their timing, vocal tones, pauses, and overall attunement to the affective style of a patient' (Halpern 2001:93), noting that empathy comes from a totality, rather than being the sum of separate actions.

Empathy is a reciprocal transaction; it is something that is both conveyed and received. Patients must receive empathy; a lack of receipt may result in signs of conversational failure such as reformulations, pausing, or an abrupt change of topic (Wynn & Wynn 2006)

An increased ability to cope with illness is correlated with patients' perception of their doctor's empathy (Mercer et al.

2001/2002). Patients undergoing homeopathic consultations consistently report a high degree of empathy (Mercer 2001, Mercer & Reilly 2004, Thompson & Weiss 2006).

Empathy has different dimensions: cognitive, affective, sharing, and behavioural components have been discussed in the literature, although there is some disagreement about the relative value of each of these, with Halpern (2003) arguing that detached concern is more valued in medicine than affective empathy. It may have a therapeutic effect in itself, deepen the therapeutic bond, and facilitate trust and disclosure (Mercer & Reynolds 2002; Wynn & Wynn 2006).

Patient-centredness

> *One of the greatest skills of a doctor, and a topic often left out of the debate around evidence based medicine, is individualisation...it is expected that any therapist who individualises his treatment will have better results, because he can harness the meaning response.* (Walach & Jonas 2004:S-109)

The concept of patient-centredness was introduced by Balint as a way to understand patients' complaints not in terms of disease, but in terms of the individuality of the patient or 'the patient's total experience of illness' (Balint 1957, Howie et al. 2004, van Dulmen 2003). Homeopathy has been described as a 'perfect example of patient-centred medicine' (Frank 2002), and indeed can only be patient-centred, due to its requirements for large amounts of patient information, symptoms, sensations etc., without which the homeopath would be unable to prescribe effectively.

A patient-centred approach is associated with reduced symptom burden, fewer referrals to other services, and higher patient satisfaction (Hartog 2009, Little et al. 2001; Maizes et al. 2009, Priebe et al 2007).

Patient-centred behaviour is related to a patient's belief in a shared understanding of health conditions and their treatment (Street et al. 2008), and patient-centred communication focuses on patients' needs, values, wishes, and preferences (Epstein et al. 2005, Epstein et al. 2008). Research shows that patients want personalised advice ('How do these figures apply to me?'), and get frustrated when their priorities are not the focus of the consultation (Goldman et al. 2009).

When consultations are not patient-centred, this leads to inadequate data gathering and non-adherence, and the patients' unvoiced agendas are more likely to lead to poorer outcomes (Barry et al. 2000; Platt et al. 2001). Non-disclosure of information may arise from off-putting health professional behaviour (hurried, not listening, blocking, arrogance), but can also be about the environment or patient factors (Bugge et al. 2006).

In modern health care, many practitioners and services claim to be patient-centred. Yet patient-centredness requires a level of individualisation that is somewhat at odds with the current tendency in health care systems to strive for standardisation. Clinical trials rightly demand fidelity of implementation in delivering interventions to ensure internal validity. The cost may well be patients (and their practitioners) who feel that the intervention is not quite tailored to their needs.

It is easier to be patient-centred if the consultation focuses on the whole person, and if the practitioner and patient reach a mutual understanding of the connection between the complaint and other pieces of information given (Rise & Steinsbekk 2009). In homeopathy the consultation is often extensive, and the patient should have a feeling of having contributed greatly during the course of the consultation; indeed, homeopaths document the patient's narrative as much as possible in his or her own words (Hahnemann 1922).

The other end of the spectrum from a patient-oriented approach is being disease focused, with less emphasis on comprehension of the patient's narrative and emotions, compassion, or more humanistic values (Schattner 2009). Interest in the patient narrative and subjective understanding of the illness experience is gaining greater attention in medicine in general (see Greenhalgh & Hurwitz 2004) with the idea of narrative competence resulting in more respectful, empathic, and nourishing care (Charon 2001).

While the elevation of evidence-based medicine (EBM) has resulted in many improvements for patients, one criticism is that it is essentially a doctor-centred approach, because it focuses on the doctor's interpretation of evidence and diminishes the importance of human relationships and the patient's role in the consultation (Sweeney et al. 1998).

Therapeutic Alliance and Compassion

Anyway, what I really wanted to email you about is that I jokingly said that I wanted a remedy that made me feel like before...you know the homeopathic magic. What actually transpired is that the consultation we had helped enormously in that area. I left feeling different and uplifted because on reflection you helped me to understand that the process that is taking place is important and a natural consequence of the experience I had, and of course it's not easy or nice but that is the nature of change, and now I am much more relaxed about the discomfort I sometimes feel and also excited about where this is taking me. (Patient quote)

I have observed, after listening to many patients describe their experiences of psychiatric care over a number of years, that often the biggest dissatisfaction comes from what is perceived as 'cold' and 'overly clinical' care or treatment. This is related to a primary focus on a disease symptom cluster, which sadly results in patients left with feelings of being 'a walking illness'. Affective neutrality (i.e., a lack of responsiveness to patients' feelings) can be a part of normal discourse in medicine (Mishler 1984).

Research clearly shows that patients value 'warmth' (Ackerman & Hilsenroth 2003). Evidence indicates that compassion is an important therapeutic factor for patients with physical illness (Di Blasi & Kleijnen 2003). Frequent emergency department attenders randomised to receive compassionate care were more satisfied and readmitted less frequently than patients receiving standard care (Redelmeier et al. 1995). Lack of compassion in conventional medical practice may be a driver for patients to seek CAM (Taylor 1997).

Research shows that physicians who adopt a warm, friendly, and reassuring manner are more effective than those who keep consultations impersonal, formal, and do not offer reassurance (Di Blasi et al. 2001, Gryll & Katahn 1978, Olsson et al. 1989, Thomas 1987). Furthermore, studies into the therapeutic alliance demonstrate that the failure of therapist and patient to form an alliance is strongly associated with increased drop-out, non-compliance with treatment plans and goals, premature treatment termination, and poorer treatment outcomes (Kossoy & Wilner 1998, Krupnick et al. 2006).

Compassion and warmth may be the most important factors in the working alliance. Studies show that therapists' experience, training, skill, and progress as therapists do not have a significant impact on the alliance as rated by patients, whereas interpersonal relationships on the cold-warm dimension have an impact on alliance ratings (Hersoug et al. 2001). Being distanced, disconnected or indifferent has a negative impact on the working alliance. Research indicates that patients tend to prefer an actively involved, responsive, and supportive therapist, rather than one who is silent, less responsive, and less engaged (Hersoug et al. 2009). This may explain why greater training is not correlated with an improvement in the patient's perception of therapeutic alliance. Patients often cite 'humaneness' as the most highly rated aspect of care (Schattner 2009).

Moreover, the quality of the alliance is a robust predictor of therapy outcome, and ratings at the end of the first session may be used to predict who will drop out of treatment prematurely (Horvath 2000). It would be interesting to see the impact of the quality of working alliance between homeopaths and patients, and if this has an impact on treatment continuation, independent of clinical outcomes. For example, a survey of cancer patients in the UK showed changes attributed to complementary medicine such as being emotionally stronger, less anxious, and more hopeful about the future, even if the cancer remained unchanged (Zollman & Vickers 1999).

Laughter can also be used in consultations to relieve anxiety, communicate caring, and enhance healing (Wender 1996). Humour that is exclusive to the patient can demonstrate the opposite, (i.e., widening interpersonal gaps) and can be used by patients as a subtle attempt to deal with various interactional problems (Haakana 2001). When mutual laughter occurs, it may be indicative of a level of warmth in the consultation.

Impact of Homeopathic Process and Philosophy of Disease

> Let us use the word 'illness' to stand for what the patient feels when he goes to the doctor and 'disease' for what he has on the way home from the doctor's office. Disease, then, is something an organ has; illness is something a man has.
> (Cassell 1995:48)

In the scientific paradigm of modern medicine, disease refers to abnormalities of the structure and function of body organs and systems. Named pathological entities, which can be identified and described by reference to certain changes, are often regarded as 'things' or independent entities. Allopathic medicine's successful focus on specific disease interventions has meant relative neglect of an emphasis on self-healing and holism. Complementary medicine's increasing popularity can in part be accounted for by this gap (Reilly 2001).

Disease is universal; aetiology, signs and symptoms, natural history, and treatment are the same in every setting (Helman 1981). The subjective response of the patient to his or her illness, the perceived significance of the event, experience of ill health, and the meaning given to the experience are given less emphasis and importance in allopathy.

The capacity for developing therapeutic relationships with patients may well be affected by different models of health and illness and treatment philosophies. Homeopathy offers a way for patients to connect different components – mental and emotional states, physical symptoms, significant life events, and the presenting problem – that may not be connected by other health practitioners (May & Sirur 1998).

Kaptchuk & Eisenberg (1998) argue that there are features of CAM that patients find persuasive; for example, the idea of benevolent 'nature', and the philosophy of vitalism or energetic medicine. Moreover, in CAM there is no rigid separation between objective phenomena and subjective experience. Our current model of health care is a disease-centric biomedical model (Maizes et al. 2009). When the focus is on disease, communication tends to be physician-centred, and is often associated with reduced patient satisfaction (Hartog 2009).

The question then arises, is there something intrinsic to homeopathy that supports the development of therapeutic relationships? In a mental health setting study that looked at recipients' views of the therapeutic relationship, exploring and validating the clients' feelings, empathy, and trust were positively correlated with a positive relationship, while poor relationships were characterised by only focusing on the pathology of the illness, with a corresponding failure to understand the meaning of the patients' illness (Coatsworth-Puspoky et al. 2006). It is hard to conceive of a homeopath being able to get adequate information to prescribe without demonstrating these positive qualities or without understanding the meaning of the patients' illness.

Consequently, it can be argued that the process of case-taking is by its very nature therapeutic. Homeopathy and allopathy diverge fundamentally in homeopathy's hunt for the non-pathognomonic symptom as the foundation of a good prescription. In-depth inquiry is necessary to find such symptoms. As Eizayaga says, 'The homeopathic physician has not yet started his clinical history while the allopath has finished it' (Eizayaga 1991:127).

Moreover, while collecting these data, the homeopath has to understand the widest meaningful totality of symptoms, and from the patient's perspective, this may contribute to the feeling that the practitioner is being holistic. Homeopathic diagnosis relies on taking into account a wide range of factors, plus the patient's subjective experience of their symptoms (Rise & Steinsbekk 2009). Just as the simillimum must reflect as closely as possible the totality of symptoms, the practitioner must use empathic inquiry to understand the patient's state; this necessarily involves a high degree of cooperation, empathy, hopefulness, enablement, and narrative competence, all of which may improve outcomes (Hartog 2009).

Patients value a non-judgmental stance from the practitioner, and the principle of similars is inherently non-judgmental (although of course its practitioners may well be judgmental); for example, tendencies to unhealthy behaviours can be seen as a sign of individual susceptibility, to be found in certain medicines, rather than simply being poor health decisions made by the patient.

Homeopathy requires longer consultations, and systematic reviews show that longer patient consultations are more likely to cover wider patient care agendas, higher patient satisfaction and enablement, and achieve better outcomes (Howie et al. 2004; Mauksch et al. 2008). So-called 'slow medicine' moves away from a model of urgent episodic care, and moves towards a pace that invites negotiating, sharing vulnerabilities, and paying attention to small things. Such care invites self-disclosure and is less driven by impersonal guidelines and decisions (Loxterkamp 1999).

Some factors that are responsible for some of the outcomes from homeopathy, such as empathy, are not specific to homeopathy, while others, such as the process of finding the simillimum, are (Thompson & Weiss 2006). In Thomson and Weiss' study, greater homeopathicity, as defined by a clear match between the homeopathic medicine and the patients' Lifeworld, appeared to result in a better outcome assessment where this occurred.

As seen in earlier chapters, homeopaths are also interested in non-verbal responses. The way in which questions are answered has additional significance for homeopaths, as a sign of pathogenesis (e.g. despairing with pain, being doubtful of recovery, weeping when narrating symptoms). These can be important diagnostic symptoms for the homeopath. Moreover, body language from the patient is not only indicative of non-verbalised or unconscious emotional responses to questions, but can also be diagnostic, as reflected in the 'gestures' section of our repertories.

In homeopathy, the disposition of the patient (Hahnemann 1922 §211) is always investigated, regardless of the presenting complaint. A biopsychosocial model may appear holistic, but often results with a set of questions based on the patient's symptom cluster, with an-add on question: 'And how are things at home?'

The identification of characteristic symptoms is central to choosing the optimal medicine, and a high degree of patient cooperation is essential for this (Marian et al. 2008). When patients realise we are seeking different types of information (both qualitatively and quantitatively) from other health care practitioners, the nature of the relationship changes. Before we start our case analysis we are required to ask questions that are often of central importance to the patient: Why are they here? What has brought about their sickness? Where are they stuck? Is this one disease or more than one disease? How are these symptoms connected in this individual? Furthermore, homeopaths are required to understand all the deviations from the patient's former healthy state (Hahnemann 1922 §6), which means, by default, the homeopath looks at the disease journey, rather than the static present state.

Despite the great improvements for patients as a result of EBM, the downside for many patients is that the resulting evidence results in care that is based on protocols and guidelines rather than the individuality of the patient. In EBM, there is no need for understanding of theories of disease or healing, only the results of well-designed, well-controlled clinical trials (Tonelli & Callahan 2001). If the individuality of the patient and the practitioner are important for healing to occur, then EBMs' need to minimise these effects (through randomisation, blinding, placebo) can often result in a seemingly disconnected experience for the patient.

It can be argued that EBM and patient-centred medicine are two different paradigms (Bensing 2000); the former resulting in a positivistic biomedical perspective (essentially disease-oriented), where the uniqueness of patients, individual needs, and emotional status are often neglected. Regardless of its ability to produce positive clinical outcomes in large populations of patients, the longevity of homeopathy may also be partially explained by its patient-centred and whole-person focus, taking account of patients' perspectives, needs, experiences and preferences, and in homeopaths' inherent need to understand the context, meaning, and coherence of the illness experience.

Chapter 11
Conclusions

- Healthy Schizophrenia
- Linear Case Taking
    - Best Practice
    - Beautiful Silence
    - Spontaneity and Transparent Responses
    - Projections, Assumptions, Speculation
    - Closing the textbooks and Analyze Later
    - Sleuthing for the Case
    - Other Case Taking Concepts
    - Fishing
    - Poker
    - Steaming the Mussel
    - Clear Education and Answering Questions
- Getting to the Centre of the Case
    - Psychoanalytic
    - Jungian
    - Synthetic Case Taking Skills
- Improving Clinical Case Taking Skills - Predilection and Practice
- The role of intuition
- Random Directives before the Case Taking
- Reflective Questions for the Homeopath
- Reflective Questions for the Client
- Patient-Centred, Person-Centred and the Relationship
    - Self Disclosure
- Final Conclusions Case Taking

Chapter 11
Conclusions

I had a sweetheart back in college, who I thought was madly in love with me. She always leaned forward, her face right in mine, when we talked. Turns out she was nearsighted. What about the patient who slides their chair up close to yours in a spacious consultation room? Do they want to connect, or did they forget their glasses? (Will Taylor)

Sometimes a cigar is just a cigar. (Freud)

Case taking in homeopathic medicine is so much more than asking questions, listening and gathering data for a prescription. While the masters of the 18th, 19th, 20th and 21st centuries gave us great guidelines for best practice in information gathering, we know that by learning from other disciplines and borrowing where appropriate we can deepen the process. Further, by re-orientating our focus back to the patient and away from the result of that process – the remedy, we can understanding and maximize the therapeutic alliance and relationship. This final chapter summarizes the exploration of the landscape. Hahnemann, Sankaran, Kent, Lippe and Bidwell who have written on case taking all wanted the same thing, better results. Some diligent students might read these authors and then Tyler, Close or Schmidt, but sadly most don't. All should be encouraged to read widely. Kaplan is compulsory. Two of the finest modern contributors have been Will Taylor and David Little, much of their work being web published.

Healthy Schizophrenia

In taking a case, we are asked to simultaneously take on two seemingly conflicting roles; these being to listen and observe carefully, free from any bias, to the spontaneous presentation of the patient, while all at once being carefully attentive to what is unusual or characterizing in the patient. This is no small or easy task and it requires that we tread a 'narrow line', from which we often inadvertently deviate if we are honest. But the task is to be the 'unprejudiced observer while keeping our eyes on the prize' (Taylor 2001). The question is how to walk this narrow line, remaining unprejudiced in our taking of a case, yet keeping our eyes always on the revealing totality?

Linear Case Taking

We started off our journey looking at the facts in the case. When a patient walks in, do this, ask that. Hahnemann did it and so did Böenninghausen. They were brilliant prescribers and those followers of that method in contemporary homeopathy get great results and the best outcomes for the patient with the issue they came in for. As I have argued in this book what is required is simply a linear style of case taking and it is characterized by and requires focus on the presenting symptoms, and understanding completeness, that is sensation, location, complaints, modalities, concomitants. In this linear process, get the information, gather the facts. Remember what

Conclusions

it is that you are looking for and go for it. The aim is to observe and hear the story of a patient.

Best Practice

We have explored those skills and techniques. The attitude of the practitioner is to be free from prejudice and have sound senses and fidelity (Hahnemann 1922 §83, §84). The principle involved is to simply let the patient talk, to write down the patient's own words, allow them to speak in their own language. One of the assumptions, about this strategy is that the patient is able to give you the information you need with very little prompting and in reality it is the case that this is not forthcoming. The value of this is that the patient delivers the information in their own words. The technique and strategy required of the listener is to maintain an attitude of silence and allow the patient to talk initially, prompt with open questions 'anything more', 'what else' and then when the questioning becomes necessary after the patient has run out of information, questions to clarify the information previously given, systematic questioning of regions of the body comes later on. Questions are required. We look for totality, peculiarity and cause. Taylor expresses it brilliantly.

> Perhaps the patient has been describing a recurrent headache. I may find myself dying to know whether it is ameliorated or aggravated by pressure, by heat, whether light or movement is bothersome, etc. I could easily interrupt to ask for this information, or take advantage of a short pause to ask more unobtrusively. But if I instead continue to listen, to allow the patient to spin their own tale, I may be somewhat surprised to hear them slide right in to talking about their relationship with

a co-worker, and their thoughts about making a career change. Now there is some logic in my patient's brain that links these things together - some richness of the patient's terrain that I would have entirely missed, in order to obtain information about some modalities that I could always have come back for. What is more interesting, more characterizing of the disharmony of this individual patient? The modalities that I think I need to know; or the story that the patient believes they need to tell me? It is much for this reason that I do not use health-history questionnaires, or review medical records before an initial interview. I do not want the patient to assume that I know anything about them before the interview, and therefore assume that they can afford to leave anything out. I want to hear their story. An elderly woman consulted me for an initial visit, and consumed the entire two-hour interview talking about seemingly everyone, except herself. Why her husband should see me, and her daughter, and what was wrong with conventional medicine, on and on for two hours, without room for any redirection from me. The few times I did manage a word in edgewise, she artfully slid off questions about herself onto other topics. All the while tugging at a stretched-out mock turtleneck sweater she was wearing. I didn't even have a presenting complaint at the end of the interview. As I sat afterwards, feeling sorry for myself for having nothing to prescribe upon - alternately dumping on myself for having taken a poor case, and upset with the obstacles to obtaining a clear case - I suddenly realized that in fact I had a great case staring me in the face: Loquacity; Desire to Hide; and Cannot tolerate tight clothing about the neck. If it was a snake, it would'a bit me! I mailed her a dose of Lachesis, and saw her in followup 4 weeks later, when she informed me that she was '100% better'. She sat silently waiting for my response (Taylor 2001).

Conclusions

The skills required of the homeopath are many, but in this technique it requires us to be silent, to shut up and to allow the patient to tell their story without interruption. It requires that the homeopath be a good observer and be very thorough. Much of the story of the case is told between the words of the delivered history.

> Some patients will rattle out a rambling two-hour narrative, as the one above. Others will deliver a carefully organized chronology of events with accurate dates and measurements. Some will name their complaint briefly, ask what homeopathy does for it, and wait for a reply. It is important to reflect not only on 'what are they telling me', but also 'how are they telling me?' and 'why are they telling me this, like that?' In addition to content, we need to make observations of context, delivery, and affect (Taylor 2001).

There are many advantages because it is relatively an objective strategy of eliciting information and often the mental and physical symptoms of the patient are equally covered. Moreover it can be taught easily and replicated over and over to develop confidence. There are few disadvantages to this style of homeopathy, but one of them is that it does not suit all patients. Closed patients can do well with it but many homeopaths who apply the strategy run into difficulty when they haven't got the flexibility to adopt another approach. Another disadvantage is that it doesn't offer much emotional support necessarily to patients. Moreover a disadvantage is that it is a strategy that does not get to the very centre of a case or the essence of a case. Rather it is useful in allowing a patient to describe their experience in the world and their symptoms, but not necessarily find the juice, the centre or the mental essence. It is linear, good and safe.

Beautiful Silence

The first part of this book identified that certain skills were mandatory. In summary, be silent, be faithful, watch for detail, observe acutely, use tact, use timing. Do not be in a hurry, have patience, have a great knowledge of human nature, be an interrogator, a detective, a criminal lawyer, be candid, have knowledge of human nature and the human heart, be quiet and cultivate silence and perception, be circumspect, have honour, be receptive, be like a photographic plate. Have a clear mind. Let them tell their own story. Develop rapport. This is the advice that comes to us down the years and generations of previous homeopaths. Another directive is to allow the client space. This requires that the practitioner is comfortable with silence. Taylor (2001) says,

> 'Pauses happen.' It is great advice. Pauses in the interview are there for a reason. They can feel uncomfortable. They can feel unproductive, and inviting of impatience. Yet, they can be the most productive element of an interview. Does the patient ask for structure ('What else do you need to know?') What direction does a patient take up spontaneously when resuming after a pause? Don't feel anxious to close pauses up with questions that could re-direct the interview; allow the patient to lead you out of them. Waiting through an extended pause is something that many of us need to practice. There's a point where we start to squirm, start to feel embarrassed. However, waiting to see where the patient will choose to go after an extended pause can be very fruitful. Even 'Well, that's about it' or 'What else do you need to know?' can offer us a great deal of insight into the case.

It is often after an extended pause, when the patient has exhausted the story they've come prepared to give you, told

Conclusions

you what they think you want to know, that they begin to be spontaneous and offer insight into what is genuinely real for them. There is a good story, sometimes attributed to Abraham Lincoln, about keeping quiet. I heard it in Law school. The purpose of the story is the value of the truth in silence. When you have the information that you need, shut up. It's a shut up, be silent story. If I remember it right, he was a lawyer before he was a politician and he was in court defending a man who was accused of having a fight with another man and in the middle of the brawl biting the other man's nose off. There was a witness. Lincoln is cross-examining the witness who claims to have seen the fight, and he says something like, 'On the night in question, do you recall what the weather was like?' The witness says, 'Yes I do, it was raining'. 'It was raining? How heavily was it raining'? 'It was really heavy'. 'And do you recall any other aspects about the weather that night'. The witness says, 'Yes, there was a fog'. 'Tell me about the fog?' 'There was a really really thick fog'. 'And do you recall if there was any moonlight that night?' He says, 'No, not an ounce of moonlight'. 'There was no moon, categorically no moon?' asks Lincoln, and he went to the meteorological records which he had on his desk and he confirmed that absolutely on that night, there was no moonlight, it was completely dark, it was pouring rain and there was thick fog. Then he says, 'How far away were you from the altercation?' The man says, 'About 200 meters'. Abraham Lincoln exclaimed, '200 metres away on a foggy night, with no moon, in pouring rain, in the middle of the night?' Abraham Lincoln asked the next question. He said, 'Well, how then sir, can you tell me then that in the middle of the night, on a foggy, wind blown night, with rain and fog everywhere, with no moon and 200 metres away you can stand there and say that my client bit that man's nose off?' The man on the stand says, 'Well when he ran past me, he spat it out!'

Spontaneity and Transparent Responses

Best practice determines we keep our clients talking. It is a great skill. The most effective responses we can make during an interview are often those in which we remain relatively transparent, and allow our patient to retain direction of the process.

> A response such as 'Well, tell me more' or 'what do you think is important for me to hear?' can move them back into elaborating or expanding on the topic. On reviewing my videotapes, I find my most common responses include simple reflective words, such as: [Patient] 'I really don't like driving over bridges'. [Taylor] 'Bridges?' A more detailed response – e.g., 'Why don't you like bridges?' - may redirect the interview away from what the patient needs to tell me. E.g. had I responded, 'Why don't you like bridges?' I might have received a useless intellectual explanation, such as, 'Well, I know better, it's really kind of silly'; while a simple 'Bridges?' might have resulted in a much more spontaneous, more useful response, such as 'Yeah, bridges. And being late - I don't like being late to things either' (Taylor 2001).

But this advice needs to be tempered with a disclaimer. The silent approach has been known to be brutal and used inappropriately. When done well, this can be a sensitive, energetic and psychic approach. Patients have often found it difficult to deal with the non interactiveness of this strategy there can be long silences which are uncomfortable. Some patients have described it as hostile.

Projections, Assumptions, Speculation

Good case taking involves knowing yourself. This is to ensure that you the case taker don't get yourself in the way of the process.

> I recall Jonathan Shore stating that the two times one can fall into the most trouble in case taking, are, first, when you hear yourself saying 'no'; and second, when you hear yourself saying 'yes'. The times that we think we understand our patient - that we think we can relate to their experience - can be very dangerous places for misunderstanding in case taking; it is here that we can too easily feel we are done listening, and move on to speculate, assume, or project our own interpretations onto a case...Abuse history is a very difficult topic re projections and speculation. Practitioners who have histories of abuse, and those who do not, all have their own personal buttons pushed by this topic when it comes up. Can we hear this in a case, and feel that we understand it as 'ailments from abuse?' I'd suggest not. 'Ailments from abuse' reminds me rather of 'Ailments from tall buildings collapsing on you'; I'd be more intrigued by the person who experienced abuse without sequellae. So, the question becomes (if an explanation does not follow spontaneously) 'If you and I were to write a book about abuse, we could fill hundreds of pages with what's wrong about it. So for you, what would be on page one?' (Taylor 2001).

Closing the Texbooks and Analyze Later

One way for us to be more effective is to be there. Really there, and in the present. We are asking ourselves to multitask at an unprecedented level when we attempt to prescribe in a chronic case at the close of an initial interview. While this is sometimes feasible, for cases of acute illness, it can be anxiety provoking and quite unreasonable in working with most cases of chronic disease.

> I arrange a second visit a few days to one week after the initial consultation, at which I suggest a remedy, having the intervening time to study the case in depth. To expect to prescribe at the close of an initial interview is to ask oneself either to prescribe 'intuitively' (a task which James Tyler Kent and Ernest Farrington agreed would require 30 years of careful experience in case taking and analysis), or to distract ourselves from unprejudiced case taking with simultaneous analysis during the interview process. Obviously there will appear to be exceptions - occasionally God and Hahnemann collaborate to send us a case that screams its simillimum at us in an unmistakable manner. However, there have been sufficient such cases screaming 'Sepia' to me that have turned out to eventually need Trillium (e.g.) to convince me that even such 'obvious' cases are deserving of formal analysis, and the focus of the initial visit on unprejudiced case taking that this permits (Taylor 2001).

Sleuthing for the Case

Irrespective of the style, one of the most important skills to develop for a case taker is the capacity to sleuth, hunt and delve for the information. Whether a criminal lawyer, an interrogator, a detective, an archaeologist or a historian the ability to observe listen and ask critical questions is invaluable. Hahnemann, Schmidt, Kent and Sankaran advocated the same thing, to understand and find fragments of the case (as you do your archaeological dig notice those fragments and include them in your homeopathic diagnosis and evaluation). The case taker who is skilled in these arts is arriving on a crime scene just like Inspector Morse, Colombo, and Sherlock Holmes, they hover on the edge and take in everything with an eagle eye. What is there and what is not there. The crime scene they arrive at, in the homeopathic context is the human body. Most bodies have been battered, bruised and abused and the health is a shambles. Your job is to understand why? How did that become this? What has gone on to enable this crime to happen? Your job is to put together the pieces from what is left, from what is there, and what is not there, what is strange, and what is incongruent. In addition, the better observers in this context are the ones that are worldly. Al Pacino does it beautifully in a scene from *Insomnia*. A woman has been murdered. He walks into the room where she once lived and takes it in. He sees everything but it is his realization that hanging in the wardrobe is a dress that is expensive as opposed to everything else that came from Wal-Mart was the first step in understanding her life and ultimately her killer.

Other Case Taking Concepts

I slowly developed the understanding and grew to know implicitly that at some level, knowing myself, addressing my prejudices, loving my prejudices and being creative in my case work were some of the ingredients that would be important if I was to thrive in practice. Over the years I have noticed other aspects of what I have been doing in the clinic room, how I take a case. I started to follow and document, as the consultation was taking place, some of these techniques that I was using. It was only when beginning to conduct the small formal exploration of case taking styles from Hahnemann to contemporary homeopathy that I began to place some of the techniques in their appropriate context and realized that some of these techniques while appropriate to some styles of homeopathy that I was using in the morning were entirely inappropriate for a case that I was taking later in the same day.

Fishing

From a personal perspective, when I am in front of a patient I shut up, I follow, I look for congruence. I also go fishing. Fishing is a technique that when I attempt to describe it in the classroom inevitably falls on deaf ears. After all how many students in a homeopathic class or seminars take delight in killing fish. It is very rare. And yet, like most metaphors in homeopathy it describes beautifully the process of what takes place in the case taking. When you are fishing you sit in the boat or on the pier, throw in your line and wait. You watch the birds, you take in the scenery, and every now and again there is a nibble. At that moment there is no need to react or do anything dramatic but simply notice. It is exactly the same in the consultation, the patient tells you about the birds and about the scenery and another story taking place in their life and every now and again they give you a small nibble on the hook, a piece of information. The fish is interested in your bait and the client is sitting in your room. You can feel the line against your finger and when you get the bite a little bit of extra pressure can be exerted, from this metaphorical perspective that is the time to begin to apply pressure and very gently start to reel it in. A homeopath might learn a lot from Hemingway. One day when you have no clients read *The Old Man and the Sea*. Failing that, take yourself off to the local pier and try some fishing. One of the things that any fishermen would tell you is that if you try and pull in a large fish by just winding it in, there is a strong statistical possibility that that fish will thrash its way off and disappear into the depths. Reeling in the homeopathic fish requires the skills of bringing it in and then letting it go, bringing it in and letting it go again. A fisherman knows that this is the way to exhaust the fish and guarantees that you will land it safely. Of course at that moment what you do is kiss it on its fishy lips, say 'Thank you', and put it back where it came from to enjoy its day. In the homeopathic context the way that we reel a patient in and let it go, reel and let it go is to focus on those aspects of the case where there is the most charge. Too much pressure and they might close up and say no more. You can do this in a consultation by talking about other mundane or unimportant matters. This is something that is very hard to teach but something that skilled homeopathic practitioners do naturally. They are able to read when a patient is uncomfortable, and rather than make the homeopathic experience miserable for them, they talk about something harmless like food cravings or their reactions to the weather. Nowhere is it said that getting to the centre of the case has to be a horrible experience for the client.

Poker

Very often I begin my consultation by asking my new client about their job or profession or what they know about homeopathy. In that way I am able to understand better how to pitch my information just right, how to engage with my clients so that I am able to describe homeopathy and ask my questions in a way which closely matches their understanding and their capacity to listen. The best way if you are playing poker and you want to win a lot of money, when betting against an opponent is to keep your cards close to your chest. But irrespective of what those cards are, the way to maximize the winnings is to meet your opponent and raise them by one.

Jeremy Sherr has lectured on this concept when taking the case. I use this daily in my practice. The idea is to stretch them a small way to keep them interested so that if they have an average hand or a good hand then they will stay in the race, keep putting their money in until you can jump over the top of them. A poker player throws in their hand every time when you, their opponent make a bid that is significantly ahead of what anyone else has been betting. This is good advice for a questioner in the homeopathic context.

Steaming the Mussel

It is easy to open a shellfish by smashing it with a hammer. Once I was at a wedding in Adelaide in Australia. A friend of mine was getting married. I had known them for a short time and so I was placed at the end table with all the extras, those people that at wedding parties no-one knows what to do with, the miscellaneous friends. We had a good time and we were drinking quite a lot when the first course arrived. It was some sort of crustacean, I think a Balmain-bug, and I was struggling to open mine. I decided to hit it with my fork. It exploded, and the whole table, men and women in their finest wedding clothes were covered in shellfish. Not a great way to meet people. Much better is to steam a shellfish and open it carefully by gently applying heat. I steam my clients in my practice. I massage information out of them, and like a frog that has been placed in the cold pot of water, sometimes they don't even realize that the temperature is rising and that they are revealing their case completely. Homeopathy is gentle medicine and I believe that the case taking should also be in that vein. It is a combination of the skills of fishing, of poker, and steaming that yields me my best results in the clinic.

Clear Education and Answering Questions

In addition, I take the time to answer all clients' questions clearly and use no jargon. Patients often have questions that they need answered, about homeopathy, about follow-up and practitioner availability, about the bag of supplements they've brought in to be gone over, about the name of their condition. They often sprinkle such questions into the initial interview. Taylor (2001) gives the best advice.

> I let folks know at the outset that I'll collect their questions, and address them all at a later time, in the second visit or in a special visit arranged for extended patient education. When questions arise in the course of the initial interview, my relationship to them is not that they are questions that need answers now, but rather that they are expressions of the patient that can lead to my understanding of the case. E.g. a patient may feel entrenched in the idea that they have 'chronic yeast syndrome', and ask numerous questions about this - could it account for this symptom, what does homeopathy do for this, etc. These are questions that may deserve to be addressed, but not in the initial interview. Return to them later - I choose to do so in a second visit - but listen to them now as expressions of the patient, as valuable as any other symptom expressed in the case. Is the focus on 'yeast syndrome' evidence of theorizing? Impressionability? Anxiety about health? Continued listening may make this clear.

Getting to the Centre of the Case

While our task is simply to ask questions and get the information, as has been argued elsewhere, sensation, location modality, experience tells us that through some simple techniques such as following the hand gesture, allowing the disease to come into the room, naming the disease or the situation we see before us, takes us straight to the centre of the case. This can happen in the blink of an eye and suddenly we are dealing with deeper information. It creates a paradox for us where we understand that on one level our job is to get information, we know that information can be deepened if we apply certain techniques and understand the patient, and further that we are required to be there fully and contactfully and that we do our best work when we make full contact with our clients and create a lasting and meaningful relationship with them.

As I have argued in Chapters 3 to 6, subsequent homeopaths to Hahnemann emphasized different aspects of homeopathy and case taking due to their own cultural sensitivities, the styles of practices that they had, and their predilections. Dunham, Kent, Lippe and the Allens were men of their times, and they practiced homeopathy within the specific social, political and financial constraints of the day. Every homeopath from 1800 to 2010 is skilled in the arts of observation. Moreover they are interesting people and these days come from all walks of life. Recently in a lecture I was giving in Malaysia I marveled at the make-up of the room. Christian, Hindu, Muslim, Indian, Chinese, Malay, English, Austrian. Doctors, PhD's, engineers, housewives, interested extras, dedicated students, blow-ins. It is such a rich family that we have. As I have argued, that richness and diversity is our greatest strength but sometimes is responsible for our disunity. What we know for sure is that that diversity creates for us a multitude of skills that come to, and are in addition to, our fundamental homeopathic skills. Many years ago I trained as a historian and use these skills every day in my practice. Homeopaths worldwide were chemists, lawyers, bankers, hippies, mothers before they reached the classroom. In other words, homeopathy since Hahnemann's time has been enriched with the skills of the people that are being drawn to homeopathy, and at times they have added depth and sophistication to the work. It is this augmentation and the borrowing of the skills from the police with their capacity for interrogation, from psychotherapy with a full array of skills that they are able to bring and a multitude of other disciplines that have pushed homeopathy further than Hahnemann's vision to the worldwide diverse phenomena that it is today. There are 550 million users of homeopathy on the planet. They are receiving their homeopathy from homeopaths from different cultures on different continents with different understandings and different styles. It is ultimately this cultural diversity that one finds when travelling around the world of homeopathy that enabled homeopathy to make a substantial change in direction as it did in the 1980's and 1990's.

During those years Sankaran, Kaplan, Castro, Norland, Sherr, Mundy and many others encouraged a generation of homeopaths at the end of the 20th century to look to the heart of the matter. The purpose, they argued was that to get to the centre was to create a better and more profound and lasting result. It was towards the psychological sciences that many turned to two general threads Psychoanalytical and Jungian.

Psychoanalytic

These days some take a psychoanalytic case taking focus to get to the centre, looking to analyse the state of the patient. The attitude of the practitioner tends to be neutral and analyzing, an intellectual process. In terms of the interview, the questioning is orientated to the areas where the patient feels some sort of emotional charge. In order to do this the listener has to be astute, has to be willing to probe and one of the skills which is crucial is that they need to be non reactive to the material that is presented to them. Ways in which such case taking can progress is through focusing on specific words and language specifics that the patient use, their expressions, their Freudian slips and the way in which they interact with the practitioner. Often the technique of the practitioner is to maintain distance, have firm boundaries, sit behind the patient, be neutral, be direct. Intellectually there is a great deal of interpretation of verbal and non-verbal signs and messages. Such a strategy requires that the homeopath remains objective and neutral, to do it well they need to be aware of their own issues, their own values, and they need to be perceptive and have sharp analytical ability. One of the major advantages of such a stance was that the patient does not necessarily have to understand their own state, it is the homeopath's job, the listener's job, to analyze, probe, suggest. The great advantage is that the listener retains control of the interaction and information and it is possible using these strategies to extract useful unconscious information. But such a strategy also has its disadvantages and often there are large power inequalities with the patient and often while the listener may think that they are being very objective, the information may be filtered through an extremely subjective lens.

Jungian

Another approach is a strategy which we have learnt from the Jungian tradition in psychotherapy to meet the patient where they're at, often in their unconscious state. The attitude of the practitioner is one of being with the patient with their full self. This is a strategy which requires of the listener to be fully present with whoever is sitting in front of them and following them to their world, the world of their unconscious parts, the unknowable parts, dreams and stories and myths, symbol and symbolic meanings, archetypes, patterns of behaviour, spiritual realms and dimensions focusing on synchronistic events and relying on the equal nature of the relationship. The listener needs to have a degree of understanding of themselves beyond the other strategies, especially an awareness of their shadow and requires self exploration and awareness, respect and an understanding of different cultures and mythology. The advantages are that this is a unique approach to explore the uncharted depths of the patient with them in an equal way, looking at the biggest picture and the spiritual aspect of a person's health dynamics. Unfortunately it also requires a huge amount from the homeopath, a commitment to themselves, knowledge of the unconscious and unknowable aspects of themselves as well.

Synthetic Case Taking Skills

While not necessarily consciously and deliberately applying these strategies above, in the last few decades, homeopaths have realized that their case taking deepens and better information emerges when they aim for the centre and follow the story to find the red line, the golden bullet, the essence, the genius, the juice, the charge, the energy. As well as the archaeological and historical skills mentioned above to find the centre of the case, homeopaths have benefited from identifying congruency, incongruency, dissonance and resonance. Looking at the verbs in a case yields results, more than the nouns of the case. By following the verbs, homeopaths are looking at those symptoms where there is more vitality, it is argued they are following the flow of energy. If a patient is a river, the nouns, the actual disease, the pathology, are the rocks in the middle of the river. To focus on these is to focus on the obstacles. The verbs are the modalities, and often more characteristic. Chinese medicine and homeopathy reminds us to focus on the flow of energy, that is the flow of water around these objects. By mapping, measuring, taking in the flow of energy, we see the true disturbance.

For those homeopaths committed to or seduced by aiming for the centre, the underlying beliefs and assumptions are important to name and articulate because at essence, practitioners of homeopathy who work in this way have broadened their definitions of health, disease and cure. Amongst the beliefs are that getting to the core creates better and longer lasting change, the body is a shadow of the mind, psyche effects substance. It is necessary to be silent and be silent on the inside. Case taking is a meditation. Required is to do nothing, follow the patient wherever they take you. More time is needed. Be a fool. Know nothing. Look for the expression of energy and, for Sankaran, look for that which is non-human specific in this case. For best practice the qualities required are empathy, unconditional positive regard, warmth, congruence, authenticity, courage, love.

Improving Clinical Case Taking Skills - Predilection and Practice

All of these strategies imply and require professional and personal self-development by the homeopath. Implicit is the need to keep studying, keep improving on the inside and outside. In some undergraduate but mostly postgraduate work and in advanced seminars I encourage homeopaths to undertake a serious and critical audit of themselves. Where have you come from? What skills have you bought from that place? What did you do prior to coming to homeopathy? What skills did you bring from that place? Wrestling with and answering these questions allows homeopaths the opportunity to get clear about their predilections, and what they are good at.

It is so easy to practice case taking skills. Everyone forgets that you don't need to have a patient in front of you to practice observation. I do my best observation work at the beach or at the café. Listening skills can be practiced in conversation with anybody, watching TV or a good movie. It is the same with congruence. You don't have to have a patient in front of you to work on this skill. But best of all watch interviewers do their work. Over the years there have been some demonstrations of brilliant and appalling interview work. Watch Parkinson or David Frost, watch sportscasters interview sports people. Watch Jon Stewart, Michael Moore and best of all if you have the opportunity watch the Australian interviewer Andrew Denton. He is a master of creating the space and then allowing the interviewee enough rope to hang themselves or to bring forward pieces of information that they didn't even know existed. Look at other professions and professionals. How do they do it? How not to do it.

The Role of Intuition

On my travels I am often asked my opinion on the role of intuition and homeopathy. Just where does intuition play a part in the homeopathic process? To my mind the only answer, is that intuition plays no role in the evaluation of the case or the selection of a remedy. I suppose it depends on one's definition of intuition. To my mind, intuition is nothing other than unconscious knowledge. Very often the most intuitive people are those people with years and years and years of practice or skills behind them. Intuition is therefore nothing other than accumulated knowledge and sometimes a great teacher cannot explain why they know something for sure or why they have selected the medicine. A really great teacher will be able to consciously articulate those required skills.

However in case taking, intuition can play a very important role. Sometimes I am asked by students why I asked a specific question and the true answer is I have no idea. I have no idea why at that time, I asked that question that led to that response, or those tears, or the deepening of the case taking. I remember many years ago I treated a lawyer. He was 57 years old and the thing about him was he had difficulty urinating. In addition to that his recently married wife who was significantly younger was intent on getting pregnant and he was having trouble maintaining and sustaining an erection. He had benign prostatic hypertrophy. He had been to see a doctor who for some reason had given him injections of testosterone for the problem of impotence and it seems that this had led to be swelling of the prostate, an iatrogenic cause. I widened my questioning and I found out that during the 1980's he had undergone some psychotherapy and had been given LSD therapeutically by his psychiatrist. This startling therapeutic intervention had left him feeling 'strange' since that time. He also mentioned feeling tired a lot of the time and on questioning the origins of that fatigue had been there since he got off the boat in Australia in the 1960's. 'Where is home for you?' I asked. He burst into tears and after composing himself, because both he and I were surprised at his reaction, he described that he'd never felt at home in Australia and longed for Europe. I have no idea why I asked that question. It had nothing to do with his prostate but it had everything to do with him. He got *Agnus castus* 12c. Within a week his prostate was down to a regular size, he was urinating perfectly and in six weeks his wife was pregnant.

Random Directives before Case Taking

In addition to the best practice directives of all the writers mentioned in Chapters 2-9, I also argue that these additional statements or reflective questions be asked, answered and addressed.

Allow yourself not to know anything
Don't meander
Examine succinctly
Allow yourself to not know what is going to happen in this case
Provide a safe and welcoming space
Be infinitely flexible
Everyone is different
Pitch your language right
Watch your jargon

Reflective Questions for the Homeopath

If it is a chronic case, and before evaluating the case and reaching for the repertory or materia medica at the end of the consultation, these are the questions (some come from Vithoulkas 2010) that I ask either myself or the patient.

What is to be cured in this patient?
What is the state of health?
What is the disease?
Is this person healthy? According to their values? My values?
What is their basic limitation to health and happiness?
What is their inner conflict or central disturbance?
What is basically wrong with them?
What is their nature?
What impression does their body type make?
What clothes do they wear?
How quickly do they answer the question?
Can they look me in the eye?
What are their hands doing?
Is there tension in the face or do they sit erect or slouch?
What can one feel from the patient? Is it neutrality, acceptance, judgement, anger, sympathy, rigidity, sexuality, anxiety, suppression of emotions, or is it a type of anxiety, a fear of some sort? Is it anger suppressed with sadness on the surface? Or anger suppressed with fear? What is cure going to look like? Very often I ask the patient this direct question as it clarifies in my mind and also in their mind just what is it that we are looking for.
Is this person really healthy on the emotional level? For example, is he/she able to express his emotions with strength and clarity? Is he/she flexible or rigid?
Is he/she finding creative solutions to problems or getting more trapped?
Does he/she have a strong sense of purpose, value and meaning in their life, or is there apathy and indifference?
How much strength of individuality is in their identity or are they weak and unassertive?
What is the balance between selfishness with a strong boundary and the over caring, over sympathetic and too selfless individual who ends up as a victim? Did he/she pass through the developmental stages easily?
What stages is he/she still trapped in?
What negative emotions are there?
What are the positive ones?
Is their health based on freedom to make choices or does the pattern of the 'subconscious' make decisions for them and restrict their freedom?

Conclusions

How are the symptoms connected to the patient's life and his development as a person?
What exactly was the way the patient perceived the stress they encountered?
How did they react to it?
Has this reaction become a rigid response?
How has this reaction continued and developed?
Identify what is diseased
Identify what is to be changed
Identify what is out of balance
What happened here; crime scene
What happened here for this to become this
What is to be cured?
What is the exciting cause?
What is the fundamental cause? Can the cause of this confusion can be untangled
Do I understand and grasp the maintaining causes in this case
What are the totality of symptoms here
Have I been free from prejudice in this case?
What are they?
What are the striking symptoms in the case?
Is this one sided?
What is the state of the mind?
What is the patient's state?
What is the essence here?
What is the delusion?
What is the verb?
Why are the symptoms represent?
What are they stopping her from doing?
What is the miasm?
What is the timeline?
What is the sensation and the function here?
How many diseases are in this body at one time?
How will I manage this case?

Do I really understand this person and their basic life dilemmas?
What projections/ role am I wearing from this patient?
How deeply do I want to know this person? What did they say? What did they not say?
What are the chances of this patient becoming involved in their healing?
What is the role of this person in their own healing?
What is the connection of the patient to the environment?
To other people?
To God or higher authority?
How and why did they get sick?
What was memorable?
How will I remember them?

Reflective Questions for the Client

In my practice a good many patients getting chronic treatment are asked these questions.

Can you visualize yourself in a state of health? If so what does that mean? (Are you going to be wearing a linen suit drinking Singapore slings? Are you going to be in your country kitchen stirring soup on the Aga? What will it feel like in your body? What does it look like? Who is there with you and around you?) Answers to these questions clarify in the mind of the case taker and then the client just what it is that we are doing here. The questions and issues below come from a number of sources and they are collated in no particular order.
Do you want to deepen the process of healing?
What are your expectations of treatment in this case?
Where is it that you want to go from this treatment?
What is cure going to look like for you?
What is the photo going to look like?
So what sort of a person are you?
Where are you at in your life?
What is to be cured?

> **What is cure going to look like for you?**
>
> When will our relationship be over? When can I discharge you? (I find this a particularly useful question at times in chronic cases and especially where the predominant issues in mental/emotional cases this question clarifies in the mind of the patient just what it is that they are wanting to be cured or fixed)

Patient-Centred, Person-Centred and the Relationship

Irrespective of the method of case taking, and or the quality of the questions asked, the argument in this book has been the need to identify the major features of the landscape and recalibrate our thinking. In Chapter 10, it was argued that the role of the relationship between the practitioner, the patient, client or the guest needs to be reevaluated and placed centrally in the homeopathic process. Gadd, myself and others have argued that the hunt for the homeopathic remedy should be re-orientated towards understanding who this ill person is here and now, and that the well selected medicine is secondary to that first important process and in fact will come easily once that person, that individual with their symptoms sitting in front of you is understood and heard by the practitioner.

It is an approach that is in the humanist tradition of listening, an alliance approach to co-explore the state of the patient by the practitioner, requiring a relationship, requiring being with the patient. The principles involved are to follow the lead of the patient wherever they go in the consultation, to respect their resistances but never avoid them, to support them as they explore themselves, to look for congruence and dissonance, to make contributions if required or to summarize and review situations when stuck. It is a technique that does not lend itself to interpretation.

The techniques and qualities needed are empathy (verbal and non-verbal), active listening strategies, paraphrasing and reflecting techniques that are often used in counseling. Feedback of feelings are also useful, as is summarizing, probing, self-disclosure at times, and the confrontation of any discrepancies which may be found from the totality of the patient's words. It requires that the homeopath is comfortable with feelings, and especially their own feelings, an awareness of their own issues in the world, and a capacity to let go of control of the consultation and let it go where the needs of the patient require. There is a level of dynamism that is created from this humanistic strategy. It requires the homeopath be fully present and a highly dynamic case taking process ensues. One of the major advantages is in the equality of power in the relationship using this humanist strategy. Generally patients feel safe and heard, it provides a good ground for intimacy and these skills are easily learned and passed on. Such skills demand that the homeopath is open and gives more input than some of the other strategies and this is often seen as a disadvantage. But not all patients or homeopaths know how to do this naturally.

Self Disclosure

The relational approach requires that we break a rule enshrined in homeopathy since the beginning. It is not really possible to fully be in relationship when one is silent, and there is a degree of self disclosure necessary for this approach to be of benefit. Well used, this can be a therapeutic tool which often helps to create intimacy and congruency, and facilitate the relationship between the client and the homeopath. There are multiple dangers in such an approach, as well as benefits. It is often that patients that are closed or reserved or wounded or in pain find the analytical, clinical, freedom from prejudice style of case taking difficult and it does not necessarily create safe, trusting and supporting environments nor encourage the exploration of that wound. There is also of course the issue of the power inequality; the inequality of the relationship between the practitioner and patient is not to be underestimated. The humanistic model relies on exploration or co-exploring issues using supportive techniques, fewer questions, empathy, congruence, paraphrasing, reflecting, summarizing, clarifying. This is a strategy that can create safety, a sense of being heard, a sense of being understood, enabling a client to move deeper into their full states. It is often taught that to self disclose, and talk about oneself in a homeopathic conversation is to be avoided. After all, why is it relevant? The patient is coming for their treatment and they are paying. Many a time I've heard the words, 'I paid all this money to...only to listen to him talk about his problems'. Surely an unprejudiced posture requires that you shut up. But it is countered in some quarters that to self disclose can be a meaningful therapeutic intervention and actually enhance a consultation. Of course it depends on if the information is relevant and whether it will enhance anything at all. The question is whether withholding information diminishes the therapeutic process. Where self-disclosure usually goes wrong is when it involves a subject that the homeopath has strong opinions about and perhaps an area of their life that the practitioner is not entirely clear of in themselves. If you have issues, then it's strongly encouraged that you don't disclose. It never goes well. 'Yes I used to have this as well', is not really what a patient wants to hear. It is rare in my practice that I talk about myself. From my limited understanding of transference and counter transference I realized that to work skillfully with this real phenomena takes years of training and appropriate therapeutic skills, skills that are not actually necessary for a homeopath to do good homeopathic work. Silence is so useful. Silence can be such a powerful tool to support or it can be interpreted as a judgment.

From this perspective best practice is based upon rapport and respect. Making the patient feel that they are respected is an important part of the process. This is a fundamental difference between orthodox medical practice and homeopathy. What is more, this difference between a stressed and busy medical practitioner and an actively listening homeopathic practitioner can be the difference between making significant progress not. Also required is courteousness, good bedside manner (Kaplan 2001) and tone of voice all to create a safe environment and space for the patient to deliver their information. When gathering feelings and mental symptoms, the best advice on eliciting emotional and mental symptoms is in Kaplan (2001:56), Taylor (2001), and P. Sankaran (1996). Give clear instructions and inform the client at all times in non-exclusive non-jargon filled language. The case taking may sometimes take two or three or even more sittings to be completed. Hahnemann said it 200 years ago. Very often, in the first sitting the patient merely becomes aware as to what sort of symptoms we expect from them and it may be only by the second or third or later interview that he or she may recall, recollect or observe and offer voluntary information about those symptoms which were omitted earlier. Here, therefore, there is often a need for great patience (P. Sankaran 1996).

Final Conclusions Case Taking

For all of our differences ultimately, as we move forward, it is inevitable that homeopaths will continue to adapt, borrow, grow in themselves, learn other techniques and share their results. What links us all as homeopaths is our love of people and the desire to relieve suffering. That which will unite us in our different opinions and ideas is reflection, listening and respect.

We are informed by the outside by our senses. We are informed from the inside by our internal bodily feelings, sensitivities and intuition. We feel strongly. Hearing some stories in our clinics gives us spaghetti in our stomachs, makes our hair stand up on end or alerts us in some way, some private way that what is being said is important, incongruent or dissonant. We are informed by the boundary between the two and perhaps the best posture of a practicing homeopath is developing the capacity to move between both of those two places. Misha Norland (1998) wrote a stunning short article about health and disease. In it he described disease as the dancer whose movements have lost flow, whose movements jar upon our senses and our aesthetics. Health is the opposite. Of course at times we don't even notice healthy people because they fly by revealing nothing for us, no hard edges, no symptoms for which our eye can catch and become fixed on.

Somewhere in the human being is a profound desire help. For very many it is a calling. For others it is an impulse. What is important is that the motives and the drivers are examined. If it is a self-esteem boosting, approval, status, power, the desire to feel useful, the desire to find intimacy, these motives need to be examined (Ram Dass 1985). Exploration of such motives and deepening your skills and understanding of yourself (Lewis 2000) are great places to start. It must be remembered that when two mammals have a conversation, a homeopathic consultation, the conversation takes place on a multitude of levels. It is worth questioning that as we move into the 21st century and further discuss case taking we will be able to retain limbic resonance when two mammals attempt to communicate through an email. After all this is the reason that emoticons were invented because of the inability to understand the intention and the feeling through the computer screen. As our technology, Skype, etc. develops and those images become clearer it might be possible to do some good work over the computer when legal and ethical considerations have been dealt with and taken into account. But there are many other more important challenges. Our patients are loaded up with toxicity making our gentle medicine work hard to break through years, decades and generations of allopathic crude medicines and shocking lifestyles. In addition, homeopathy faces significant legal obstacles in many countries and it is an imperative that these are addressed. There are challenges in education and in the media and significant threats from the outside as we move further into the 21st century from the medical profession keen to hold on to its vested interests and question the validity of anything which is outside its own understanding of evidence-based medicine. Those are high hurdles. But by keeping our tools sharp, and by understanding our materia medica, by grounding that in our philosophy, we know that the technical parts of homeopathy can be practiced well and taken care of. Our clinical results will continue to be effective. But by deepening our understanding of the relationship between patient and the practitioner and truly realizing the significant depth of that relationship, by teaching and harnessing the skills of best practice in homeopathic case taking our clinical results can only improve. If this is coupled to the effective communication of those results and our research skills continue to develop, that represents a bright future. If homeopathy wasn't effective, if homeopathy wasn't making significant improvements in people's lives, if homeopathy was bland, then it would have gone away a long time ago. But it hasn't. And it won't.

Our true challenge as we move into the next decade, is that our worst weakness could be exploited. The broad church that is homeopathy has split apart before. By understanding the landscape of our profession, identifying and celebrating what is common and unifying, starting with the most important part of that, which is our capacity to take cases and be in a relationship with our clients, we can walk forward into the 21st century with our diversity and with our flexibility. In keeping with our philosophy of health and disease, that is a truly healthy posture.

Appendices

- Appendix 1 : Examples of general questions from Hahnemann
- Appendix 2 : Examples of some specific questions from Hahnemann
- Appendix 3 : The Life of Hahnemann
- Appendix 4 : Kent's Questionnaire

Appendices

Appendix 1

Chapter 2

Examples of general questions from Hahnemann

1.	How are the bowel movements?
2.	How does the urine pass?
3.	How is sleep both during the day and at night?
4.	How are the emotions, temper, mental power constituted?
5.	How is the appetite, the thirst?
6.	How is the taste in the mouth, all by itself?
7.	What foods and drinks taste the best? Which ones are the most epugnant to the patient?
8.	Does each food have its full natural taste or some other strange taste?
9.	How is the patient after eating or drinking?
10.	Is there anything to recall about the head, the limbs, the abdomen?
11.	How frequent are his bowel movements? What is the exact quality of the stools? Was the whitish bowel movement, mucous or fecal matter? Were there any pains upon defecation, or not? Exactly what kind of pains and where?
12.	What did the patient vomit?
13.	Is the vile taste in the mouth putrid, bitter, sour, or something else? Does it come before, during or after eating or drinking? At what time of the day is it the worst? What is the taste of any eructations?

14. Does the urine become cloudy on standing or is it cloudy immediately upon being passed? What is its color when it is first passed? What color is the sediment?
15. How does the patient gesticulate and express himself in his sleep? Does he whimper, groan, talk or cry out in his sleep? Does he get frightened during sleep? Does he snore on breathing in or breathing out? Does he lie only on his back, or on his side; which side? Does he cover up snugly, or can he not stand being covered? Does he wake easily, or does he sleep too soundly? How does he feel immediately after waking?
16. How often does this or that ailment occur?
17. What occasions the ailment? Does it come on while sitting, lying, standing, or with movement? Only on an empty stomach, or at least early in the morning; Only in the evening, or after a meal, or when does it usually occur?
18. When did the chill come? Was it only a chilly sensation or was the patient cold at the same time? In what parts was the patient hot to the touch during the chilly sensation? Was it merely a sensation of cold without shivering? Was he hot without being flushed in the face? What parts were hot to the touch? Or did he complain about heat without being hot to the touch? How long did the chill last; how long the heat? When did the thirst come? With the chill? With the heat? Before or after the heat or the chill? How strong was the thirst and for what? When did the sweat come? At the beginning or at the end of the heat? Or how many hours after the heat? While asleep or while awake? How strong was the sweat? Was it hot or cold? On which parts? What was the odor? What ailments did the patient complain of before or with the chill? With the heat? After the heat? With or after the sweat?
19. With respect to the female gender, how are the menses or other discharges? etc. (Hahnemann 1921 footnote § 89)

Appendix 2

Chapter 2

Examples of some specific questions from Hahnemann

(If they have not been told by the patient spontaneously.)
1. How does the patient gesticulate during the visit?
2. Is he vexed, quarrelsome, hasty? Inclined to weep, anxious, despairing or sad; or is he comforted, calm, etc.?

3.	Is he drowsy or generally dull witted?
4.	Does he speak in a demanding manner, very faintly? Inappropriately, or in any other way?
5.	How is the colour of his face and eyes, and the color of his skin in general?
6.	How is the vivacity and energy of his expression and eyes?
7.	How is the tongue?
8.	How is the smell of the mouth?
9.	How is the respiration?
10.	How is the hearing?
11.	How much are the pupils dilated or constricted? How rapidly do they alter in the dark or light?
12.	How is the pulse?
13.	How is the abdomen?
14.	How damp or dry, cold or hot to the touch is the skin in general, or this or that part of it?
15.	Does the patient lie with his head bent back? With his mouth half or wide open? With his arms placed over his head? Does he lie on his back or in another position?
16.	With what exertion does the patient straighten himself up?
17.	Anything else the physician can perceive about him that is strikingly noticeable.

Appendix 3

Chapter 2

Hahnemann's Life

Samuel Friedrich Christian Hahnemann was born on 10 April, 1755, just before midnight in Meissen, Saxony. At the age of 20 he finished at the St. Afra's School and left for Leipzig for higher studies in medicine. He supported himself by teaching French and German and by translating books from English into many languages. From Leipzig he went to Vienna to witness the practice of medicine in the hospitals. Soon he went to Herrmannstadt accepting the family-physician cum librarianship role for the Governor of Transylvania. After 2 years he went to Erlangen to complete his studies and graduated in 1779. After getting his M.D. he went back to Hettstadt, Saxony to practice, only to move soon to Dessau in 1783. Quickly he moved to Gommern as the District Physician and married his first wife Leopoldine Henriette.

In the meantime he had become disillusioned with the uncertainty and barbarity of medical practice and devoted himself to the study of chemistry and other allied subjects. In 1789 he moved to Leipzig. Here in 1790 (Joardar 2002) he translated Cullen's materia medica. Struck by the comment of the author that Peruvian bark cured ague because it was bitter, he, to verify the claim for some reason deliberately took 4 drams of its extract, twice daily for a few days. He observed that the results of this self poisoning produced were very similar to not only the general symptoms but also the characteristic symptoms of the ague. This necessitated further experiments on others, for verification and thereafter provings conducted with other medicinal substances.

He took the charge of an asylum for the insane in Georgenthal in 1792, and he was the first who pleaded for and practiced the moral (mild instead of coersive) treatment of the insane. He was soon on the move again, Walschleben, Pyrmont, Brunswick, Wolfenbuttel and Koenigslutter and it was the hostility of the apothecaries and physicians of Koenigslutter in particular that drove him on further. His comments, writings, letters, severe criticisms and scathing remarks on the practices of venesections, blood letting and massive doses of drugs in single prescriptions contributed to the displeasure and hatred of the apothecaries and the physicians towards him.

Numerous publications were published in the various places he lived along with equally numerous children born. Articles, booklets and books began to establish him as a great reformer in medicine. Most important was the Organon of Medicine in 1810. At this time be was back in Leipzig. He published his Materia Medica Pura in 1811. Then in order to give lectures in the medical college he had to defend a thesis before the faculty of medicine. The Thesis De Helleborismo Veterum in Latin was enthusiastically received by the faculty members and he was allowed to lecture and to practice. His lectures attracted many followers. From these he chose a few to further assist him in proving medicines. This was carried on without a break till 1821, when he was again driven out of Leipzig by the apothecaries and doctors.

He moved to the small town of Coethen under the patronage of the prince Anhalt Coethen. There he published The Chronic Diseases in 1828, also the 3rd, 4th and 5th editions of The Organon. In 1829 a large number of admirers assembled to celebrate his 50th anniversary of his getting the M.D. degree. He had lost his wife in 1830. In 1835 he left Coethen for Paris, marrying his second wife Melanie de Hervelie. It was here he received not only the authorization to practice but all the freedom, recognition and honour that had been denied him for so long. His fame, spread throughout Europe to the US and he attracted many patients. He died on 2nd July 1843 (Winston 1999, Wikipedia).

Appendix 4

Chapter 4

Kent's Questionnaire

What The Doctor Needs To Know In Order To Make a Successful Prescription (Kent 1957).

Section 1:
Every case must be individualized, every symptom from head to feet. This complete picture of the disease cannot always be given in a written communication, and hence, it is best for the physician to see the patient at least once. But many patients wish to be treated by correspondence. The following pamphlet was suggested by Kent for written correspondence by patient who cannot visit the doctor:
1. When you add to the general statement 'I have the headache,' the individual peculiarities, sharp shooting pains in the left side of the head and temple,' you simplify the selection of a remedy very much. When you further add that the pains 'always come on when the slightest cold air strikes the head,' the pains are 'much less when lying down and covering up the head warmly,' and 'much worse when rising up, walking about, or when the head becomes cool,' you then state just what the physician needs to guide him. This is what is called 'individualizing the case.'
2. Write name and address in full; give the age, occupation, married or single (how long married).
3. The colour of your hair and eyes, the complexion, height, weight and any peculiarity of the patient as to form, appearance, size, etc.
4. Write whether any near relative on father's or mother's side has died of, or been troubled with, consumption, asthma, cancer, tumors, scrofula, hives, erysipelas, skin diseases of any kind, or any other chronic complaint; also any peculiarity of the family on either side.
5. Give history of trouble- how it commenced and how long it has been troubling, and any changes which may have taken place.
6. Any medicine which have been used extensively.
7. What you think caused the trouble? What name has been given to the disease?
8. Whether gaining or losing flesh or weight in the past few months
9. How often you have been vaccinated and the effect.

Section 2: After the first prescription

Always write when you began the last medicine; state any changes in the conditions or symptoms since taking the medicine, and the time of the change; mention the symptoms which are entirely gone, or are better, since taking the medicine, and all new ones. Specify the new symptoms, and the old ones which return since treatment.

Section 3: Mental symptoms

The symptoms of the Mind and Disposition are most important and should be carefully considered and reported.

How is your memory? For what is it poor? At what time is it poor? Do you remember what you read? Do you read with interest and pleasure? Can you apply your mind easily? In what way is your disposition changed during sickness? Are you mild, easy, gloomy, hopeless, obstinate, irritable snappish, petulant, 'real ugly' or sullen, cheerful, happy, or in what way is the disposition affected? Do you comprehend easily? Do you answer the questions of others promptly or slowly? Do you have anxiety, apprehension of the future, aversion to being looked at or touched, aversion to people, company or things; bashfulness, desire for company or solitude; desire for death; confusion of mind, delirium, discontent, disgust; dread of the future, of people, of animals or things; any peculiar feeling; mind full of crowding ideas, ill-humor, impatience, indecision, indifference, jealousy, too easily excited to tears or laughter, laziness, loquacity (inclined to much talking); disappointed love, melancholy, easy to be offended, feel like quarrelling, sadness, scolding, screaming, sighing, taciturnity (silent mood), bad or persistent thoughts, or crowding of ideas, aversion to work, play, or anything else? How does the future look to you? Have you any delusions of any kind, or do you imagine you see things that have no existence, that your family has turned against you, that a man is under the bed or in the house, that some one is following or hounding you, that you are rich or poor, or will die in the poor house, hear voices, or that you are called, or anything else in this line?

The questions and language here used are merely suggestive, being intended to lead you to give all your symptoms. Give your case in your own language carefully and fully.

Section 4: Sensations

Give the sensation in your own language to ex-matter how simple, or even ludicrous, it is necessary to give it.

It may be like a mouse or bug crawling; like wind blowing into the ears or eyes; as if someone was pulling a hair; as of a blow on the back; as if the heart was grasped by an iron hand; as if claws were grasping the bowels; as of a splinter in the throat or flesh; like a string or thread on the tongue or in the throat; as if a joint were dislocated; as of a band or cord around the head; as though you had a cap on or hat; as of a plug in the ear or in some other place. Always give the location as well as the sensation.

Section 5 : Better or worse

This section refers to each disease, each sickness and to every symptom. No matter the trouble may be it is necessary to refer to this section. Be sure that the aggravation or amelioration you notice is from the cause given.

The time of an aggravation or amelioration refers to the year, the month, the week, the day, the night, or the hour. State at what time your trouble, or any single symptom, is better or worse. State what season of the year, what time in the month, whether the phases of the moon cause either, what part of the week, what hour of the day or night the trouble or single symptom comes on, or is made better or worse.

Is there any position which you may assume that causes the trouble or any single symptom to be better or worse? It may be when you first lie down, or after lying down awhile, or rising up after lying down; on sitting down, after sitting awhile, or on rising after sitting; standing, after standing awhile, or on sitting after standing; walking much, walking in the house or in the open air, or in cold or warm air, or at night; running rapidly or slowly; when stooping over, after stooping, or on rising from stooping; leaning the head backward, forward, to one side, or leaning the head on the table or the hand; lying with the head high or low; lying in some particular position; crawling on the hands and knees; or some other of many possible positions.

Does anything cause the trouble or a single symptom to be better or worse? It may be reading, writing, music, ascending or descending the stairs or a hill, biting the teeth together, blowing the nose, before or after one of the meals, breathing deeply, when chewing food, when eating or drinking, closing or opening the eyes, looking up, down or sideways, from heat, cold, from warm or cold air, heat of the stove or sun, dry or moist air, going into a warm room, sunlight or lamplight, from excitement, fright, grief, sorrow, fasting, some kind of food or drink, motion or quiet, when nose is discharging or is dry, from gratification of the passions, scratching, rubbing, beginning of sleep, during or after sleep, loss of sleep, sneezing, before or during a storm, thunder storm, snow storm, swallowing food, drink or saliva, talking, singing, hearing others talk or sing, music, touch, turning over in bed, covering up or uncovering, wet, dry, windy, or clouding weather.

Section 6: Pain

Give the exact location on the head, body, arms, hands, legs, feet, etc. right side or left side; make this location as minute as you can.

State whether the pain remains in one place, or whether it changes places; if moving or changing place state just how and to what place it goes. Always mention the place where it starts and then where it goes and how it goes. State how the pain makes you feel; the effect on you; how you act during the pain? Is there anything, any act, any position, any part of the day or night, application of cold or warm water, or dry heat or cold, any change in the weather, cold or warm air, or any other circumstances that causes the pain to be easier or worse, or removes it entirely (see Section 5). Is there any change in the appearance or feeling of the skin, flesh or bone after the pain leaves? What is your general feeling after the pain leaves? How does the pain come, quickly or slowly? Anything that seems to bring it on? How does the pain leave, quickly or slowly? What seems to cause it to leave? What kind of pain is it? What does it seem like to your feeling or imagination? This is very important as there are various kinds of pain, such as cutting, boring, digging, bruised, sore, aching, biting, burning, cramp-like, dull, drawing, gnawing, jerking, labor-like, oppressive, paralytic, piercing, pinching, pressing, pricking, pulsative, stitching, shooting, tearing, violent, wandering (changing place), as from ulceration, as from excoriation or a raw place. Express the sensation of pain in your own language – just as it feels to you.

How much of the time do you have the pain? When is it likely to come on? When are you likely to be free from it? Is there any sore, eruption or swelling at the seat of the pain? Any change in the colour of the place or in the usual appearance of the skin? Mention anything else about the pain that occurs to you, especially anything that appears to be unusual or singular.

Section 7: Discharges of all kinds

This refers to discharges from open sores, boils, fistulas, ulcers etc., from the eyes, nose, ears, mouth, private parts, lungs the skin, etc.

Give the quantity and the time or condition under which the quantity varies. (Section 5.) Give the consistency, whether thin or thick, stringy, clotted like jelly, white of an egg, gruel, water, etc. The appearance, just what it looks like, the colour, and the time or condition when the appearance varies.

The odor, what it reminds you of; whether the odor varies and the time and circumstances of the variation.

Appendices

Whether it makes the parts sore, and in what way; whether the discharge has any effect on your feeling or strength; how long it has continued; whether the discharge comes and goes, and the time and circumstance of this variation. Whether it is sticky, forms a scab, etc. Mention anything else about it that you may notice.

Section 8: Head

Describe any pain as in Section 6. Describe any sores, lumps, or skin disease as in Section 7 and 32. For Sensation in head see Section 4.

Is the hair very dry or naturally moist? Does it split at the ends? Does it tangle easily, - how? Does it came out badly? Any dandruff? Quantity, shape and appearance. Is the hair oily or greasy? Does it break off or mat together? Does it come out in spots or bunches. Be sure to give the exact location of any trouble of the head and whether internal or external.

Dizziness. Describe as in Section 5. What position, motion, or cause brings on the dizziness? What is the sensation? Do you feel like falling in any particular direction? Does it affect the sight? Do you feel as if swaying to and fro, in a circle, falling, rising, floating, as if bed were sinking, things about you were moving, etc. Give all the particulars.

Section 9: Ears

Describe pain as in Section 6. Describe discharges as in Section 7. Sores as in Section 32.

Is the trouble inside, in the canal, or on the external ear? Right or left ear? Are you deaf? When and how can you hear best? When is your hearing poorest? How far from the right ear and the left ear can you hear a watch tick? Is your hearing getting better or worse? Can you hear better in a noise, on the cars, or riding? Is the hearing poor for the human voice or other noises or sounds? Have you too acute hearing? Do sounds hurt the ear or feel unpleasant? Have you any noises in the ear? Which ear? State minutely what the noise is like. Give any sensations in the ears as in Section 4. How does your own voice sound to you?

Section 10: Eyes

Describe pain in the eyes as in Section 6. Discharges as in Section 7. Sensation as in Section 4.

Is the trouble in one eye or both? Which eye? Upper or lower lid? Inner or outer corner of the eye? Under the lid or on the outer side? Does one eye or both water? When? How much? Does the water make the eye or cheeks sore? How does reading or sewing affect the eyes? Are the eyes weak? Does the light of the sun or of a lamp hurt them or cause them to water? At what time are your eyes worse? Have you any peculiar feeling about the eyes? (See Section 4.) How long have you had the trouble? Have you or has any near relative ever had any trouble of the eyes? Have you ever used any eye-washes or salves? Can you refer the trouble to any cause? What appearance has lamp light to you? Has lamp light any peculiar circle around it? Are you near or far-sighted? Any swelling above or below the eyes? Any coloured rings around the eyes? What colour? Do you wear glasses? At what age did you begin to wear glasses? In case you do wear glasses, what would be the result if you did not? Have you had styes? On which lid and how many? Have you ever had a blow or other injury to the eyes?

Section 11: Nose

Is the trouble inside or outside, in forepart or back? For discharge, see Section 7.

Do you blow out scabs or plugs? Give the size, colours, odors, consistency, and any other information about the scabs. Do the discharges make the nose or lip sore? Is the nose painful, swollen, or sore? (See Section 6 and 32.) Do you catch cold easily? Do colds always affect the nose? Under what circumstances do you usually catch cold? For cold and catarrh report fully as in Section 5 and 7.

Section 12: Mouth and tongue

State whether the trouble is with the tongue or mouth, and what part of the mouth.

Any sores? Give the location, appearance, colour and size of the sores. Whether depressed or elevated? For the pain in the sores see Section 6. Is mouth or tongue dry or moist? Much or little saliva? Character, colour, appearance and any peculiarities of the saliva? Thirst. (See Section 15.) Is the breath bad or foul? When does foul breath occur and what is it like? Any bad taste? When does it occur and what is it like? Any peculiar taste? Any peculiar sensation? See Section 4. Is the tongue moist or dry? What is the coating on the tongue, its colour and appearance? What part of the tongue is coated? Is there any peculiarity about the coating? How are the edges of the tongue? How is the tip? How is the back part? Does the tongue show the imprint of the teeth? Can you put it out of the mouth easily? When putting it out does it turn to one side or tremble? Any swelling or soreness under the tongue? Give direction and location of any fissures or cracks on tongue.

Appendices

Section 13: Teeth

Are the teeth sound or decayed? When did they begin to decay? Which teeth are decayed? What part of the teeth decay? What kind of fillings have you in the teeth? On what kind of plate are your false teeth? Are the front teeth smooth or rough on the edges like a saw? Are the teeth dirty-looking, yellow, black or covered with mucus? Do they ache? (See Section 6.) Which teeth ache? What causes the teeth to ache? Cold air, warm or cold food or drink, when the body is cold or warm, when lying down, at night, etc.? What relieves the aching? (See Section 5.) Is there any abscess at the root of a tooth? Do the teeth break off easily or crumble? Also consult Section 4.

Are the gums healthy? Do the gums bleed or recede from the teeth? Do you have gum boils? Are the teeth loose in the gums? Have you ever been salivated? Have the gums or teeth been in good condition since being salivated?

Section 14: Throat

Are you subject to throat troubles? Have you had quinsy, diphtheria, croup or sore throat? Have you had the throat burnt out, tonsils cut or lanced, or have used strong gargles? Have you pain in the throat? (See Section 6.) Is there pain on swallowing solid food drinks or saliva (empty swallowing)? Is the pain during swallowing or after? Have you pain when not swallowing? Have you any sensation or peculiar feeling about the throat; (Section 4.) Have you a desire to keep swallowing? At what time or from what cause do throat troubles come on? On which side of the throat is the trouble? Is it in the upper or lower part of the throat? Is there mucous causing hawking? When do you have to hawk the most? What causes the hawking? Do colds usually affect the throat? Is there any rattling in the throat? What is the appearance, colour and condition of the throat? For swelling on the outer throat or neck see Section 32.

Is your voice clear? State what may be wrong with the voice? What is the effect of talking or singing on the voice? Is voice low, high or hoarse? Is the voice certain in speaking? Are you hoarse much of the time? Is the hoarseness painful? When does the hoarseness come on? What causes the hoarseness?

Section 15: Eating and drinking

Have you a craving for any special article of food? (Not merely a desire, but a feeling that you must have it). Any aversion to any special article of food? Name the article in either case. Are you hungry much of the time or at any special time? Is the hunger or craving for food excessive? Have you no desire for food? Do you eat without hunger? Does the food taste good? Has the food a natural taste? How do you feel food taste good? Has the food a natural taste? How do you feel before eating? Have you any bad effect from eating much or little? Do you desire little or much food at a time? Is there any special food that disagrees? Do you desire solid or liquid food? Do you crave you don't know what? Do you crave substantial food or dainties, candy, cakes, sweet things, sour things, etc.? Is the appetite even or variable? Does food satisfy you? Any trouble that always comes on after eating all you want, or after a little food? Do you eat hastily or slowly? Do you have sick stomach or vomiting after eating? Does eating aggravate other complaints? Are you sleepy after eating? Have you pain anywhere after eating? (See Section 6). Do you suddenly lose your appetite or relish for food while eating, or at any time?

Are you very thirsty or thirstless? Do you wish to drink often or seldom? Do you want to drink much at a time, or little? What effect has drinking on you? Any trouble that always comes on after drinking? Do you crave any special drink. Do you wish hot or cold, or ice cold drinks? Do you feel badly after drinking? Does drinking satisfy you? Do you use tea or coffee? How much? Do you use alcoholic or other liquors? Do you use much milk? Does milk agree? Do you have sick stomach or vomiting after drinking? Does drinking aggravate other complaints? How does water, or other drinks, taste?

Section 16: Nausea, vomiting, eructations, etc.

These terms stand for different things. It is necessary to make the distinction in writing your case.

Eructations. (belching of wind). Is it frequent? When does it usually come on? Does it last long at a time? What relieves it? What makes it worse? Does it relieve the stomach, pain in any place, the throat, or do you feel better generally after belching? Have you pain anywhere before or during belching. Is the amount of wind great or small? Does it come up easily or with difficulty? Is there any other trouble that always accompanies it? Is there any other trouble that always accompanies it? Is there any bloating of the stomach or abdomen? Do you try to belch but cannot? Any nausea with it? Any taste with it? Acid, like almonds, like apples, bitter, greasy, fetid or foul, of food eaten, hot, rancid, salty, sweetish, etc.? State in your own language what the taste is like. Have you gagging? When and under what circumstances? Any accompanying troubles? How does it affect you? Have you at any time heartburn (an uneasy, burning feeling in the stomach)? Any accompanying troubles? How does it affect you? Have you at any time hiccoughing? When does it come on? How often? Any pain? Any accompanying troubles? How does it affect you? What relieves it? Have you at any time regurgitation of food (spitting up food) in small quantity without vomiting? Give particulars. Nausea (qualmishness, squeamishness, loathing, sickness at the stomach). Where is the nausea located, or from where does it seem to come? Does it come and go, or is it constant when present? Does it always come on at a particular time? What seems to cause it? Is there any other trouble or pain that always comes before it or with it? How does it affect you? Describe the feeling in your own words? Does it come on suddenly or gradually? What relieves it? What makes it worse? Is there with it any faintness, fainting, dizziness, paleness, weakness? Do you vomit or retch with the nausea? Is there any sweating with it? Where is the sweat? Is the sweat warm or cold? Do you feel that it would relieve you to vomit? Is there simple nausea, or do you feel deathly sick?

Retching (to make an effort, or straining to vomit without vomiting). What causes it? When does it come on? Does it cause pain anywhere? How does it affect you? (Consult Nausea and Vomiting). Vomiting (emptying the stomach of its contents; puking). Give a minute description of what you vomit as to the appearance, consistency, colour, taste, quantity, etc.

Is it acid, acrid, like white of an egg, bilious, bitter, black, bloody or blood, bluish, brown, clayey, like coffee grounds, cold, curdled, fecal, fetid or foul, fluid, frothy, glaimy, greasy, green, jelly-like, milk, milky, mucous, musty, of pus or matter like rice water, salty, sweetish, watery, white, of worms, yellow?

Is it constant, copious, what you drink, what you eat, difficult, painful, periodic, spasmodic, violent, forcible, slow in coming on, sudden, coming on quickly? When does it come? After eating, after drinking, after chill, from choking, from coffee, from cold, with colic, in convulsions, with cough, with cramps, during teething, with eructations, with eruptions on the skin, after exercise, during expectoration, in fever, from pain, from colic, when hawking, with heat, with hiccough, lying down, rising up, sitting up, standing, from motion, in the morning, when riding, after sleep, from smoking, before stool, on stooping, with sunstroke, swallowing, with thirst, with weakness? Is there anything, any position, food or drink, or application that aggravates the vomiting, or relieves it? Are there any accompanying troubles? How does it affect you? Make a full statement of anything else that may occur to you regarding the vomiting. Water brash (pain or hot feeling in the stomach with a rising of water to the mouth). When does it come on? What is the amount? What is the taste? How does it affect you?

Section 17: The stomach
The stomach is situated below the lower part of the breastbone, or beneath the depression known as the pit of the stomach.
In stomach troubles, indigestion, dyspepsia, etc., it is necessary to consult Sections 4, 6, 15, 16. For the part external to the stomach consult Section 32. For bloating consult Section 18.

Section 18: Abdomen
The abdomen is the belly, that part of the body between the chest and the pelvis. In troubles of the abdomen consult Sections 4, 6, 15, 16. For the external abdomen consult Section 32.
Is there any bloating? When does the bloating come on? Is the bloating much or little, or tense, painful, etc.? Is the bloating over the whole abdomen or only in one place? What effect has it on you? Describe carefully any rumbling? When does it come? How much of the time is the rumbling present? Is the abdomen depressed or full? Is there any soreness of, or oozing from the navel?
Describe rupture or hernia fully as in Section 4, 5, 6, 32. How long as the rupture been present? How did it start? Is there any known cause of the rupture? Have you worn a truss or other appliance?

Section 19: Urine and urination
The bladder is situated behind and extends a little above the bone in the middle lower abdomen. If painful describe as in Section 6. Describe any feeling or sensation as in Section 4.
Have you ever had any blow or injury in this region? Have you ever retained the urine too long, or till it became painful? Any swelling or distension? Is it hot or inflamed? Any soreness or tenderness? Any bearing down pressure? Any sense of weakness? Any sense of uneasiness? Describe any trouble, pain or sensation in the urethra (the canal through which the urine passes). Describe any discharge from the urethra as in Section 7. Consult also the questions in Section 36 and 37.
The kidneys are located on either side of the backbone (spinal column) in front of and more to the upper part of the small of the back, a little above the level of the navel. Describe any pain, sensation or trouble in the region of the kidneys as in Section 6, 4 and 5.

Urination (the act of passing urine). Does the desire to pass urine come on at any particular time, or from any known cause? Is there any pain with the desire? (Section 6). Does the urine flow easier in any particular position or under any special circumstances? Do you have desire to pass urine but cannot? Does it flow freely in a stream, or in drops? Does it flow at once or must you wait? Is there any thing that you must do to help the flow start? Does it flow slowly or come in a gush? Is the desire urgent or can you easily wait? Have you involuntary urination during the day, at night, while coughing, sneezing, or at any time? What part of the night do you wet the bed? Is there any dribbling or leakage? At what time do you have most desire to urinate? Do you have to get up at night? How after? Can you pass urine without stool or stool without urine? Have you no desire to pass urine? Have you no passage of urine and yet no inconvenience? Do you feel the stream when passing? Does the flow intermit, start and stop? Any straining to pass? Is the stream even or divided?

Before urination. Describe any trouble, pain, etc., that always comes on just before the flow starts. Describe pain as in Section 6. Is there any burning before the flow starts? Describe and locate it? Is there any pressure? Any discharge other than urine? Be as explicit as you can as to these troubles.

During urination. Describe every trouble that accompanies the flow, or that comes on during the flow. Describe every trouble that accompanies the flow, or that comes on during the flow. Describe pain as in Section 6. Describe the burning minutely and locate it. Give the peculiar sensations as in Section 4. Do you have any chill, chilliness any discharge other than the urine, faint feeling, pain anywhere, shuddering, etc.

After urination. The same as above.

The urine. Is the urine acrid (corroding), black, bloody, brown, burning, changeable in colour, clear (limpid, no sediment or colour), cloudy, like coffee, cold when passed, pellicle or cuticle or scum on it, dark, decomposes rapidly, decreased in quantity, flaky, foamy, frothy, like thin glue, dirty grey, greenish, high coloured, hot, increased in quantity (profuse), jelly-like, light coloured, milky, muddy, pale, red, scalding, scanty, smoky, straw-coloured, suppressed, thick, turbid, violet colour, watery, like whey, white, yellow.

Mention any difference when first passed and after standing? What is the smell or odour? Do you pass gravel? Describe the sediment (the substance that falls to the bottom of the vessel) very carefully as to the amount, colour, consistency, appearance, whether it varies, and other facts that you may notice. Does the sediment adhere tightly to the vessel? What is the colour, consistency and appearance of that which adheres?

Section 20: Stool, diarrhoea, constipation

Stool (whether diarrhoea, dysentery or constipation).

Character of Stool: Acrid (excoriating), with air bubbles, balls, beaded, bilious, bloody, burning the parts, as if burnt, chalky, changeable, chopped, clayey, coffee grounds, copious, crumbling, curdled, diarrhoeic, difficult to expel, dry, dysenteric, fatty, fecal, fermented, fetid or foul, flaky, flat, fluid, foamy, forcibly expelled, frothy, glassy, like glue, granular, greasy, green scum, gritty, gushing out, hard, full of holes, hot, insufficient, involuntary, irregular, jelly-like, knotty, too large in size, lienteric (with undigest food), liquid, long, loose, lumpy, membranous, mixed, mucus, mushy, narrow in form, noisy (with wind), odourless, oily, painful, painless, pappy, pasty, like pea soup, periodic (at stated times other than each morning), pouring out, profuse, purulent (like matter), recedes (slips back), retained, retarded, like rice water, rough, like cooked sago, sandy, scaly, scanty (too little), like scrapings of intestines, sheep dung, shreddy, slender in size, slow, small in form, soaps suds, soft, passes better when standing, passes better when leaning back, starchy, square, sticky, stringy, sudden in explosion, tar-like, tenacious, thin, thready, triangular, urging desire (cannot wait), watery, white, with worms.

Colour of stool: Ash coloured, black, bluish, brown, changeable, dark, green, grey, liver coloured, reddish, variegated, yellow, white.

When do you have stool? Afternoon, when coughing, after drinking, after eating, frequent, morning, on motion, from least movement, at night, at noon, before or during urination, after washing.

What trouble before stool? For pain see Section 6. For any other trouble locate and describe minutely. Chilliness, colic, faint feeling, fainting, flatulence (gas in bowels), passing wind, heat, piles come down, languor, lazy, nausea, sweat, tenesmus (pressing down in rectum), thirst, trembling, urging to stool (more than natural), vertigo (dizziness), vomiting.

What trouble during stool? For pain see Section 6. For any other trouble locate and describe minutely. Anxiety, bleeding, breathing affected, chill, chilliness, coldness, colic, disagreeable sensation, fainting, faintness, flatulence (gas in bowels), passing wind, heat, piles come down, hunger, nausea, nervousness, loss of fluid from privates sleepy, straining at stool, sweat, bad taste, tenesmus (involuntary straining), thirst, urination, vertigo (dizziness), vomiting, weakness.

What trouble after stool? Same as during stool.

Constipation. See Stool in this Section. For pain anywhere describe as in Section 6. To what extent and when are you constipated? Are there any troubles that come on during or that accompany the constipation? Describe all troubles and locate. Do you feel better or worse during constipation? How often do you have a stool? Have you any desire for stool? How does the constipation affect the mind, the disposition, the head and the breathing? How long have you been costive? Has it followed any sickness, other trouble, or physic? Is it habitual or temporary? Does it always come on before or during any particular trouble, or at any particular time? Is the child teething? Does it alternate with diarrhoea? Have you taken much physic or many pills? If so, state what kind. Have you used Hall's treatment of injections of hot water? Have you indigestion? Much wind in the bowels? The piles (see Section 21)? Liver or spleen trouble? A bad taste? Sore mouth? Nausea? Any skin disease (Section 32)? Vertigo or dizziness? Vomiting? What kind of appetite? What kind of thirst (Section 15)?

Diarrhoea. See Stool in this Section. Is it painful or painless? For pain Section 6. Consult Section 7. Most of the questions under Constipation (n this Section) are suitable for diarrhoea.

What aggravates or ameliorates the diarrhoea? (Section 5). What seems to cause it? Acids, bathing, from cold, after drinking, during or after eating, exertion or work, riding, during sleep, after vaccination, after washing, any kind of weather?

Does it come on at any particular time of the year, month, day or night? Does it alternate with constipation? Is it chronic? Is the child teething? Does it weaken much? Do you lose flesh? Have you fever?

Dysentery (bloody flux). Same question as under Stool and Diarrhoea. Describe more minutely the quantity of blood and mucus, and the character of the tenesmus (involuntary pressing down in bowels).

Section 21 : Anus, rectum, piles

Anus.

Have you any trouble of the anus? abscess, aching, beating, bleeding, boil, boring, bruised pain, burning, clawing, constriction, spasmodic contraction, cramping, crawling, cutting, darting, discharge (other than stool), dragging, drawing, dryness, eruptions, excoriated (chafed, raw), fissures (cracks), fistula (an opening beside the anus with constant discharge), dullness heat, heaviness, inflamed (sore), injured, itching, jerking, pain (see Section 6), pinching, feeling as of a plug, pressure, pricking, prolapsed (protruding) : state when and the effect, relaxed, sensitive, shooting, smarting (when?), soreness, sticking, stinging, stitches, straining, sweat, swelling, throbbing, tickling, tingling, ulcers, warts.

Rectum. *(The intestine just within the anus.)*
Same questions as under Anus.
Piles. *(Haemorrhoids).*
Describe the appearance of them. Colour and shape. When do they come down? What causes them to come down? What relieves the pain in them? What aggravates them? How long have you had them? For the pain; see Section 6. For the discharge, see Section 7. Any peculiar feeling in them (Section 4)? Any bleeding? How much and when? Any pain or trouble anywhere else that accompanies the piles? Do they come with diarrhoea or constipation? Any itching, burning, smarting, soreness? Are they large or small? When and under what circumstances did you first have them? Have you ever had an operation for the piles? Have you ever had an injection of medicine into the piles?

Section 22: Lungs and breathing

Is the pain or other trouble in the chest muscles or deep in the lungs? For pain see Section 6. For cough and expectoration see Section 24.

Do colds usually affect the lungs? Do you cough up anything? Do you have any difficulty in lying on either side or the back in lung troubles? Is there any rattling in the chest? Is there any consumption or lung disease in father's or mother's family? How many near relatives have died of lung troubles? Is there any soreness of the lungs? Any sensitiveness? Have lungs been injured by excessive exercise, running, etc? Do you have any trouble in breathing? By what is the breathing affected? In what position is the breathing affected? What position do you assume when breathing is affected? Do you have difficulty in breathing outward or inward (exhalation or inhalation)? Is breathing affected during or after sleep? While drinking? For troubles of external chest see Section 32.

Section 23: Heart

Does the heart palpitate? At what time or under what circumstances does palpitation come on? Any trouble of heart after eating or sleeping? What kind of palpitation? Is heart beat regular, loud, prolonged, purring, intermitting or skipping? Any other sound in the heart beside the beat? For pain in the heart see Section 6. Do heart and pulse beat together? How many beats per minute? Have you blueness of lips or fingers? Any difficulty in breathing in heart troubles? Any sensation in region of the heart? (Section 4.) Does motion or quiet affect the heart? Has heart ever been strained by excessive exercise, mountain climbing, etc.?

Section 24: Cough and expectoration

What kind of cough have you? Constant, croupy, crowing, deep, dry, explosive, fatiguing, forcible, frequent, gagging, hacking, harassing, hard, harsh, hissing, hoarse, hollow, jerking, labored, loose, loud, moist, muffled, nervous, noisy, painful, in paroxysms (spells), periodic (at certain times), racking, rapid, rattling, ringing, rough, scraping, screeching, shaking, sharp, short, shrill, in single coughs, spasmodic, sudden, suffocative, tearing, teasing, tickling, (where?), tight, tormenting, violent, wheezing, whistling).

What causes the cough? Acids, anger, anxiety, coffee, from cold, crying, teething, while drinking, after drinking, as from dust, while eating, after eating, emotions, excitement, exertion or working, in fever, liver troubles, least motion, mucus in throat or lungs, music, from nausea, odors, playing the piano, running, from smoke, stooping, talking, tickling (where?), dry weather, wet weather, windy weather, from warm room into open air, when thinking of it, during study, sensation of sulphur fumes, feather, or what?

When does cough come on? Afternoon, evening, forenoon, lying down, sitting up, morning, night, noon, during sleep (does it waken you?) before arising in the morning, just after arising, before midnight, after midnight, early evening, when going to bed, just after going to beds in company, when alone, during the day, only at night, etc.?

Where does cough seem to come from? Abdomen, chest (lungs), back of mouth, windpipe, stomach, throat, etc.?

Where does it hurt you when you cough? How does it hurt you? What effect has the cough on you? Must you hold your throat, chest, head, stomach, or any other part while coughing? For pain while coughing see Section 6.

Expectoration. Do you cough up anything? Describe it as in Section 7. What does it taste like? Can you spit it out? Does it fly out of the mouth while coughing? Does it float in water or sink? Does it vary as to quantity, colour, consistency, taste, etc?

When do you expectorate and when not? Morning, noon, afternoon, evening, forepart of night, after part of night, at bed time, on arising in the morning, after arising in the morning? Under any other circumstance?

Section 25: Joints

Locate the joint affected and the side the joint is on. For pain see Section6. Describe any sensation or feeling as in Section 4.

Any cracking on movement? Has it been out of place or dislocated? Has it ever been injured? Does it feel as if dislocated? Any eruption or sore about it? (Section 32.) Is it inflamed, hot, swollen, sore, painful? Does it move easily? It is stiff or is there no motion? Does the inability to move come from pain, or from what cause? Is it numb? Have you rheumatism now, or have you had it? Has it ever been sprained? Is it weak? Have you corns or bunions? Locate and describe as to pain and other particulars. Any trouble in walking?

Section 26: Muscles

For pain in muscles see Section 6. For discharge from muscles (sores of any kind) see Section 7.

Are muscles contracted, knotted, sore, stiff, any numbness, pricking, tickling? Report the sensation as in Section 4.

Section 27: Bones

Describe pain in bones as in Section 6. Locate the bone affected.

Has the place affected ever been injured, bruised or broken? Do your bones break easily? Is there any swelling of the bone? Describe the trouble carefully in all particulars.

Section 28: Back

For pain see Section 6. Also consult Section 5 and 32.

Especially describe the time or position in which the pain comes on. Also what position or act (like pressure, lying on hard bed, etc.) makes the pain better or worse. State carefully the part of back affected. Describe the sensations as in Section 4. Have you ever had the back injured in any way?

Section 29: Wounds and injuries

Have you had severe wounds or injuries in the past? Was your general health good after the injury? Have you had a hard fall? Describe it carefully. Is the wound a cut, tearing of the flesh, punctured, gunshot, sting of insect, a strain, or what? For discharge see Section 7. For pain see Section 6.

Give exact location. What caused the wound or injury? Did it bleed much, little or any? Did the wound heal readily? What is the appearance, colour and shape of the scar? Does the sear give you any trouble? Does the scar change colour at any time? What kind of insect stung you (if bad effect from insect sting)? What bruised the place? What is the colour, appearance, extent of the bruise? What produced the burn (steam, hot water, fire, hot wax, etc.)? What is the extent and appearance of the burn? Is the burn deep or only on the skin? What produced the cut or laceration? Was either deep or shallow? Is the wound cold, or very hot?

Section 30: Bleeding

Give the cause of bleeding. Give the location or where the bleeding is from.

Does the blood ooze, flow, or come in gushes? Is the blood thin or thick, clotted, lumpy, stringy, hot? Give colour and appearance of the blood. Are you subject to bleeding? From what place? Have you ever been subject to bleeding? Does the bleeding weaken you? Are there any peculiar sensations or feelings that accompany the bleeding? Give all other known particulars.

Section 31: Morbid growths, tumors, cancers, etc.

In the treatment of these every symptom from head to feet must be known, therefore nearly every part of this pamphlet must be consulted and symptoms given as directed. These troubles can all be cured by the internal homeopathic remedy when taken in time. To cut them out does note cure them. Cutting them out removes the effect of disease, but does not remove the disease itself. It is like cutting off the tops of weeds-they will grow again, either as the same place or in another place. Month of careful treatment are required for their cure. When thus cured they will remain cured.

Give the exact location. Describe pain as in Section 6. Describe discharges as in Section 7. Describe the appearance, if on the outside. Describe the feeling to the hand, if on the inside. Give the size and general form. How long has it been coming? Is it hard, soft, yielding, movable? Any sensation in it? (Section 4) Have you ever had any injury or blow on or near the place? Describe how it began and the growth. Has the growth been slow or rapid? Is it fast to the skin (if within)? Does it grow at any particular time or from any cause? What has it been called by other physicians? What treatment have you had for it? Ever had a surgical operation for this or any similar trouble? Have you applied any medicine to it locally? Has the treatment or local application made any change in it? Has any near relative on father's or mother's side had the same, or a similar trouble?

Section 32: Skin diseases

This includes all eruptions, pimples, sores felons, abscesses, ulcers, carbuncles, boils, warts, morbid growths, tumors, cancer, and all kindred diseases, as these are all amenable to the homoeopathic internal treatment. Consult Sections 4, 5, 6, 7, and 31.

Does the skin heal readily after an injury? Any roughness chapping, sores from washing or cold weather? Are you subject to skin diseases, and for how long? Have any of your near relatives been troubled in the same way, or with any other skin trouble? Have you been vaccinated? How did it take, and what was the effect? Have you had the itch? What treatment was used for it? Have you had measles, scarlet fever, chicken pox, small pox, mumps, or other similar diseases, and how did you get along during the sickness and afterwards? And how did you get along during the sickness and afterwards? Have you ever had a surgical operation for the removal of tumors, morbid growths, etc.? (Section 31.) How do your nails differ from healthy nails? Have you hang-nails? Ingrowing toe nails? Have you foul, sweaty feet? (Section 7) How long has the skin trouble been present? How did it first start? Is the trouble sensitive to touch or pressure? Give the exact location of places affected. Has the trouble been treated by local applications? Has any skin disease ever been suppressed or apparently cured by local applications? If so, what and when? What does the disease or sore look like? What is the appearance of the skin around the sore or under the sore? Is there any itching of the sore? What effect has scratching? Any scabs? What is the appearance and general form of the scabs? Any matter under scabs? (Section 7.) Describe any discharge from the sores as in Section 7. Describe pain as in Section 6. Any roughness of the skin? In what way is the skin different from healthy skin? Is there itching of the skin? (Section 5.) Give location, color and character of any spots or blotches on the skin where very small or large. Give location, color and appearance of any moles or warts. What is the location, color, size, shape and appearance of any swelling? Any sensations on skin as itching, burning, pinching, crawling, of insects or bugs, stinging or anything else? See Section 4 and 5. Is the skin oily, shining, scaly? What is the color of the skin? Is the color permanent or natural? Describe pimples, little blisters, etc., as to location size, contents, appearance, etc., Describe corns and bunions as to appearance, location and pain as in Section 6.

Section 33: Fever, chill and sweat

Where have you flashes of heat? Have you flashes of heat and chill intermingled or alternating? Give location and time when either comes on. Is there shuddering? Are you inclined to be chilly generally, or in special parts? Where does the chilliness, or chill, begin and what course does it take? Do you like or desire the warmth or heat of the stove, sun or wraps? Do you feel better when warm or cold? Do you have thirst with the chill, fever or sweat? Do you have hunger with the chill, fever of sweat? At what time of the day or night does the chill, fever or sweat come on? At what time is either the highest? At what time is either the lowest? What seems to cause the chill, fever or sweat? Have you coldness (other than chill) internally or externally? Does any other complaint or sickness come on during the chill, fever or sweat? How long does the chill, fever or sweat continue? In intermittent fever (ague) do you have a distinct stage of chill, fever and sweat? How do you feel generally between the chill, fever and sweat, or after either? When having intermittent fever (ague) do you have hours or days when feeling perfectly well? Is one part is cold? Do you have a chill as to any specified hour or day? Which predominates, or is worse, the chill, fever or sweat? Is the skin hot, dry, moist, red, pale, cool or purple with the fever? Is there goose flesh with the chill or chilliness?

What is the condition of the flesh during the sweat? What is the pulse rate? Is the pulse full, bounding, thready, skipping a beat, imperceptible, compressible.

Is sweat local or general over the body? Does any particular part or place sweat at any time? Do the covered or uncovered parts sweat? Is the sweat warm, cold, sticky, musty, clammy, foul, greasy, pungent smell, sour? What is the color? What color does it stain the clothing? Is sweat weakening? How do you feel during and after sweat? Do you sweat easily? Where, on what part do you sweat most?

Mention any other peculiarity of the chill, fever or sweat. Have you ever had ague? When, how long, and what medicine was taken for the ague? Have you been well since having the ague?

Section 34: Sleep and dreams

State when and under what circumstances you are abnormally drowsy or sleepy. State when and under what circumstances you have yawning. Is the yawning painful or spasmodic? State all troubles or symptoms occurring before, during or after sleep, or when just falling to sleep? State all troubles that come on just as you waken, and how you awaken; what awakens you during the night? Are you a sound, deep or a light sleeper? What causes the sleeplessness? When and under what circumstances are you sleepless? What seems to keep you awake when first going to bed, or when awaking during the night? Do you awaken often during the night? Is the sleep restful refreshing? How do you feel when first awaking and on first arising in the morning? Do you take a nap or sleep during the day? Do you feel well after a sleep during the day? Are you easy or hard to awaken? Do you sleep quietly or toss and roll about during sleep? Do you like to sleep with the head high or low? Do you have the nightmare? Do you snore loudly? Do you moan, scream, or make other noises during sleep? Have you sweat during sleep? Have you grating or grinding of the teeth during sleep?

Do you dream much? Do you remember your dreams? Do the dreams trouble you after waking? In what part of the night do you dream? Do you dream the same dream over the same night, or later? Are the dreams confused, pleasant, horrible, frightful, disgusting, disagreeable, vexatious, vivid? Do you dream of accidents, animals, cats, dogs, blood, business, church, death or corpses, dancing, danger, drinking, drowning, eating, falling, fire, flying, fruit, ghosts, horses, houses, being hungry, lightning, misfortunes, money, murder, of people, praying, being pursued, of quarrelling, riding, robberies, sexual pleasure, shooting, sickness, snakes, snow, talking, being thirsty, trees, urinating, vomiting, of water, weeping? Do you have day dreaming?

Section 35: For women only

In the treatment of diseases peculiar to women all symptoms from head to feet, and previous history should be given. Local examinations and local treatment are seldom required and will only be made by the homoeopathic physician when really necessary.

Mammae (the breasts).

For pain see Section 6. For discharges see Section 7. For skin eruptions, spots, hard lumps, morbid growths cancer, etc., consult Sections 31 and 32. Have you ever had abscess of the breasts? Have breasts ever been injured? Are breasts cold? Are breasts hard, swollen, inflamed, hot, sensitive, sore? Are breasts undeveloped (too small) or too large? Do breasts itch? Is there pain when nursing the child (Section 6)? Is there any fluid or milk in breasts other than when nursing?

Is there any trouble with the nipples or the part around them? Such as bleeding, burning, cracks, eruptions, gummy secretions, hard, inflamed, inverted or retracted, itching, pain (Section 6), redness, sensitiveness, soreness, swelling, ulcers?

Genitals (external sexual parts).

Consult especially Sections 4, 6, 31 and 32.

Is there any trouble of the genitals? Biting, burning, congested, cracks, dryness, enlarged, eruptions, loss of hair, heat (feels hot), inflammation, irritation, itching, moisture, rawness, sensitiveness, smarting, soreness, stinging, stitching, sweat, swelling, tickling,

Appendices

tumors, ulcers, voluptuous sensation, warts. For any trouble, pain, etc., state all the facts as to aggravation and amelioration, Section 5.
Vagina.
Especially consult Section 4, 6, 7, 31. State all the troubles of the vagina fully and particularly. Do not allow modesty to prevent a full statement. These matters are held in the strictest confidence.
There may be want of all feeling in the vagina, bearing down in the vagina, biting, burning, coldness congestion, constriction and contraction of the walls, discharges (see Leucorrhoea), dragging, drawing, dryness, flatus or wind from vagina, fullness, granulations, undue heat, heaviness, inflammation, irritation, itching, jerking, pain, pressing, pitching, prolapse or falling of the walls of the vagina, rawness, sensitiveness, smarting, soreness, stitches, swelling, ulcers, warts.
Ovaries (the ovarian region is to either side of the womb and above the groins).
Especially consult Section 4, 5, 6. Always state on which side the trouble is. If an enlargement or a tumor state pains minutely (Section 6), whether it increase or decreases, its relation to discharges from the vagina and menses, how long present, whether growth is rapid or slow, whether movable, and about the size. Have you ever been injured in the ovarian region? Did you have any trouble before marriage? Have others of your family, or your mother, had the same or similar trouble?
State all others troubles. There may be aching, bearing down, boring, burning, cramping, dragging, drawing, gnawing, grinding, heaviness, hardness, inflammation, itching (internal), jerking, numbness, pain, pinching, pressing, pushing, sensation, sensitiveness, tenderness, shooting, soreness, stinging, stitching, swelling, throbbing or beating, twitching, twisting, etc.
The uterus (the womb is situated in the middle lower abdomen, behind and extending a little above the bladder).
In this place it will be well to ask some very delicate, but important questions. A true answer to these may throw much needed light on the case. With these, as with all questions, no reply is to be made unless there should be something abnormal. Were you led into the habit of masturbation (self-abuse) when a child, or later? To what extend did you practice it? Is there undue sexual desire? Is the sexual desire lost? Is sexual embrace painful or distasteful? Has sexual embrace been excessive? Are there any bad results following (within a few hours) sexual embrace? If married, how many children? If no children, do you do anything to prevent them? How do you prevent having children? It

will be well to fully state everything abnormal about these things, and ask any questions that may give you needed light. Especially consult Section 4, 5, 6, 31, for womb troubles. Do you have a consciousness of a womb? State the sensation if the womb seems not to be in the proper position. If there is pain or other trouble in any other part of the body which seems to be connected with the womb, state particulars and mention what relation there seems to be, have you falling of the womb? If so, give the extent, the accompanying troubles, the time and cause, what relieves or aggravates (Section 5), and the effect upon you generally. To what extent have you worn a pressary or support, and what would be the effect if you did not wear any? For haemorrhage see Section 7 and 30, and 'Flow' under Menses in this Section. Have you ever received an injury in the region of the womb? Have you been ruptured or torn in childbirth? In womb trouble there may be aching, bearing down (or a pushing as though everything would come out), burning, bursting, feeling, contraction, congestion, cramps, cutting, discharge (see Vagina in this Section), distress, drawing, enlargement, fullness, heaviness, hardness, inflammation, labor-like pains, motion, neuralgia, pain, pressure, sensitiveness, soreness, spasms, squeezing, sensation, swelling, throbbing, etc.

Menses

To insure a prompt cure it is necessary for patients to be very observing and report all symptoms as directed in other Sections. The interval between the menstrual periods is 28 days, counting from the beginning of one period to the beginning of the next. At what age did you have your first menses? Had you any trouble before or during the first period? Have you, at any time, had your menses stopped or deranged by getting feet wet, from a general wetting, from cold, fright, sickness, or from any cause? Have menses been irregular or painful since a particular time? Are your menses too frequent, too seldom, delayed, regular, early, late? How often do they come? For pain at the period describe as directed in Section 6, and Before, During, and After, in this Section. Do you have menses during the nursing of your child? Do you have the whites or nose bleed instead of the menses? How long do menses last? Does excitement or overexertion bring menses on? When does the flow increase, decrease, or cease? Afternoon, day only, evening, lying down, morning, motion, at night only, walking. Mention anything that affects the flow.

Character of the flow. Describe the flow very carefully. Acrid black, bright red, brown, changeable, clotted or lumpy, copious, dark, excoriating (making parts sore), fetid or foul, greenish, gushing, hot (unduly so), intermitting as to flow, membranous (shreds), milky, mucous, odor (what is the odor?), pale, profuse, protracted (lasts too long), scanty, stringy, tenacious, thick, too thin, viscid, watery, dark clots in bright blood, etc. Give exact appearance and odor of the flow. Before the menses. It is very necessary to state whether the accompanying trouble of the menses are before, during or after the flow. We mention some of the more frequent troubles occurring at these times. Various troubles of the abdomen. Loss of or a very great appetite. Troubles of the back. Difficulty in breathing. Troubles of the chest. Chill. Chilliness. Costiveness. Convulsions. Cough. Delirium. Diarrhoea. Ear trouble. Eructations. Eruptions. Eye trouble. Face trouble. Fainting. Cold feet. Head troubles; headache. Leucorrhoea. Pain in arms or legs. Swelling, itching and soreness of the breasts. Mental changes (Section 3). Nausea or vomiting. Bleeding of nose. Ovarian troubles. Pain (Section 6). Restlessness. Sexual excitement. Urinary troubles. Great weakness or weariness. Describe all such troubles, and others, as directed in the various Sections.

During the Menses. This refers to the time from the starting to the ending of the flow. All the troubles mentioned as occurring 'Before the Menses' may occur during the period, and many others. Describe everything as directed in other sections. Consult especially Section 3, 4, 5, 6. After the Menses. Many of the troubles referred to above may occur after the menses. Give all the complaints carefully as above.

Leucorrhoea (the whites)

At what time does it come on? Is it all the time? Describe the colour, consistency, odor and appearance of the discharge, and all accompanying complaints. Does it make the pats sore, raw or itch? What color does it stain the napkin or clothing? Notice what other complaints always come on or are worse when the leucorrhoea comes on, or is worse. Does it corrode the clothing? Does it come an, or is it worse, before or after the menses? Are you excessively weak?

It may be acrid (corroding), albuminous (like white of an egg), briting, black, bloody, brown, burning, clear, cold, cream-like, dark, fetid or foul, like jelly, greenish, in gushes, honey-colored, lumpy, mild or bland, milky, mucous, opaque, profuse, purulent (mattery), ropy, scalding, scanty, smarting, causing soreness, starchy, sticky, stiffening the linen, suddenly coming and going, tenacious, thick, thin, thready, transparent, watery, white, yellow.

Pregnancy (during and after)

Treatment during this period is not only best for the mother, but is also best for the future health of the coming child, as well as for future pregnancies. The healthy woman will have no trouble and the minimum of pain in bearing children; normal labor is easy labor.

Report all these complaints as in the various section of this pamphlet, but especially consult Section 3, 4, 5, 6, 7. Nearly every abnormal condition of the pregnant woman will be found in the preceding sections. Have you ever miscarried? How often, and what was the condition of your health afterward? At what month of pregnancy was the miscarriage? What caused the miscarriage?

For morning sickness consult Sections 15 and 16 and state how long pregnant.

How did you get along at your last confinement? Were instruments used? How long were you in labor? Was there any trouble with the after birth or with the lochia (discharge)? How was your recovery from childbed? Describe any complaints you may have had following it. Have you had milk leg? Do you nurse your child? If not, why not? Was the milk good and sufficient? How long after childbirth before having your menses? Describe any trouble you may have had during pregnancy or after childbirth.

Climacteric (the charge of life)

Describe any trouble which may arise during this period as directed in the various section preceding, and especially consult Section 3, 4, 5, 6, 7. At what age did your mother or older sister pass this period? If you are now passing it, at what age did it begin? Do you have flashes of heat? If profuse flooding, describe as directed in 'Flow' in this section and as in Section 30. If past the period, how long since? Did you have any trouble during the climacteric?

Section 36: For men only

For all complaints, whether local or general, the preceding sections should all be consulted and every symptom reported as herein directed. For all complaints, whether local or general, consult especially Section 3, 4, 5, 6, 7, 32.

Answer the following questions, when suited to your case, fully not by 'yes' or 'no', nor by a mere acknowledgement. Have you been addicted to the practice of masturbation (self-abuse) in the past? To what extent? Have you excessive sexual desire? Is sexual desire diminished or lost? Is there an aversion or repugnance to sexual embrace, or to women? Do thoughts of the sexual relation, or the desire for sexual gratification, crowd upon your mind? Does the presence of women cause sexual thoughts, or erections? Are your dreams persistently of sexual gratification, or of lewd women? Do you have sexual desire or teasing without erection? Are the erections incomplete or too soon lost? Has sexual embrace any bad effect on you mentally or physically? Is sexual embrace thrilling or has it no pleasure? Is sexual embrace complete or does the erection fail? Is the semen discharged too soon, or too late? Is the discharge of the semen painful? Do you have erections when riding in a carriage, or on the cars? Are you prompted to expose your private parts? Are you inclined to handle or manipulate your private parts? For pain in the parts locate and describe as in Section 6. Is there any unpleasant odour from the parts? Is there warm or cold sweat on the parts? Are there warts or growths on the parts? (Section 31 and 32.) Do the parts feel natural and healthy, or do they feel weak? Is the penis shrunken, retraced, relaxed, lifeless, small, swollen, etc? State the part of the penis affected as well as the trouble. Is the scrotum (bag) sweaty, contracted, itching, swollen, relaxed, or hanging loose, etc.? State any affection of the testicle (seeds). Describe any eruption or sores on the privates as in Section 32. Have you loss of semen (spermatorrhoea) at night, during stool, or at any time? What is the effect of this seminal loss? Is there a thrill with the seminal loss? Is the seminal loss during lewd dreams? Have you indulged your sexual appetite extensively? Have the parts been injured by a fall or a blow? Have you ever had a gonorrhoea (clap)? State the time and treatment, and the state of your health since. Have you ever had syphilis (pox)? State the time and treatment, and the condition of your health since. Have you had buboes, chancre, or ulcers? Have you had eruptions, sores, warts, etc., since having gonorrhoea or syphilis? Locate, state the character and the result. Have you gleet or any discharge from the penis? Describe as in Section 7.

References

Ackerman, S.J. & Hilsenroth, M. J. (2003), A review of therapist characteristics and techniques positively impacting the therapeutic alliance, *Clinical Psychology Review*, 23:1-33.

Adams, P. (2009), Where is homeopathy going?, *Homeopathy*, 28(1):26-29.

Allen, T.F. (1889), *Handbook Of Homoeopathic Materia Medica*, EE Boericke: Philadelphia, (accessed Encyclopaedia Homeopathica, 2010).

Allen, H.C. (1881), Prejudice the chief obstacle to the scientific investigation of posology in clinical medicine, *American Institute Of Homoepathy*, (accessed Encyclopaedia Homeopathica, 2010).

Allen, H.C. (1903), The Keystone Of A Prescription, *American Institute Of Homoepathy*, (accessed Encyclopaedia Homeopathica, 2010).

Allen, J.H. (2001), *The Chronic Miasms*, B. Jain Publishers, New Delhi.

Asay, T.P. & Lambert, M. J. (1999), The empirical case for the common factors in therapy: Quantitative findings, in Hubble MA, Duncan BL & Miller SD (eds.), *The Heart and Soul of Change: What Works in Therapy*, 33-56, American Psychological Association.

Bailey, P.M. (1995), *Homeopathic Psychology*, (accessed Encyclopaedia Homeopathica, 2010).

Bakshi, J.P.S. (1998), *Manual of Psychiatry: for homoeopathic students and practitioners*, Cosmic Healers: New Delhi.

Baldwin, S.A., Wampold, B.E. & Imel, Z.E. (2007), Untangling the Alliance-Outcome Correlation: Exploring the Relative Importance of Therapist and Patient Variability in the Alliance, *Journal of Consulting and Clinical Psychology*, 75(6):842-852.

Balint, M. (1957), *The Doctor, His Patient & The Illness*, Tavistock Publications: London.

Ball, J. (2004), *Understanding Disease A Health Practitioner's Handbook*, Random House.

Banerjee, P.N. (1984), *Chronic Disease, Its Cause And Cure*, Pratap Medical Publishers Pvt. Ltd: New Delhi.

Barry, C., Bradley, C., Britten, N. & Stevenson, F. (2000), Patients' unvoiced agendas in general practice consultations: qualitative study, *BMJ*, 320:1246-1250.

Barry, C.A., Stevenson, F.A., Britten, N., Barber, N. & Bradley, C.P. (2001), Giving voice to the lifeworld. More humane, more effective medical care? A qualitative study of doctor-patient communication in general practice, *Social Science & Medicine*, 53:48.

Beck, R.S., Daughtridge, R. & Sloane, P.D. (2002), Physician-Patient Communication in the Primary Care Office: A Systematic Review, *J Am Board Fam Pract*, 15:25-38.

Benedetti, F. (2008), Mechanisms of Placebo and Placebo-related Effects Across Diseases and Treatments, *Annual Review of Pharmacology and Toxicology*, 48:33-60.

Bensing, J. (2000), Bridging the gap. The separate worlds of evidence-based medicine and patient-centered medicine, *Patient Education and Counseling*, 39(1):17-25.

Bidwell, G.I. (1911), *The Indicated Homoeopathic Remedy: How To Find It,* Transactions of the Homeopathic Medical Society of the State of New York, (accessed Encyclopaedia Homeopathica, 2010).

Bidwell, G.I. (1915), *How To Use The Repertory*, Boericke & Tafel: Philadelphia (accessed Encyclopaedia Homeopathica, 2010).

Blow, A. & Sprenkle, D.H. (2001), Common Factors Across Theories of Marriage and Family Therapy: a Modified Delphi Study, *Journal of Marital and Family Therapy*, 27(3):385-401.

Blow, A.J., Sprenkle, D.H. & Davies, S.D. (2007), Is who delivers the treatment more important than the treatment itself? The role of the therapist in common factors, *Journal of Marital and Family Therapy*, 33(3):298-317.

Böenninghausen, C. (1908), *The Lesser Writings of Boenninghausen,* Boericke & Tafel: Philadelphia, (accessed Encyclopaedia Homeopathica, 2010).

Boericke, G. (1929), *A Compend of the Principles of Homoeopathy for Students in Medicine*, Boericke & Tafel: Philadelphia, (accessed Encyclopaedia Homeopathica, 2010).

Boger, C.M. (1939), *The Study Of Materia Medica And Taking The Case*, Roy: Bombay.

Bohart, A.C. (2000), The Client is the most important common factor: clients' self-healing capacities and psychotherapy, *Journal of Psychotherapy Integration*, 10(2):127-149.

Borland, D.M. (2003), *Pneumonias*, B. Jain Publishers (P) Ltd: New Delhi.

Bradford, T.L. (1895), *The Life and Letters of Dr. Samuel Hahnemann*, Roy Publishing House: Calcutta.

Bridger, M. (1998), Up the Swanee to Atlantis, *Homeopath*, 68:835-839.

References

Buck, H. (1865), *The Outlines Of Materia Medica*, Leath and Ross: London, (accessed Encyclopaedia Homeopathica, 2010).

Budd, S. (1994), Transference revisited, in Budd S & Sharma U, *The Healing Bond: The Patient-Practitioner Relationship and Therapeutic Responsibility*, Routledge: London, 153-170.

Bugge, C., Entwistle, V.A. & Watt, I.S. (2006), The significance for decision-making of information that is not exchanged by patients and health professionals during consultations, *Social Science & Medicine*, 63(8): 2065-2078.

Burnett, J.C. (1881), *Diseases Of The Veins* (accessed Encyclopaedia Homeopathica, Archibel 2010).

Burnett, J.C. (1901), *Curability Of Tumours* (2nd edn.), Boericke & Tafel: Philadelphia, (accessed Encyclopaedia Homeopathica, 2010).

Burnett, J.C. (1898), *The Change Of Life In Women*, Boericke & Tafel: Philadelphia, (accessed Encyclopaedia Homeopathica, 2010).

Burt, W.H. (1873), *Characteristic Materia Medica*, Boericke & Tafel: Philadelphia, (accessed Encyclopaedia Homeopathica, 2010).

Busse, W.W. & Lemanske, R.F. (2009), The placebo effect in asthma: far more complex than simply 'I shall please', *Journal of Allergy and Clinical Immunology*, 124(3):445-446.

Candegabe, E.F. (1997), *Comparative Materia Medica, The Value Of Symptoms*, Beaconsfield Bucks: Beaconsfield, (accessed Encyclopaedia Homeopathica, 2010).

Cape, J. (2000), Patient-rated therapeutic relationship and outcome in general practitioner treatment of psychological problems, *British Journal of Clinical Psychology*, 39:382-395.

Carlston, M. (2003), *Classical Homeopathy*, Elsevier Churchill Livingstone.

Case, E.E. (1916), *Some Clinical Experiences of Erastus E. Case*, The Emerson Publishing co: Ansonia.

Cassell, E.J. (1995), *The Healer's Art* (3rd edn.), MIT Press: Cambridge, Mass.

Castro, J.B.D. (1998), *Logic of Repertories*, B. Jain Publishers: New Delhi.

Catty, J. (2004), 'The vehicle of success': Theoretical and empirical perspectives on the therapeutic alliance in psychotherapy and psychiatry, *Psychology and Psychotherapy*, 77:255-272.

Chauhan, D. *(2010), A Wander with Little Wonder: Child Centric Case Witnessing.*

Charon, R. (2001), Narrative Medicine: A Model for Empathy, Reflection, Profession and Trust, *JAMA*, 286:1897-1902.

Chatterjee, T.P. (1988), *Fundamentals Of Homoeopathy And Valuable Hints For Practice*, B. Jain Publishers: New Delhi.

Cheraghi-Sohi, C., Holem A.R., Mead, N., McDonald, R., Whalley, D., Bower, P. & Roland, M. (2008), What Patients Want From Primary Care Consultations: A Discrete Choice Experiment to Identify Patients' Priorities, *Annals of Family Medicine*, 6:107-115.

Chhabra, D. (2002), Interview, *Simillimum*, XV(4), Winter.

Chitkara, H. (1921), *Best of Burnett*, (accessed Encyclopaedia Homeopathica, 2010).

Cicchetti, J. (2003), *Dreams, Symbols and Homeopathy: Archetypal Dimensions of Healing*, North Atlantic Books: California, USA.

Cicchetti, J. (2004), Interview with Jane Cicchetti by Elaine Lewis, published on *Hpathy Ezine*, August, available online at http://www.hpathy.com/interviews/janecicchetti.asp.

Clarke, J.H. (1885), *The Prescriber: A Dictionary of the New Therapeutics*, Keene & Ashwell. London, (accessed in Encyclopaedia Homeopathica Archibel 2010).

Clarke, J.H. (1895), *Diseases Of The Heart Arteries*, E. Gould & Sons: London, (accessed Encyclopaedia Homeopathica, 2010).

Clarke, J.H. (1908), *The Cure Of Tumours By Medicine*, (accessed in Encyclopaedia Homeopathica Archibel 2010).

Clarke, J.H. (1927), *Constitutional Medicine With Especial reference To The Three Constitutions Of Von Grauvogl*, Homoeopathic Publishing Co: London, (accessed in Encyclopaedia Homeopathica Archibel 2010).

Close, S. (1924), *The Genius Of Homoeopathy; Lectures And Essays On Homoeopathic Philosophy*, Boericke & Tafel: Philadelphia.

Coatsworth-Puspoky, R., Forchuk, C. & Ward-Griffin, C. (2006), Nurse-client processes in mental health: recipients' perspectives, *Journal Psychiatric and Mental Health Nursing*, 13(3):347-355.

Coulter, H.L. (1973), *Divided Legacy: The Conflict Between Homeopathy And The American Medical Association*, Wehawken Press & North Atlantic Books: Washington.

Cousins, N. (1980), *Anatomy of an illness as perceived by the patient: reflections on healing and regeneration*, GK Hall: Boston.

Currim, A. (1996), Guide To Kent's Repertory And The Collected Writings Of Arthur Hill Grimmer, *New England Journal Of Homoeopathy*, (accessed Encyclopaedia Homeopathica, 2010).

References

D'Aran, K. (1997), Totality of the Whole Person or Totality of the Whole Diseased Person *HANSW*, 1(1), April, Australia.

D'Aran, K. (2008), Lecture, AHA Case Conference, Sydney.

D'Aran, K. (2010), Private correspondence with the author.

Danciger, E. (1987), *The Emergence of Homeopathy. Alchemy to Medicine*, Century: London.

Das, A.K. (1998), *A Treatise on Organon of medicine*, Souvik Kumar Das: Calcutta.

De Schepper, L. (1996), *Hahnemann Revisited*, New Mexico Full of Life: Sante Fe.

Desai, B.D. (1988), *How To Find The Similimum With Boger-Boenningshausen's Repertory*, (accessed Encyclopaedia Homeopathica, 2010).

Detlefsen, T. (1990), *The Healing Power of Illness Element*, London.

Di Blasi, Z., Harknes, E., Ernst, E., Georgiou, A. & Kleijnen, J. (2001), Influence of context effects on health outcomes: a systematic review, *Lancet*, 357(9258):757-762.

Di Blasi, Z. & Kleijnen, J. (2000), *Consultations at Glasgow Homeopathic Hospital*, Department of Health Sciences and Clinical Evaluation and NHS Centre for Reviews and Dissemination: University of York, UK.

Di Blasi, Z. & Kleijnen, J. (2003), Context Effects: Powerful Therapies or Methodological Bias?, *Evaluation and the Health Professions*, 26:166-179.

Dimitriadis, G. (1993), On Observation, *Homoeopathic Links*, 1/93:20.

Dimitriadis, G. (2000), *The Bönninghausen Repertory: Therapeutic Pocket Book Method*, Hahnemann Institute: Sydney, Australia.

Dixon, A.C. (1943), How Good Are You At Case Taking, *Homoeopathic Recorder*, March Vol Lviii (accessed Encyclopaedia Homeopathica, 2010).

Dunham, C. (1877), *Homoeopathy The Science Of Therapeutics*, Francis Hart & company, New York (accessed Encyclopaedia Homeopathica, 2010).

Dunham, C. (1878), *Lectures On Materia Medica*, Francis Hart & company: New York (accessed Encyclopaedia Homeopathica, 2010).

Eccles, R. (2007), The power of the placebo, *Current Allergy and Asthma Reports*, 7(2):100-104.

Eisler, I. (2006), The heart of the matter—A conversation across continents, *Journal of Family Therapy*, 28:329–333.

Eizayaga, F.X. (1991), *Treatise on Homeopathic Medicine*, Ediciones Marecel: Buenos Aires.

Elkins, D. (1995), Psychotherapy and Spirituality: Toward a Theory of the Soul, *Journal of Humanistic Psychology*, 35(2):78-98.

Enck, P., Benedetti, F. & Schedlowski, M. (2008), New insights into the placebo and nocebo responses, *Neuron*, 59:195-206.

Epstein, R., Franks, P., Fiscella, K. & Shields, C. (2005), Measuring patient-centered communication in patient–physician consultations: theoretical and practical issues, *Social Science & Medicine*, 61:1516-1528.

Epstein, R., Mauksch, L., Carroll, J. & Jaén, C. (2008), Have You Really Addressed Your Patient's Concerns?, *Family Practice Management*, 35-40, March.

Epstein, R.M. (2006), Making communication research matter: What do patients notice, what do patients want, and what do patients need?, *Patient Education and Counseling*, 60:272-278.

Evans, M.A., Shaw, A.R.G., Sharp, D.J., Thompson, E.A., Falk, S., Turton, P. & Thompson, T. (2007), Men with cancer: is their use of complementary and alternative medicine a response to needs unmet by conventional care?, *European Journal of Cancer Care*, 16(6).

Eyles, C., Walker, J. & Brien, S. (2009), Homeopathic Practitioner's Experiences of the Homeopathic Consultation: A Protocol of a Grounded Theory Study, *The Journal of Alternative and Complementary Medicine*, 15(4):347-352.

Farrington, E.A. (1890), *Clinical Materia Medica*, FE Boericke Hahnemann Publishing House: Philadelphia, (accessed Encyclopaedia Homeopathica, 2010).

Farrington, H. (1940), Homoeopathic Philosophy, *Homoeopathy Herald*, Vol iii, November, (accessed Encyclopaedia Homeopathica, 2010).

Farrington, H. (1955), *Homoeopathy and Homoeopathic Prescribing*, American Institute of Homeopathy: Philadelphia, (accessed Encyclopaedia Homeopathica, 2010).

Feller, C.P. & Cottone, R.R. (2003), The Importance of Empathy in the Therapeutic Alliance, *Journal of Humanistic Counseling, Education and Development*, 42(1):53-62.

Ford, S., Fallowfield, L. & Lewis, S. (1996), Doctor-Patient Interactions in Oncology, *Social Science & Medicine*, 42(11):1511-1519.

Foubister, D.M., *Homoeopathy and Paediatrics*, (accessed Encyclopaedia Homeopathica, 2010).

Foubister, D.M. (2001), *Significance of past history in Homoeopathic prescribing*, B. Jain Publishers (P) Ltd: New Delhi.

References

Frank, R. (2002), Homeopath and patient – a dyad of harmony?, *Social Science and Medicine*, 55(8):1285-1296.

Freeman, W.H. (1906), *The Malarial Similimum*, Transactions of the Homeopathic Medical Society of The State of New York, (accessed Encyclopaedia Homeopathica, 2010).

Gafoor, A. (2010), *The Art of Case Taking in Homeopathy*, available online at: http://www.similima.com/Rep38.html (last accessed 9 March 2010).

Gaskin, A. (1985), *Comparative Study On Kent's Materia Medica*, B. Jain Publishers: New Delhi.

Gibson, D.M. (1940), Value Of Symptoms In The Selection Of The Remedy, *Homoeopathy Herald*, vol iii, July, (accessed Encyclopaedia Homeopathica, 2010).

Goldman, R., Sullivan, A., Back, A. & Alexander, S. (2009), Patients' reflections on communication in the second-opinion hematology–oncology consultation, *Patient Education and Counseling*, 76:44-50.

Grauvogl, E.V. (1870), Text Book Of Homoeopathy, Halsey Bros: Chicago, (accessed in Encyclopaedia Homeopathica, 2010).

Gray, A. (2009), *Thriving Homeopathic Practice in Australian and New Zealand*, Sydney, Australia.

Gray, A. (2010a), Private Correspondence to the author.

Gray, A. (2010b), *Crossing the Bridge*, Sydney, Australia (unpublished).

Gray, B. & Shore, J. (1989), Seminar, Burgh Haamstede, (accessed Encyclopaedia Homeopathica, 2010).

Gray, B. & Shore, J. (1994), Case Taking: Penetrating The Essence, *Homoeopathic Links*, (accessed Encyclopaedia Homeopathica, 2010).

Gray, B. (1999), An Interview With Bill Gray, *American Homoeopaths*, (accessed Encyclopaedia Homeopathica, 2010).

Greenhalgh, T. & Hurzitz, B. (2004), Narrative Based Medicine, *BMJ Books*: London.

Grimmer, A.H. (1955), Hindrances To The Homoeopathic Prescription, *Homoeopathy Herald*, vol xvi, June, (accessed Encyclopaedia Homeopathica, 2010).

Grimmer, A.H. (1997), *The Collected Works*, Norwalk Conn & Greifenberg: Germany, Hahnemann International Institute for Homœopathic Documentation, (accessed Encyclopaedia Homeopathica, 2010).

Gryll, S.L. & Katahn, M. (1978), Situational factors contributing to the placebo effect, *Psychopharmacology (Berl)*, 47:253–261.

Guernsey, H.N. (1873), *Application Of Principles Of Homeopathy To Obstetrics*, Boericke & Tafel: Philadelphia, (accessed Encyclopaedia Homeopathica, 2010).

Guild-leggett, S.L. (1920), Why Take The Case 'And Make An Anamnesis', *International Hahnemann Association*, (accessed Encyclopaedia Homeopathica, 2010).

Gunavante, S.M. (1994), *The 'Genius' Of Homoeopathic Remedies*, B. Jain Publishers: New Delhi.

Haakana, M. (2001), Laughter as a patient's resource: Dealing with delicate aspects of medical interaction, *Interdisciplinary Journal for the Study of Discourse*, 21(1-2):187–219.

Haehl, R., *Samuel Hahnemann His Life & Works*, (accessed Encyclopaedia Homeopathica, 2010).

Hahnemann, S. (1922), *Organon of Medicine (6th edn.)*, Boericke & Tafel: Philadelphia, (accessed Encyclopaedia Homeopathica, 2010).

Hahnemann, S. (1999), *The Lesser Writings of Samuel Hahnemann* (reprint edn.), Jain Publishers: New Delhi.

Hahnemann, S. (2007), *The Chronic Diseases* (reprint edn.). Vol. 1, B. Jain Publishers: New Delhi.

Haidet, P. & Paterniti, D. (2003), 'Building' a history rather than 'taking' one: a perspective on information sharing during the medical interview, *Archives of Internal Medicine*, 163:1134-1140.

Halpern, J. (2001), *From Detached Concern to Empathy: Humanizing Medical Practice*, Oxford University Press: New York.

Halpern, J. (2003), What is Clinical Empathy?, *Journal of General Internal Medicine*, 18(8):670-674.

Harry, V.D.Z. (1906), *Miasms In Labour*, Transactions of The Homeopathic Medical Society of The State of New York, (accessed Encyclopaedia Homeopathica, 2010).

Hartog, C. (2009), Elements of effective communication -Rediscoveries from homeopathy, *Patient Education and Counseling*, 77:172-178.

Helman, C. (1981), Disease versus illness in general practice, *Journal of the Royal College of General Practitioners*, 31(230):548-552.

Hemmerdinger, J.M., Stoddart SDR & Lilford RJ (2007) A systematic review of tests of empathy in medicine, *BMC Medical Education*, 7(1):24.

Hering, C. (1865-1866), Hahnemann's Three Rules Concerning The Rank Of Symptoms, *Hahnemannian Monthly*, (accessed Encyclopaedia Homeopathica, 2010).

Heritage, J., Robinson, J., Elliott, M. & Beckett, M. (2007), Reducing patients' unmet concerns in primary care: the difference one word can make, *Journal of General Internal Medicine*, 22(10):1429-1433.

Hersoug, A.G., Høglend, P., Havik, O., Von Der Lippe, A. & Monsen, J. (2009), Therapist characteristics influencing the quality of alliance in long-term psychotherapy, *Clin. Psychol. Psychother.*, 16(2):100-110.

Hersoug, A.G., Høglend, P., Monsen, J.T. & Havik, O.E. (2001), Quality of working alliance in psychotherapy: Therapist variables and patient/therapist similarity as predictors, *Journal of Psychotherapy Practice and Research*, 10(4):205.

Heudens-mast, H. (1998), An Interview With Henny Heudens-Mast, *American Homoeopaths*, (accessed Encyclopaedia Homeopathica, 2010).

Hillman, J. (1975), *The Dream and the Underworld*, Harper and Row: New York, USA.

Hillman, J. (1997), *A Blue Fire*, HarperPerennial: New York, USA.

Hoffman, T., Bennett, S. & del Mar, C. (2010), *Evidence Based Practice Across the Health Professions*, Churchill Livingstone.

Horvath, A.O. (2000), The therapeutic relationship: From transference to alliance, *Journal of Clinical Psychology*, 56(2):163-173.

Horvath, A.O. & Symonds, B.D. (1991), Relationship between working alliance and outcome in psychotherapy: A meta-analysis, *Journal of Counseling Psychology*, 38:139–149.

Howie, J.G.R., Heaney, D. & Maxwell, M. (2004), Quality, core values and the general practice consultation: issues of definition, measurement and delivery, *Family Practice*, 21(4):458-468.

Hughes, R. (1868), *On Pharmodynamics* (accessed Encyclopedia Homeopathica Archibel 2010).

Hyland, M.E. (2005), A tale of two therapies: psychotherapy and complementary and alternative medicine (CAM) and the human effect, *Clinical Medicine*, 5(4):361-367.

Jacobs, J. (1990), A Case of Chronic Constipation International Foundation for Homeopathy: Case Conference Proceedings (accessed Encyclopaedia Homeopathica, 2010).

Jaisoorya, N.M. (1946), The Basic Principles Of Case Taking, *Homoeopathy Herald*, vol vii, June, (accessed in Encyclopaedia Homeopathica Archibel 2010).

Joardar, R.R. (2002), *The Dictionary Of Organon* (3rd edn.), Chhaya Joardar: Calcutta.

Johannes, C. & Lindgren, C. (2009), Homeopathy as a Transpersonal and Transformative Practice, *Homoeopathic Links*, 22:128, Autumn.

Julian, O. (1997), *Materia Medica of Nosodes with Repertory*, B. Jain Publishers, New Delhi.

Jung, C.G. (1974), *Dreams*, Princeton University Press: New Jersey, USA.

Jung, C.G. (1990a), *Man and his Symbols*, Arkana: England.

Jung, C.G. (1990b), *The Archetypes and the Collective Unconscious*, Princeton University Press: New Jersey, USA.

Kalff, D.M. (1991), Introduction to Sandplay Therapy, *Journal of Sandplay Therapy*, 1(1).

Kanjilal, J.N. (1977), *Writings on Homoeopathy*, Das: Calcutta.

Kaplan, B. (2006), Homeopathy, contrarianism and Provocative Therapy, *Homeopathy in practice*, 38-43, Summer.

Kaplan, B. (2001), *The Homeopathic Conversation: The Art of Taking the Case*, Natural Medicine Press.

Kaplan, H. (2005), How do art therapy and homeopathy work, *Homeopathy in Practice*, 14-17, Autumn.

Kaplan, S.H., Greenfield, S. & Ware, J.E. (1989), Assessing the effects of physician-patient interactions on the outcomes of chronic disease, *Med Care*, 27(3 Suppl):S110-127.

Kaptchuk, T.J. (2002), The Placebo Effect in Alternative Medicine: Can the Performance of a Healing Ritual Have Clinical Significance?, *Ann Intern Med*, 136:817-825.

Kaptchuk, T.J. & Eisenberg, D.M. (1998), The Persuasive Appeal of Alternative Medicine, *Annals of Internal Medicine*, 129(12):1061-1065.

Karver, M.S., Handelsman, J.B., Fields, S. & Bickman, L. (2005), A Theoretical Model of Common Process Factors in Youth and Family Therapy, *Mental Health Services Research*, 7(1):35-51.

Kendall, A. & Bend, G. (1911), The Anamnesis, *Homoeopathic Recorder*, (accessed in Encyclopaedia Homeopathica Archibel 2010).

Kent, J.T. (1905), *Materia Medica*, (accessed in Encyclopaedia Homeopathica Archibel 2010).

Kent, J.T. (1900), Lectures On Homoeopathic Philosophy, Ehrhart & Karl: Chicago, (accessed in Encyclopaedia Homeopathica Archibel 2010).

Ehrhart & Karl: Chicago, (accessed in Encyclopaedia Homeopathica Archibel 2010).

Kent, J.T. (1921), *Lesser Writings,* (accessed in Encyclopaedia Homeopathica Archibel 2010).

References

Kent, J.T. (1957), *What The Doctor Needs To Know In Order To Make a Successful Prescription*, Sett Dey: Calcutta, (accessed in Encyclopaedia Homeopathica Archibel 2010).

Kishore, J. (2004), Evolution of homoeopathic repertories and repertorisation (2nd edn.), B. Jain Publishers: New Dehli.

Kossoy, A. & Wilner, P. (1998), The Therapeutic Alliance in Randomized Controlled Clinical Trials, *Forschende Komplementarmedizin*, 5L(Suppl S1):31-36.

Krauss, J. (1922), *Hahnemann Introduction to Doctor Boericke's translation of sixth edition of Hahnemann's Organon*.

Krichbaum, P.E. (1923), The Remedy And The Dose?, *North American Journal Of Homeopathy*, (accessed in Encyclopaedia Homeopathica Archibel 2010).

Krupnick, J.L., Sotsky, S.M., Elkin, I., Simmens, S., Moyer, J., Watkins, J. & Pilkonis, P.A. (2006), The role of the therapeutic alliance in psychotherapy and pharmacotherapy outcome: findings in the National Institute of Mental Health Treatment of Depression Collaborative Research Program. Focus; 4 (2): 269-277.

Krupnick, J.L., Sotsky, S.M., Simmens, S., Moyer, J., Elkin, I. & Watkins, J. et al. (1996) The role of therapeutic alliance in psychotherapy and pharmacotherapy outcome: Findings in the National Institute of Mental health Treatment of Depression Collaborate Research Program. Journal of Consulting and Clinical Psychology; 64: 532-539.

Lambert, M.J. (1992), Psychotherapy outcome research: Implications for integrative and eclectic therapists, in Norcross JC & Goldfried MR (eds.) *Handbook of psychotherapy integration*, Wiley: New York, 94-129.

Lewis, T. (2000), *A General Theory of Love*, Random House.

Lindfors, P. & Raevaara, L. (2005), Discussing patients' drinking and eating habits in medical and homeopathic consultations, *Communication and Medicine*, 2(2):137-149.

Little, P., Everitt, H., Williamson, I., Warner, G., Moore, M., Gould, C., Ferrier, K. & Payne, S. (2001), Observational study of effect of patient centredness and positive approach on outcomes of general practice consultations, *BMJ*, 323(7318):908-911.

Logan, R. (1998), *The Homeopathic Treatment Of Eczema*, Beaconsfield Bucks: Beaconsfield, (accessed in Encyclopaedia Homeopathica Archibel 2010).

Loxterkamp, D. (1999), The old duffers' club, *Annals of Family Medicine*, 7(3):269-272.

Luff, D. & Thomas, K. (2000), 'Getting somewhere', feeling cared for: patients' perspectives on complementary therapies in the NHS, *Complementary Therapies in Medicine*, 8:253-259.

Maizes, V., Rakel, D. & Niemiec, C. (2009), Integrative Medicine and Patient-Centered Care, *Explore: The Journal of Science and Healing*, 5(5):277-289.

Malhotra, H.C., *Care And Treatment - Fistula, Piles*, (accessed in Encyclopaedia Homeopathica Archibel 2010).

Mangialavori, M. (1999), An Interview With Massimo Mangialavori, *American Homoeopaths*, (accessed in Encyclopaedia Homeopathica Archibel 2010).

Mansoor, A. (2010), Seminar paper '*Case taking - A developmental approach*', available online at: http://www.similima.com/Rep1.html.

Marian, F., Joost, K., Saini, K.D., von Ammon, K., Thurneysen, A. & Busato, A. (2008), Patient satisfaction and side effects in primary care: An observational study comparing homeopathy and conventional medicine. *BMC Complementary and Alternative Medicine*; 8 (1): 52.

Marnocha, M. (2009), What Truly Matters: Relationships and Primary Care, *Annals of Family Medicine*, 7(3):196-197.

Martin, D.J., Garske, J.P. & Davis, M.K. (2000), Relation of the therapeutic alliance with outcome and other variables: A meta-analytic review, *Journal of consulting and clinical psychology*, 68(3):438-450.

Marvel, M., Epstein, R., Flowers, K. & Beckman, H. (1999), Soliciting the patient's agenda: have we improved?, *JAMA*, 281(3):283-287.

Master, F.J. (2007a), *Homoeopathy In Cervical Spondylosis*, (accessed in Encyclopaedia Homeopathica Archibel 2010).

Master, F.J. (2007b), *Perceiving Rubrics Of The Mind*, (accessed in Encyclopaedia Homeopathica Archibel 2010).

Master, F.J. (2007c), *The Bed side Organon of Medicine*, (accessed in Encyclopaedia Homeopathica Archibel 2010).

Mattoli, D., *The Totality Of Symptoms*, Quinquennial Homoeopathic International Congress, RADAR, (Encyclopaedia Homeopathica, 2007).

Mauksch, L.B., Dugdale, D.C., Dodson, S. & Epstein, R. (2008), Relationship, communication, and efficiency in the medical encounter: creating a clinical model from a literature review, *Archives of Internal Medicine*, 168(13):1387-1395.

May, C. & Sirur, D. (1998), Art, science and placebo: incorporating homeopathy in general practice, *Sociology of Health & Illness*, 20(2):168-190.

McIntosh, C. & Ogunbanjo, G.A. (2008), Why do patients choose to consult homeopaths? An exploratory study, *SA Fam Pract*, 50(3):69-69c.

Mercer, S. (2001), *Enablement and the Therapeutic Alliance: An evaluation of the Consultation at the Glasgow Homoeopathic Hospital.* Accessed online at: http://www.adhom.com/adh_download/enablement.pdf (accessed 10 February 2008).

Mercer, S., Watt, I. & Reilly, D. (2001), Empathy is important for enablement, *BMJ*, 322:865.

Mercer, S.W. (2005), Practitioner empathy, patient enablement and health outcomes of patients attending Glasgow Homeopathic Hospital: a retrospective and prospective comparison, *Wien Med Wochenschr*, 155(21-22):498-501.

Mercer, S.W. & Reilly, D. (2004), A qualitative study of patient's views on the consultation at the Glasgow Homoeopathic Hospital, an NHS integrative complementary and orthodox medical care unit, *Patient Education & Counseling*, 53(1):13-18.

Mercer, S.W., Reilly, D. & Watt, G. (2001), *Enablement and the Therapeutic Alliance: An evaluation of the Consultation at the Glasgow Homoeopathic Hospital*, accessed at http://www.adhom.com/adh_download/enablement.pdf on 11 February 2008.

Mercer, S.W., Reilly, D. & Watt, G. (2002), The importance of empathy in the enablement of patients attending the Glasgow Homoeopathic Hospital, *British Journal of General Practice*, 901-905, November.

Mercer, S.W. & Reynolds, W.J. (2002), Empathy and quality of care, *British Journal of General Practice*, 52(Suppl):S9-12.

Messer, S.B. & Wampold, B.E. (2002), Let's face the facts: Common factors are more potent that specific therapy ingredients, *Clinical Psychology: Science and Practice*, 9:21-25.

Mishler, E. (1984), The Discourse of Medicine, *Dialectics of Medical Interviews*, Ablex Publishing Corporation: Norwood, New Jersey.

Mishler, E.G., Clark, J.A., Ingelfinger, J. & Simon, M.P. (1989), The language of attentive patient care, *Journal of General Internal Medicine*, 4(4):325-335.

Mohanthy, N. (1983), *Textbook of Homœopathic Materia Medica*, Namita Mohanty: Bhubaneswar.

Mohanty, N. (1999), *Case Taking Receiving and Recording*, IBPP Indian Books & Periodicals Publishers, New Delhi.

Morrison, R. (1987), *Seminar Burgh Haamstede*, (accessed in Encyclopaedia Homeopathica Archibel 2010).

Mundy, D. (1997), Interview With David Mundy, *American Homoeopaths*, (accessed in Encyclopaedia Homeopathica Archibel 2010).

Narasimhamurti, K.L. (1994), *Handbook Of Materia Medica And Therapeutics Of Homeopathy*, B. Jain Publishers: New Delhi.

Nash, E.B. (1913), *Leaders In Homoeopathic Therapeutics* (4th edn.), Boericke & Tafel: Philadelphia, (accessed in Encyclopaedia Homeopathica Archibel 2010).

Nash, E.B. (1995), *Nash Expanded Work*, B. Jain Publishers: New Delhi.

Neesgaard, P., *Hypothesis Collection - Primary Psora And Miasmatic Dynamic*, (accessed in Encyclopaedia Homeopathica Archibel 2010).

Neumann, M., Bensing, J., Mercer, S., Ernstmann, N., Ommen, O. & Pfaff, H. (2009), Analyzing the "nature" and "specific effectiveness" of clinical empathy: A theoretical overview and contribution towards a theory-based research agenda. *Patient Education and Counseling;* 74: 339-346.

Norland, M. (1999), A Day in the Life of Misha Norland, *The Homoeopath*, 76, November.

Norland, M. (2008), *Interview with Misha Norland*, available online at: http://www.wholehealthnow.com/teleconferences.html.

Norland, M. (1998), In Sickness and in Health, *The Homeopath*, 70, accessed http://www.alternative-training.com/uploads/in_sickness_and_in_health_1.pdf.

Olsson, B. & Tibblin, G. (1989), Effect of patients' expectations on recovery from acute tonsillitis, *Fam Pract*, 6:188–192.

Ortega, P.S. (1977), *Notes On The Miasms*, NP: Mexico, (accessed in Encyclopaedia Homeopathica Archibel 2010).

Patel, R.P. (1998), *Art of case taking and practical repertorisation*, Sai Homoeopathic Book Corporation: Kerala.

Paterson, J. (2003), *The Bowel Nosodes*, B. Jain Publishers (P) Ltd: New Delhi.

Peräkylä, A., Ruusuvuori, J. & Vehviläinen, S. (2005), Introduction: Professional theories and institutional interaction, *Communication & medicine*; 2(2):105-109.

Piaget, J. (1997), *Moral Judgment of the Child*, Simon and Schuster.

Plant, R. (1999), An Interview With Bill Gray, *American Homoeopaths*, (accessed in Encyclopaedia Homeopathica Archibel 2010).

Platt, F.W., Coulehan, J.L., Fox, L., Adler, A.J., Weston, W.W., Smith, R.C. & Stewart, M. (2001), The Patient-Centered Interview, *Annals of Internal Medicine*, 134(11):1079-1085.

Platt, F.W. & Platt, C.M. (1998), Empathy: a miracle or nothing at all?, *Journal of Clinical Outcomes Management*, 5(2):30-33.

Porter, R. (1997), *The Greatest Benefit to Mankind: A Medical History of Humanity*, Harper Collins: London.

Porter, R. (2004), *Flesh in the Age of Reason. How the Enlightenment Transformed the Way We See Our Bodies and Souls*, Penguin Books: London, England.

Price, D.D., Finniss, D.G. & Benedetti, F. (2008), A Comprehensive Review of the Placebo Effect: Recent Advances in Current Thought, *Annual Review of Psychology*, 59:565-590.

Priebe, S., McCabe, R., Bullenkamp, J., Hansson, L., Lauber, C., Martinez-Leal, R., Rossler, W., Salize, H., Svensson, B. & Torres-Gonzales, F. (2007), Structured patient clinician communication and 1-year outcome in community mental health care: Cluster randomised controlled trial. *British Journal of Psychiatry;* 191 (5): 420-426.

Pulford, D. (1931a), Why Do We Take The Case?, *Homoeopathic Recorder*, Vol Li, March, (accessed in Encyclopaedia Homeopathica Archibel 2010).

Pulford, D. (1931b), Taking the case, *Homoeopathic Recorder*, Vol XLVI, June, (accessed in Encyclopaedia Homeopathica Archibel 2010).

Quinn, J.F., Smith, M., Ritenbaugh, C., Swanson, K. & Watson, M.J. (2003), Research guidelines for assessing the impact of the healing relationship in clinical nursing, *Alternative Therapies in Health and Medicine*, 9(3;SUPP):65-79.

Quirk, M., Mazor, K., Haley, H., Philbin, M. & Fischer, M. (2008), How patients perceive a doctor's caring attitude, *Patient Education and Counseling*, 72:359-366.

Rabe, R.F. (1883), *Remedy Selection As An Art*, Homeopathic Medical Society: Pennsylvania, (accessed in Encyclopaedia Homeopathica Archibel 2010).

Ram, Dass & Groman, P. (1985), *How Can I Help*, Random House.

Rastogi, D.P. (1995), *Homeopathic Gems*, (accessed in Encyclopaedia Homeopathica Archibel 2010).

Ratcliffe, J., van Haselen, R., Buxton, M., Hardy, K., Colehan, J. & Partridge, M. (2002), Assessing patients' preferences for characteristics associated with homeopathic and conventional treatment of asthma: a conjoint analysis study, *Thorax*, 57:503-508.

Redelmeier, D.A., Molin, J.P. & Tibshirani, R.J. (1995), A randomised trial of compassionate care for the homeless in an emergency department, *Lancet*, 345:1131-1134.

Reilly, D. (2001), Enhancing human healing: Directly studying human healing could help to create a unifying focus in medicine, *BMJ*, 322:120-121.

Rice, P. (1908), *The Taking Of A Case*, (accessed in Encyclopaedia Homeopathica Archibel 2010).

Ring, A., Dowrick, C.F., Humphris, G.M., Davies, J. & Salmon, P. (2005), The somatising effect of clinical consultation: What patients and doctors say and do not say when patients present with medically unexplained physical symptoms. *Social Science and Medicine;* 61: 1505-1515.

Rise, M.B. & Steinsbekk, A. (2009), How do parents of child patients compare consultations with homeopaths and physicians? A qualitative study, *Patient Education and Counseling,* 74(1):91-96.

Risquez, F. (1995), *Psychiatry And Homeopathy,* B. Jain Publishers: New Delhi.

Roberts, H.A. & Wilson, A.C. (1935), *The Principles And Practicability Of Boenninghausen's Therapeutic Pocket Book,* Boericke & Tafel: Munster, (accessed in Encyclopaedia Homeopathica Archibel 2010).

Roberts, H.A. (1936), *The Principles and Art of Cure by Homoeopathy,* Homœopathic Publishing Co: London, (accessed in Encyclopaedia Homeopathica Archibel 2010).

Rogers, C. (1951), *Client-centered therapy: Its current practice, implications and theory,* Constable: London.

Rogers, C. (1957), The necessary and sufficient conditions of therapeutic personality change, *Journal of Consulting Psychology,* 21:95-103.

Rogers, C. (1961), *On becoming a person. A therapist's view of psychotherapy,* Mifflin: Boston, MA.

Ruusuvuori, J. (2005a), Comparing homeopathic and general practice consultations: The case of problem presentation, *Communication and Medicine,* 2(2):123-135.

Ruusuvuori, J. (2005b), 'Empathy' and 'Sympathy' in Action: Attending to Patients' Troubles in Finnish Homeopathic and General Practice Consultations, *Social Psychology Quarterly,* 68(3):204-222.

Saine, A. (1997), *Psychiatric Patients,* Eindhoven: Lutra, (accessed in Encyclopaedia Homeopathica Archibel 2010).

Sankaran, P. (1996), *The Elements of Homoeopathy,* Homoeopathic Medical Publishers, Mumbai, Volume 1.

Sankaran, R. (1991), *The Spirit Of Homoeopathy,* (accessed in Encyclopaedia Homeopathica Archibel 2010).

Sankaran, R. (1999), Glimpses Of A System, *American Homoeopaths,* (accessed in Encyclopaedia Homeopathica Archibel 2010).

Sankaran, R., *The System Of Homeopathy,* (accessed in Encyclopaedia Homeopathica Archibel 2010).

Sankaran, R. (2008), *The Other Song* Homeopathic Medical Publishers: Mumbai.

Sankaran, R. (2010), http://www.homeopathyworldcommunityu.com/video/case-taking-dr-rakams-method.

Sardello, R. (1996), *Love and the Soul. Creating a Future for Earth*, HarperPerennial: USA.

Schadde, A. (1997), Anna Schadde Takes A Case, *American Homoeopaths*, (accessed in Encyclopaedia Homeopathica Archibel 2010).

Schadde, A. (1995), Intuition, And Dream-Work, *American Homoeopaths*, (accessed in Encyclopaedia Homeopathica Archibel 2010).

Schattner, A. (2009), The silent dimension: expressing humanism in each medical encounter, *Arch Intern Med*, 169(12):1095-1099.

Schmidt, P. (1996), *The Art Of Case Taking* (reprint edn.), B. Jain Publishers: New Delhi, (accessed in Encyclopaedia Homeopathica Archibel 2010).

Schmidt, P. (1997), *The Art Of Interrogation* (reprint edn.), B. Jain Publishers: New Delhi, (accessed in Encyclopaedia Homeopathica Archibel 2010).

Scholten, J., *Homoeopathy And Minerals*, (accessed in Encyclopaedia Homeopathica Archibel 2010).

Scholten, J., *Homoeopathy And The Elements*, (accessed in Encyclopaedia Homeopathica Archibel 2010).

Scott, A. & Vick, S. (1999), Patients, doctors and contracts: an application of principal-agent theory to the doctor-patient relationship, *J Polit Econ.*, 46(2):111-134.

Shah, J. (1993), Face to face with Misha Norland, *National Journal of Homeopathy*, 11(2):57-61, March-April.

Shang, A., Huwiler-Muntener, K., Nartey, L., Jüni, P., Dörig, S., Sterne, J.A.C., Pewsner, D. & Egger, M. (2005), Are the clinical effects of homoeopathy placebo effects? Comparative study of placebo-controlled trials of homoeopathy and allopathy. *Lancet*, 366: 726–32.

Sherr, J. (2000), An Interview With Jeremy Sherr, *American Homoeopaths*, (accessed in Encyclopaedia Homeopathica Archibel 2010).

Sherr, J. (1994), Lecture, Dynamis School: London.

Sherr, J. (2007), Interview with Jeremy Sherr by Manish Bhatia, published on *Hpathy Ezine*, November, Available online at: http://www.hpathy.com/interviews/jeremy-sherr.asp.

Shore, J. (1999), The Salt Of The Essence: An Exploration Of The Relationship Between Totality, Essence, And Central Delusion, *American Homoeopaths*, (accessed in Encyclopaedia Homeopathica Archibel 2010).

Spalding, R.W. (1931a), Taking The Case And Its Analysis, *Homoeopathic Recorder*, Vol Li, March, (accessed in Encyclopaedia Homeopathica Archibel 2010).

Spalding, R.W. (1931b), The Relation Of Case Taking To Repertory And Materia Medica Study, *Homoeopathic Recorder*, Vol Xlvi, June, (accessed in Encyclopaedia Homeopathica Archibel 2010).

Spence, D.S., Thompson, E.A. & Barron, S.J. (2005), Homeopathic treatment for chronic disease: a 6-year, university-hospital outpatient observational study, *J Altern Complement Med*, 11:793-798.

Stankowitch (1896), Taking The Case, *Hahnemannian Advocate*, volume xxxv, Chicago, (accessed in Encyclopaedia Homeopathica Archibel 2010).

Stearns, G.B. (1917), *Case-Taking*, International Hahnemann Association, (accessed in Encyclopaedia Homeopathica Archibel 2010).

Steinsbekk, A. (2005), Empowering the Cancer Patient or Controlling the Tumor? A Qualitative Study of How Cancer Patients Experience Consultations With Complementary and Alternative Medicine Practitioners and Physicians, Respectively. *Integrative Cancer Therapies*; 4 (2): 195-200.

Stevens, G.B. (1914), *Case Taking*, International Hahnemann Association, (accessed in Encyclopaedia Homeopathica Archibel 2010).

Stewart, M.A. (1995), Effective physician-patient communication and health outcomes: a review, *CMAJ*, 152(9):1423-1433.

Stewart, R. (1995), Taking The Case, *American Homoeopaths*, (accessed in Encyclopaedia Homeopathica Archibel 2010).

Street, R.L., O'Malley, K.J., Cooper, L.A. & Haidet, P. (2008), Understanding Concordance in Patient-Physician Relationships: Personal and Ethnic Dimensions of Shared Identity, *Annals of Family Medicine*, 6(3):198-205.

Stroebe, M., van Son, M., Stroebe, W., Kleber, R., Schut, H. & van den Bout, J. (2000), On the classification and diagnosis of pathological grief, *Clinical Psychology Review*, 20(1):57-75.

Suchman, A.L., Markakis, K., Beckman, H.B. & Frankel, R. (1997), A model of empathic communication in the medical interview, *JAMA*, 277:678-682.

Sutherland, A.D. (1930), Editorial, *Homoeopathic Recorder*, Vol xlv, June, (accessed in Encyclopaedia Homeopathica Archibel 2010).

Sutherland, A.D. (1944), The Similimum Case Taking, *Homoeopathic Recorder*, Vol Lix, May, RADAR, (Encyclopaedia Homeopathica, 2007).

References

Swash, M. & Glynn, M. (2007), *Hutchison's Clinical Methods*, Saunders Ltd.

Sweeney, K.G., MacAuley, D., & Gray, D.P. (1998), Personal significance: the third dimension, *Lancet*, 351(9096):134-136.

Taylor, M.B. (1997), Compassion: its neglect and importance, *The British Journal of General Practice*, 47(421):521-523.

Taylor, W. (2001), *Taking the Case*, available online at: http://www.wholehealthnow.com/homeopathy_pro/wt1.html.

Thomas, K.B. (1987), General practice consultations: is there any point in being positive?, *BMJ*, 294:1200–1202.

Thompson, T.D.B. & Weiss, M. (2006), Homeopathy - What are the active ingredients? An exploratory study using the UK Medical Research Council's framework for the evaluation of complex interventions, *BMC Complementary and Alternative Medicine*, 6:37.

Thomson, J.W. (1924), *A Clinical Case- Rhus Tox Bureau Of Homoeopathy*, (accessed in Encyclopaedia Homeopathica Archibel 2010).

Tiwari, S.K. (2000), *Essentials Of Repertorization* (2nd edn.), B. Jain Publishers (P) Ltd: New Delhi.

Tonelli, M.R. & Callahan, T.C. (2001), Why alternative medicine cannot be evidence-based, *Academic Medicine*, 76(12):1213-1220.

Townsend, I. (2002), Before the Actualising Tendency: Putting body into the person-centred process, *Person-Centred Practice*, 10(2):81-87.

Townsend, I. (2001), Manning the Lifeboats or Sailing the Seas with Confidence? Supervision in the Service of a Profession, *NASH News*, Spring, 10-14.

Tumminello, P.L. (2001), *The child's mind and behaviour: a repertory: how to take the case*, Medicine Way: Bondi Junction, Sydney.

Turner, J.A., Deyo, R.A., Loeser, J.D., Von Korff, M. & Fordyce, W.E. (1994), The importance of the placebo effects in pain treatment and research, *JAMA*, 271(20):1609-1614.

Tyler, M.L. (1927), *How Not To Do It*, Quinquennial Homoeopathic International Congress (Transactions of the ninth congress, The science and art of homoeopathy), (accessed in Encyclopaedia Homeopathica Archibel 2010).

Tyler, M.L. (1928), Different Ways Of Finding The Remedy, John Bale, Sons and Danielsson ltd: London, (accessed in Encyclopaedia Homeopathica Archibel 2010).

John, Bale, Sons and Danielsson ltd: London, (accessed in Encyclopaedia Homeopathica Archibel 2010).

van Dulmen, S. (2003), Patient-centredness, *Patient Education and Counseling*, 51:195-196

van Weel, C. (2001), Examination of context of medicine, *The Lancet*, 357:733.

Vick, S. & Scott, A. (1998), Agency in health care. Examining patients' preferences for attributes of the doctor-patient relationship, *J Health Econ.*, 17(5):587-605.

Vickers, A. & de Craen, A. (2000), Why use placebos in clinical trials? A narrative review of the methodological literature, *Journal of Clinical Epidemiology*, 53:157-161.

Vincent, C. & Furnham, A. (1996), Why do patients turn to complementary medicine? An empirical study, *British Journal of Clinical Psychology*, 35:37-48.

Vithoulkas, G. & Olsen, S., *Winning Strategies Of Case Analysis,* (accessed in Encyclopaedia Homeopathica Archibel 2010).

Vithoulkas, G. (1980), *Talks On Classical Homoeopathy*, The Esalen Conferences, (accessed in Encyclopaedia Homeopathica Archibel 2010).

Vithoulkas, G. (1980), *The Science of Homeopathy*, Grove Press.

Vithoulkas, G. (1999), An Interview With George Vithoulkas, *American Homoeopaths*, (accessed in Encyclopaedia Homeopathica Archibel 2010).

Vithoulkas, G. (2010), *Strategies of Case Taking*, http://www.wholehealthnow.com/ homeopathy pro/strategies.html last acessed March 2010.

Wagner, M.W. (2006), *Exploring the Therapeutic Relationship: Practical Insights for Today's Clinician*, Aardvark Global Publishing: USA.

Walach, H. & Jonas, W.B. (2004), Placebo research: The evidence base for harnessing self-healing capacities, *Journal of Alternative and Complementary Medicine*, 10(Suppl. 1):S103-S112.

Ward, J.W. (1917), Taking The History Of The Case, Pacific Coast, *Journal Of Homoeopathy*, Volume xxviii, April, (accessed in Encyclopaedia Homeopathica Archibel 2010).

Weinberger, J. (1995), Common factors aren't so common: The common factors dilemma, *Clinical Psychology: Science and Practice*, 2:45-69.

Weir, J. (1927), *The Science And Art Of Homoeopathy*, Quinquennial Homoeopathic International Congress (Transactions of the ninth congress), (accessed in Encyclopaedia Homeopathica Archibel 2010).

Weir, M. (2007), *Complementary Medicine Ethics and Law,* Promethius: Australia.

Wells, P.P. (1988), The Examination Of The Patient For A Homoeopathic Prescription, *Homoeopathic Physicians*, vol viii, (accessed in Encyclopaedia Homeopathica Archibel 2010).

Wender, R. (1996), Humor in Medicine, *Primary care*, 23(1):141-154.

Wensing, M., Jung, H.P., Mainz, J., Olesen, F., & Grol, R. (1998), A systematic review of the literature on patient priorities for general practice care. Part 1: Description of the research domain, *Social Science & Medicine*, 47(10):1573-1588.

Wheeler, C.E., *Introduction To The Principles Of Homeopathy*, (accessed in Encyclopaedia Homeopathica Archibel 2010).

Whitmont, E.C. (1991), *The Symbolic Quest, Basic Concepts of Analytical Psychology*, Princeton University Press: New Jersey, USA.

Whitmont, E.C. (1999), *Dreams, A Portal to the Source*, Routledge: New York, USA.

Whole Health Now, http://www.wholehealthnow.com, (accessed March 2010).

Wikipedia http://en.wikipedia.orm, (accessed March 2010).

Winston, J. (1995), Kent - a modern biography of James Tyler Kent, *American Homoeopaths*, (accessed in Encyclopaedia Homeopathica Archibel 2010).

Winston, J. (2001), The Böenninghausen Method, *American Homoeopaths*, (accessed in Encyclopaedia Homeopathica Archibel 2010).

Winston, J. (1999), *The Faces of Homeopathy*, Tawa, Wellington, New Zealand.

Witt, C.M., Lüdtke, R., Mengler, N. & Willich, S.N. (2008), How healthy are chronically ill patients after eight years of homeopathic treatment? – Results from a long term observational study, *BMC Public Health*, 8(1):413.

Wodward, A.W. (2003), *Constitutional Therapeutics*, B. Jain Publishers (P) Ltd: New Delhi.

Wright-Hubbard, E. (1999), *A Brief Study Course In Homoeopathy*, B. Jain Punlishers (P) Ltd, New Delhi.

Wynn, R. & Wynn, M. (2006), Empathy as an interactionally achieved phenomenon in psychotherapy. Characteristics of some conversational resources, *Journal of Pragmatics*, 38(9):1385-1397.

Yasgur, J., *Homeopathic Dictionary*, (accessed in Encyclopaedia Homeopathica Archibel 2010).

Zaren, A. (1989), Seminar, Lelystad Netherlands, (accessed in Encyclopaedia Homeopathica Archibel 2010).

Zaren, A. (1993), Casetaking And Materia Medica Of Infants, *New England Journal Of Homoeopathy*, Vol 2, RADAR (Encyclopaedia Homeopathica, 2007).

Zaren, A. (1997), Pioneering Women Homeopaths: Interview With Ananda Zaren, *American Homoeopaths*, (accessed in Encyclopaedia Homeopathica Archibel 2010).

Zee, V.D. (1906), *Miasms in Labour*, Transactions of The Homeopathic Medical Society of the State of New York, (accessed in Encyclopaedia Homeopathica Archibel 2010).

Ziv, R.B. (2000), Who am I? A case of Hydrogen, *American Homoeopaths*, (accessed in Encyclopaedia Homeopathica Archibel 2010).

Zollman, C. & Vickers, A. (1999), Complementary Medicine and the Patient, *BMJ*, 319: 1486-1489.

Index

A

Acute Case Taking 203
Allen, H.C. 47, 105
Allen, T.F. 425
Alternating Disease 68
Anxious patients 7, 189, 211
Aphorisms 23, 28, 39, 91, 116, 201
Archetypes 219, 237, 434, 447
Art Therapy 219, 235
Attention in observing 28, 329
Attitude 59, 61, 143, 145, 160, 162, 168, 178, 183, 189, 300, 361, 375, 376, 439
Authenticity 267, 268, 271, 378

B

Best Practice 3, 5, 23, 72, 107, 134, 135, 170, 171, 175, 251, 275, 357, 361
Bidwell 81, 85, 93, 107, 359, 426
Böenninghausen 6, 9, 10, 13, 46, 47, 81, 86, 87, 88, 89, 90, 91, 93, 100, 103, 105, 107, 139, 141, 215, 231, 313, 360, 426, 429, 445, 447
Boger 13, 52, 53, 81, 85, 88, 100, 101, 215, 426, 429, 447
Burnett 47, 81, 97, 99, 100, 107, 156, 427, 428, 447

C

Case 1, 3, 12, 13, 14, 15, 16, 17, 23, 46, 65, 68, 78, 79, 81, 87, 94, 100, 107, 109, 119, 120, 122, 152, 155, 165, 171, 181, 183, 195, 200, 203, 219, 223, 228, 247, 250, 251, 277, 286, 287, 291, 304, 323, 357, 359, 360, 368, 369, 373, 377, 378, 381, 389, 426, 427, 429, 431, 432, 433, 434, 436, 437, 439, 441, 442, 443, 444, 447, 449
Cause 36, 37, 39, 43, 44, 47, 48, 49, 50, 51, 75, 98, 107, 134, 144, 157, 159, 161, 179, 180, 185, 199, 201, 211, 224, 232, 271, 285, 302, 337, 361, 380, 383, 401, 402, 403, 404, 405, 407, 408, 409, 411, 414, 415, 417, 420, 422
Centre of the Case 357, 373, 447
Children 7, 100, 101, 156, 190, 204, 205, 206, 237, 238, 243, 248, 267, 398, 419, 421
Cicchetti 13, 232, 238, 246, 428, 447
Clarke 14, 47, 81, 97, 98, 99, 100, 428, 447
Classical 13, 14, 17, 109, 114, 427, 444, 447
Close 12, 27, 39, 48, 49, 62, 87, 91, 114, 120, 128, 143, 146, 159, 228, 260, 270, 307, 322, 359, 364, 367, 368, 371
Compassion 327, 347, 349, 443, 447
Complementary medicine 209, 247, 332, 349, 444, 451
Complete symptom 6, 47, 88, 90, 176, 199, 204
Concomitant Symptoms 89, 447

Congruence 253, 267, 275, 447
Cooper 81, 97, 100, 442
Critical audit 379
Critical thinking 323

D

D'Aran 27, 46, 89, 175, 181, 284, 285, 306, 429, 447
Delusion 277, 294, 295, 298, 300, 301, 441, 447
De Schepper 179, 187, 188, 191, 193, 194, 195, 196, 202, 203, 209, 211, 429, 447
Dimitriadis 55, 56, 88, 89, 118, 190, 429, 448
Dream 144, 219, 231, 232, 233, 234, 237, 238, 296, 418, 433, 441
Dunham 14, 41, 47, 81, 91, 92, 93, 103, 107, 374, 429, 448

E

Education 8, 103, 118, 140, 249, 306, 312, 373, 390
Eizayaga 240, 352, 429, 448
Elderly 201, 209, 211, 362
Empathy 263, 268, 330, 334, 335, 336, 339, 343, 344, 345, 351, 352, 353, 378, 386, 387, 432, 437, 438
Endeavour College of Natural Health xv, 451, 453
Endings 171, 198
Evidence 3, 9, 39, 125, 159, 180, 209, 257, 323, 325, 331, 340, 341, 345, 347, 354, 373, 390, 426, 443, 444
Evidence based medicine 325, 345

F

Fairy Tales 237
Farrington 14, 48, 81, 95, 368, 430, 448
Fidelity 28, 38, 39, 57, 65, 250, 346, 361
Flexner report xii
Freud 8, 225, 227, 231, 260, 273, 359, 448

G

Gadd 325, 327, 329, 385
Gafoor 14, 56, 63, 65, 167, 199, 201, 202, 431, 448
Gestalt therapy 270
Google xiii
Grimmer 14, 52, 144, 428, 431, 448
Guernsey 81, 95, 214, 432, 448

H

Hahnemann 8, 9, 11, 12, 13, 14, 15, 16, 17, 23, 27, 28, 29, 30, 31, 33, 35, 36, 37, 38, 39, 40, 41, 42, 43, 44, 45, 46, 47, 49, 50, 53, 55, 56, 57, 58, 62, 63, 64, 65, 66, 67, 68, 69, 70, 72, 78, 79, 81, 85, 87, 88, 90, 93, 94, 95, 96, 97, 98, 99, 100, 106, 107, 114, 116, 119, 122, 127, 133, 140, 141, 142, 144, 152, 156, 175, 177, 178, 194, 199, 200, 201, 205, 213, 214, 215, 224, 225, 226, 227, 230, 231, 248, 257, 259, 261, 281, 286, 309, 310, 329, 337, 347, 353, 354, 359, 360, 361, 368, 369, 374, 375, 388, 393, 395, 396, 397, 426, 429, 430, 431, 432, 433, 435, 442, 448
Hahnemann's Main Writings 23, 78, 448
Health 11, 35, 36, 37, 48, 56, 59, 65, 66, 68, 70, 71, 73, 124, 145, 161, 177, 180, 182, 199, 202, 205, 225, 229, 239, 250, 266, 269, 303, 305, 330, 331, 332, 333, 334, 335, 336, 339, 346, 350, 351, 352, 354, 362, 369, 373, 377, 378, 382, 384, 389, 391, 414, 421, 422, 423, 427, 428, 429, 435, 437, 438, 439, 442, 444, 451
Hering 96
Hughes 47, 81, 96, 99, 103, 107, 139, 433, 448
Human Resources 253, 260, 448
Humour 253, 270, 350, 448

I

Indisposition 66, 448
Infants 190, 205, 206, 263

Intermittent Diseases 68, 448

J
Julian 47, 96, 434, 448

K
Kaplan 15, 114, 117, 140, 175, 181, 184, 185, 187, 192, 199, 203, 205, 206, 207, 209, 228, 233, 236, 251, 258, 260, 261, 262, 263, 265, 266, 267, 268, 269, 270, 271, 273, 274, 289, 331, 360, 375, 388, 434, 448
Kent 9, 12, 15, 27, 30, 41, 47, 62, 85, 101, 106, 107, 109, 113, 115, 116, 117, 118, 119, 120, 122, 123, 124, 125, 126, 127, 128, 131, 132, 133, 134, 135, 139, 140, 141, 142, 143, 144, 164, 166, 167, 175, 195, 199, 215, 224, 225, 231, 248, 257, 258, 262, 281, 359, 368, 374, 393, 399, 428, 431, 434, 435, 445, 448, 449
Kent's Questionnaire 393, 399, 449

L
Legalities 171, 197, 449
Literature Review 3, 12
Local Affections 66
Loquacious Patients 209

M
Male patients 209, 210
Mental Diseases 67
Metaphor 219, 237, 449
Method 5, 6, 10, 19, 41, 61, 87, 89, 95, 99, 100, 101, 106, 107, 114, 115, 124, 125, 139, 141, 155, 159, 180, 213, 214, 215, 216, 228, 235, 236, 249, 263, 281, 283, 284, 287, 304, 306, 308, 309, 312, 313, 314, 315, 317, 319, 323, 360, 385, 441, 449
Myths 230, 237, 238, 377, 449

N
Nash 16, 47, 81, 85, 97, 102, 438, 449
Neuro-linguistic programming xi

Neutrality 29, 61, 132, 267, 339, 348, 382
Non-human Specific 277, 302, 449

O
Observation 43, 56, 61, 63, 64, 70, 72, 85, 86, 93, 104, 123, 131, 156, 162, 163, 189, 190, 194, 200, 212, 292, 297, 309, 374, 379
One Sided Disease 66
Organon of Medicine 14, 15, 16, 17, 27, 79, 398, 432, 436, 449
Own words 65, 119, 161, 184, 192, 196, 228, 347, 361, 407

P
Paracelsus 43, 44, 449
Patient-centredness 345, 444, 449
Peculiarity 43, 53, 55, 56, 57, 92, 291, 297, 361, 399, 404, 417
Physical examination 62, 91, 120, 123, 141, 158, 159, 167, 181, 192, 193, 194
Placebo 122, 130, 133, 156, 157, 170, 214, 263, 330, 335, 340, 341, 342, 343, 354, 427, 429, 430, 432, 436, 441, 443
Police 253, 259, 375
Psychology 62, 152, 228, 235, 258, 334, 436
Psychotherapy 6, 8, 10, 11, 32, 219, 235, 246, 258, 266, 327, 330, 333, 334, 336, 375, 376, 380, 426, 427, 430, 433, 435, 445
Purpose of Case Taking 171, 181

Q
Questioning 171, 191, 219, 242, 449

R
Recording 171, 194, 437, 449
Research 19, 210, 269, 323, 330, 334, 340, 391, 430, 435, 438, 443, 444, 445, 451
Roberts 16, 41, 113, 135, 139, 157, 160, 162, 167, 178, 440, 449

Rogers 253, 262, 263, 264, 267, 268, 335, 344, 440, 449

S

Sandplay 219, 235, 237, 434, 449

Sankaran, P. 48, 49, 51, 52, 168, 178, 179, 180, 181, 182, 183, 184, 186, 188, 189, 195, 196, 202, 388, 440

Sankaran, R. 114, 168, 178, 179, 180, 181, 182, 183, 184, 186, 188, 189, 195, 196, 202, 213, 215, 253, 261, 262, 267, 274, 275, 277, 281, 282, 283, 285, 287, 288, 289, 290, 292, 293, 295, 296, 297, 298, 299, 301, 302, 303, 304, 305, 306, 307, 308, 309, 310, 312, 313, 314, 315, 316, 317, 318, 319, 320, 321, 322, 359, 368, 375, 378, 388, 440, 441

Schmidt 10, 12, 17, 41, 113, 116, 135, 139, 140, 141, 142, 143, 144, 146, 147, 148, 152, 167, 199, 281, 359, 368, 441, 450

Scope of practice 193, 246

Self Audit 275

Self Disclosure 357, 386

Sensation 19, 32, 41, 74, 88, 141, 180, 192, 203, 204, 210, 214, 228, 238, 268, 299, 300, 301, 302, 303, 304, 306, 308, 309, 312, 313, 314, 316, 321, 323, 360, 373, 383, 396, 400, 401, 402, 403, 404, 405, 408, 410, 412, 413, 414, 415, 419, 420

Sherlock Holmes 140, 162, 179, 180, 368, 450

Sherr 18, 27, 195, 228, 250, 251, 289, 296, 372, 375, 441, 450

Silence 29, 31, 171, 191, 211, 296, 306, 309, 338, 357, 361, 364, 365, 388, 450

Similar and Dissimilar Disease 204

Skeptics xii

Soul 67, 70, 219, 223, 224, 225, 226, 227, 228, 229, 231, 234, 235,

Sound Senses 23, 62

Spirit of homeopathy 5

Stream of Consciousness 219

Swedenborg 109, 116, 117, 257, 450

T

Tact 38, 39, 71, 73, 122, 128, 133, 154, 158, 159, 168, 201, 248, 364

Tattoos 219, 234, 450

Teens 207, 450

The Levels 277, 299, 450

Therapeutic Alliance 327, 347, 430, 435, 437, 450

Therapeutic Relationship 327, 329, 331, 333, 444

Time Management 171, 198

Timing 38, 39, 128, 248, 323, 344, 364

Totality 6, 43, 44, 45, 46, 47, 48, 49, 50, 53, 54, 68, 77, 94, 105, 122, 123, 160, 167, 177, 178, 194, 213, 225, 248, 249, 289, 296, 340, 344, 352, 360, 361, 383, 386

Tyler 17, 41, 47, 113, 115, 135, 142, 144, 155, 156, 157, 214, 215, 359, 368, 443, 445, 450

U

Unconditional positive regard 29, 58, 263, 266, 267, 268, 335, 378

Underlining 171, 197, 450

V

Vithoulkas 12, 17, 113, 212, 213, 246, 309, 315, 381, 444, 450

W

Wright-Hubbard 17, 101, 113, 135, 157, 160, 184, 445, 450

About the Author

MSc (UK) BAHons (NZ) ADH (NZ) DSH (UK) PCH (UK) PCHom (Malaysia)

Alastair Gray works in Australia as the National Academic eLearning Manager at Endeavour College of Natural Health. Prior, he headed up the homeopathy department, a dual-sector role that involved running an advanced diploma in the vocational education sector and a degree in the higher education sector. He was responsible for quality of the curriculum, management of all staff, and the academic integrity of the programs.

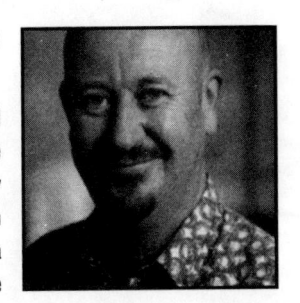

He has lectured under and post-graduate naturopathy for 17 years, philosophy, case taking and management, ethics, business practices and scope of practice. A regular seminar and conference presenter in far-flung places from New Zealand to Malaysia, the USA, Ireland, Belgium, Germany, Spain, Canada, the UK, India, Thailand and Australia, he also delivers webinars worldwide.

Author of 22 books and numerous articles on primary research in natural medicine, his latest is a text book for homeopaths Case Management (2014) to complement Case Taking (2010), Volume I in The Landscape of Homeopathic Medicine series and Method (2011). He is passionate about eLearning, instructional design, educational technology in his academic and teaching work. Clinical practice (25 years in NZ, the UK and Australia) remains a significant focus especially the treatment of anxiety, depression, addiction and men's health.

Reviews

'When an author begins a thoughtful and thorough work on a complex topic with the statement that the book is the first of seven, the reader knows that they are dealing with someone who is tenacious, with vision, and with a genuine passion for their subject. Alastair Gray has all of these qualities, and more. He is an outstanding practitioner, a teacher with international credentials, and an accomplished author. This book offers the reader both a thorough description of the history of homeopathy, and a glimpse into its future. The author faces contentious issues directly, and questions existing standards with rigour. He begins his seven-part series with the topic of case taking which, in my opinion, is completely appropriate. If a practitioner cannot take a complete and accurate case, if the true intellectual, psychological and physical characteristics of the patient are not discovered, and if the fundamental causes of the patient's condition are not found, then a successful prescription cannot be guaranteed in chronic conditions. The author offers the reader an insight into homeopathic case-taking that is conceptually as well as practically complete. The book leaves the reader impatient to discover what gems the remaining six books in the series will contain.'

—**Dr Isaac Golden**, Endeavour College of Natural Health Australia

'Al Gray has produced a thorough and magnificent new resource for students and practitioners of Homeopathy on the art of case taking. The scope is ambitious! He weaves together the insights of homeopaths to those of the psychotherapeutic tradition in a way that is both accessible and mind expanding. He navigates the often turbulent waters of allegiances to different homeopathic gurus in a refreshing way. No doubt those whose systems he describes will find a sympathetic yet critical examination of their approaches. He even gives them 'voice' / right of reply by including extracts from extensive interviews with contemporary leading lights. This is a breadth of fresh air - it is not the voice of the apologist or sycophant but rather a considered critical examination of some of the greatest influences upon modern homeopathic practice.'

—**Susanna Shelton**
Principal, Bay of Plenty College of Homeopathy and New Zealand Director of Operations for Endeavour College of Natural Health

'Even for those of us who disagree with newer approaches this is an impressive overview of thoughts on case taking and an interesting source of questions.'

—**Dr Joe Kellerstein**, Canada

'Alastair Gray's new book should be required reading for ALL students of homeopathic medicine. Gray provides an exhaustive overview of the history and diversity of homeopathic case taking, with the academic citations to the original sources, with reference to the slight and significant changes in case taking that have evolved over the past 200 years, and with specific and practical applications to the varying styles of homeopathic practice that have emerged since homeopathy's inception. Besides being of value to students of homeopathy, this book is also a valuable resource for practicing homeopaths who often need to be reminded of the origins of the case taking process as well as its most recent developments as a means of creatively and effectively understand the patients who we see.'

—**Dana Ullman**, USA